Instructor's Manual

to accompany

ABNORMAL PSYCHOLOGY
CURRENT PERSPECTIVES

Eighth Edition

Lauren B. Alloy

Temple University

Neil S. Jacobson

University of Washington

Joan Acocella

Prepared by
Gregory H. Cutler
Bay de Noc Community College

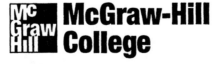

Boston Burr Ridge, IL Dubuque, IA Madison, WI New York San Francisco St. Louis
Bangkok Bogotá Caracas Lisbon London Madrid
Mexico City Milan New Delhi Seoul Singapore Sydney Taipei Toronto

McGraw-Hill College

A Division of The McGraw-Hill Companies

Instructor's Manual to accompany
ABNORMAL PSYCHOLOGY: CURRENT PERSPECTIVES, EIGHTH EDITION

Copyright © 1999 by The McGraw-Hill Companies, Inc. All rights reserved.
Previous editions copyright © 1972, 1977, 1980, 1984, 1993, 1996 by The McGraw-Hill Companies, Inc.
Printed in the United States of America.

The contents of, or parts thereof, may be reproduced for use with
ABNORMAL PSYCHOLOGY: CURRENT PERSPECTIVES, EIGHTH EDITION by
Lauren B. Alloy, Neil S. Jacobson, Joan Acocella, provided such reproductions bear copyright notice and
may not be reproduced in any form for any other purpose without permission
of the publisher.

    2 3 4 5 6 7 8 9 0 QPD/QPD 9 0 9

ISBN 0-07-303462-2

www.mhhe.com

Table of Contents

Preface

This Instructor's Manual accompanies the Eighth Edition of Alloy, Jacobson, and Acocella's *Abnormal Psychology: Current Perspectives* and is designed to help you to help students maximize their understanding of the principles and research of abnormal psychology. The manual has several components to support instructors in developing and expanding their lectures and classroom activities.

Chapter Map

The Chapter Map provides a quick overview of the chapter headings alongside the major components of the instructor's manual. Instructors will find this helpful as they integrate activities and other instructor manual components with their lectures.

Chapter Outline

The Chapter Outline is a detailed outline of the major content areas of the chapter. Key terms are embedded in the outline and are boldfaced.

Learning Objectives

The learning objectives are coordinated with the *Student Study Guide*. These chapter objectives are intended to allow the instructor to formulate lectures that are coordinated to the text in the chapter. The numbers in parentheses correspond to the page numbers of the material in the chapter.

Lecture Leads

Each chapter includes a number of supplemental lecture ideas that instructors can use as starting points. Each lecture lead includes a citation of source materials.

Talking Points

Talking Points are intended to provide instructors with ideas to stimulate class discussion and effective examples to illustrate important concepts and principles. Talking Points can be used as lecture lead-ins, homework questions, or small-group discussion questions.

Cross Cultural Teaching

Each chapter in the Instructor's Manual includes a list of idioms and colloquialisms that English as a Second Language students may have difficulty understanding. The purpose of the list to alert instructors so that they may provide additional support in the form of definitions and examples.

Activities and Demonstrations

Activities and Demonstrations are projects that instructors can use to reinforce key points in the chapters and have been developed for use both in and out of the classroom. These activities range from very short to relatively long-term activities and from small group activities to large group activities.

Films and Videos

This section is an annotated list of films and videos that are appropriate for the content of the course. The Appendix A lists the addresses where these resources can be located.

Movies and Mental Illness

This new feature of the manual provides a link to Wedding and Boyd's *Movies and Mental Illness: Using Films to Understand Psychopathology.* In this resource, Wedding and Boyd describe movies that illustrate abnormal behavior. This section of the instructor's manual identifies the movies most useful in presenting the behaviors described in each of the chapters. Instructors may wish to show these movies in class or at least make references to them since many students have seen these movies.

Classroom Assessment Techniques

In recent years a set of techniques have been developed by K. Patricia Cross and Tom Angelo that give instructors and students opportunities to provide ungraded, formative feedback. The techniques (e.g., One-Minute Paper, Directed Paraphrasing) are typically completed by students anonymously and turned in to the instructor who uses them to determine if the students have understood the concept or principle. If the feedback suggests that students did not grasp the material, the instructor may elect to provide supplemental assignments, activities, or lectures. These techniques of assessment are also pedagogical as students evaluate their own learning of the material. Many of the Classroom assessment techniques are further described in Angelo and Cross (1993) and instructors are encouraged to review this very valuable resource.

Suggestions for Essay Questions

Three to four essay questions designed to encourage critical thinking are included in each chapter. Instructors may wish to use them as exam questions, discussion questions, or small group work.

Acknowledgments

A number of people deserve my thanks for their helpful comments and guidance. I would like to thank the editorial staff at McGraw-Hill, specifically Meera Dash, Kristen Mellitt, Susan Kunchandy, and Lai Moy. I want to recognize the work of Todd Zakrajsek, Timothy P. Tomzcak, and Anita Rosenfield, authors of other McGraw-Hill ancillaries, as providing the foundation for many ideas used in this instructor's manual. And of course, thank you Denise, Alyssa, Miranda, Katelyn, Noelle, and Bethany for putting up with it all and reversing the lock on my den door.

Gregory H. Cutler
Bay de Noc Community College
Escanaba, Michigan

August 1998

Chapter 1

Abnormal Behavior: Historical Perspectives

Chapter Map

Section	Instructor Manual Components
Abnormal Behavior and Society • Defining Abnormal Behavior • Relating Abnormal Behavior to Groups • Explaining Abnormal Behavior • Treating Abnormal Behavior	*Norms influencing behavior and perception (LL 1-1)* *Cultural differences in nonverbal communication (LL 1-2)* *Taijin Kyofusho (LL 1-3)* *Student-generated examples (TP 1-1)* *Culture-specific abnormalities: Fact or Fiction? (TP 1-2)* *Eating a bug and other things (TP 1-3)* *Statistical rarity (TP 1-4)* *Group differences (TP 1-5)* *Relating etiology to treatment (TP 1-6)* *What is normal and abnormal here? (TP 1-7)* *Real people (TP 1-8)* *Scientific journals in abnormal psychology (TP 1-9)* *Background knowledge probe (ACT/DEMO 1-1)* *Defining abnormal behavior (ACT/DEMO 1-2)*
Conceptions of Abnormal Behavior: A Short History • Ancient Societies: Deviance and the Supernatural • The Greeks and the Rise of Science • The Middle Ages and the Renaissance • The Eighteenth Century and After: The Asylums • Foundations of Modern Abnormal Psychology • Non-Western Approaches to Abnormal Behavior	*Abnormal behavior and treatment in art (LL 1-4)* *Careers in mental health (LL 1-5* *Medical student syndrome (LL 1-6)* *Help with terms (TP 1-10)* *Bedlam (TP 1-11)* *Survey of psychological disorders (ACT/DEMO 1-3)* *Role playing (ACT/DEMO 1-4)*

A Multiperspective Approach	*Do something abnormal (ACT/DEMO 1-5)*

Chapter Outline

I.   Abnormal Behavior and Society
      A.   Defining Abnormal Behavior
            1.   Norm Violation
                 a.   **Norms** as rules of "right" and "wrong"
                 b.   Abnormal behavior as a violation of cultural norms
                 c.   Limitations include variability of norms and rewarding of conformity
            2.   Statistical Rarity
                 a.   Abnormal behavior as a deviation from the average
                 b.   Normal behavior as falling within the average
                 c.   Diagnosing mental retardation using statistics
                 d.   Limitations include a lack of values
                 e.   Not all rarities should be identified as abnormal
            3.   Personal Discomfort
                 a.   Abnormality as distressing thoughts or behaviors
                 b.   People are their own judges of their own normality
                 c.   Limitations include no standard for evaluating the behavior itself and individuals may still need help if behavior is not harmful
            4.   Maladaptive Behavior
                 a.   Abnormality exists if behavior pattern prevents the demands of life from being met
                 b.   Related to norm violation
                 c.   Focuses on behavior relative to life circumstances
            5.   A Combined Standard
                 a.   Should standard of abnormality be based on facts or values?
                 b.   Both facts and values are used
                 c.   Most societies identify the same categories of abnormal behavior such as harmful behavior, poor reality contact, inappropriate emotional reactions, and erratic behavior
      B.   Relating Abnormal Behavior to Groups
            1.   Cultural and Ethnic Group Differences
                 a.   Psychological disorders affect different cultures at different rates
                 b.   Psychological disorders are experienced and managed differently among different cultures
                 c.   Cultures have differing idioms of distress--ways that illness is signified
                 d.   Diagnosis should take into account individual's cultural background
            2.   Gender Differences

          a.   Gender affects the expression of psychological disorders
          b.   Gender affects susceptibility to psychological disorders
          c.   Diagnosis should take into account individual's gender
  B.   Explaining Abnormal Behavior
        1.   The Medical Model
              a.   The **medical model** argues that abnormal behavior is comparable to disease
              b.   Each abnormal behavior has causes and set of symptoms
              c.   Abnormal behavior is **biogenic**
              d.   Long history of biogenic theories of abnormal behavior
              e.   Biogenic theories supported by early discoveries of brain pathologies
              f.   Conceptualization of abnormal behavior influenced by medical model
              g.   Criticisms of model include labeling effects
              h.   **Biological perspective** focuses on physical components of abnormal behavior, but not necessarily agrees that all abnormal behavior are merely symptoms of biological abnormalities
        2.   A Multiperspective Approach
              a.   Psychological theories attribute abnormal behavior to psychological process from interaction between person and environment
              b.   Psychodynamic, behavioral, cognitive, humanistic-existential, interpersonal, and sociocultural perspectives are examples of psychological theories
  C.   Treating Abnormal Behavior
        1.   Nature of society affects the treatment of abnormal behavior
        2.   Way in which abnormal behavior is defined influences its treatment
        3.   Suspected causes of abnormal behavior influences its treatment

II.   Conceptions of Abnormal Behavior: A Short History
  A.   Ancient Societies: Deviance and the Supernatural
        1.   Belief in supernatural forces influenced treatment such as **exorcism**
        2.   Undramatic treatments were probably common in ancient societies
  B.   The Greeks and the Rise of Science
        1.   Evolution of naturalistic approach to abnormal behavior
        2.   Hippocrates suggested all illness as due to natural causes
              a.   Importance of observing cases of abnormal behavior
              b.   Developed first biogenic theory suggesting abnormalities of **humors**
              c.   Developed one of the first classification systems

3. Plato argued that care of mentally ill was a family responsibility and influenced the treatment located in retreats

C. The Middle Ages and the Renaissance: Natural and Supernatural
1. Medieval Theory and Treatment
   a. Abnormal behavior thought to be caused by supernatural forces
   b. Treatment reflects belief in the supernatural
   c. Many cases were seen as caused by intervening factors of physical or emotional mishaps
2. The Witch Hunts
   a. The stage was set to perceive anyone behaving strangely as a witch
   b. Papal bull declaring church's intention of seeking and punishing witches
3. Renaissance Theory and Treatment
   a. Accusations of witchcraft were often used for political and economic reasons
   b. Many of those alleged to be witches were psychologically disturbed
   c. Many were institutionalized or cared for at homes

D. The Eighteenth Century and After: The Asylums
1. The Early Asylums
   a. Hospitalizing mentally ill is an old idea
   b. Public hospitals became "madhouses"
   c. Conditions of mental hospitals, such Bethlehem Hospital in London, were often terrible
   d. Bedlam reported in many asylums was due to violent patients
2. The Reform of the Asylums
   a. Pussin, superintendent at La Bicête in Paris, established new rules that were later extended by Pinel
   b. Tuke attempted similar reforms in England
   c. New approach to treatment known as **moral therapy** designed to treat patients like human beings
3. The Reform Movement in America
   a. Rush is known as the "father of American psychiatry"
   b. Rush moved the treatment of mentally disturbed toward human therapy
   c. Dix traveled country and became an advocate calling for humane treatment of mentally ill in appropriate facilities
4. Hospitalization and the Decline of Moral Therapy
   a. Lack of enough advocates of moral therapy to staff growing number of mental hospitals
   b. Prejudice against Irish Catholics by Protestant-staffed mental hospitals reduced likelihood of using moral therapy

        c.   Medical model rising directed efforts toward biological treatment

        d.   Custodial care was replacing moral therapy

        e.   **Prefrontal lobotomy** used on patients considered uncontrollable

    5.   The Exodus from the Hospitals

        a.   Deinstitutionalization movement led to many individuals being discharged

        b.   Cost of care and development of phenothiazines contributed to deinstitutionalization movement

        c.   Community Mental Health Centers Act (1963) led to different types of care--**outpatient, inpatient**

        d.   Different types of programs were available, such as **day hospital** and **night hospital**

        e.   **Halfway houses** were developed to help patients with readjustment to community life

        f.   Insufficient funds have led to inadequate and nonexistent services; some patients are homeless

        g.   "Revolving door syndrome" results from a lack of services

E.   Foundations of Modern Abnormal Psychology

    1.   The Experimental Study of Abnormal Psychology

        a.   Methods developed by Wundt were applied to the study of abnormal behavior

        b.   Kraepelin studied **psychopathology** in his laboratory

    2.   Kraepelin and Biogenic Theory

        a.   Kraepelin developed classification system based on biogenic perspective

        b.   **Syndrome** is a distinct cluster of symptoms and is used in classification

        c.   Neurological research made significant progress in linking syndromes with brain pathologies such as **general paresis**

        d.   **Psychogenic theory** suggests that psychological disturbances are due primarily to stress and not organic dysfunction

    3.   Mesmer and Hypnosis

        a.   Mesmer applied knowledge of magnetism and electricity to study of mental states

        b.   Mesmer believed that "animal magnetism" could treat hysteria

        c.   Success was actually due to the power of suggestion

        d.   **Hypnosis** was originally known as "mesmerism"

    4.   The Nancy School

        a.   Liebeault and Bernheim used hypnosis as treatment

        b.   Argued that **glove anesthesia** was a form of hysteria caused by self-hypnosis

    c.   The Nancy school suggested that mental disorders were caused by psychology factors

    d.   Charcot criticized the Nancy school

5. Breuer and Freud: The Beginnings of Psychoanalysis

    a.   Breuer, in treating Anne O., found the talking cure to be useful

    b.   Freud and Breuer argued that disorders were due to unconscious conflicts and were to be drawn out under hypnosis

    c.   **Free association** was used to examine unconscious conflicts

    d.   This form of therapy is called psychoanalysis and has had profound influence

F. Non-Western Approaches to Abnormal Behavior

    1. Africa

        a.   Family plays an important role in dealing with disturbed people

        b.   Causes of abnormal behavior often linked to individual's relationship with spirit world

        c.   Many principles common in the West are used, such as the goal of insight

    2. Asia

        a.   Religion emphasizes self-awareness through meditation

        b.   Meditation is used to treat variety of psychological problems

        c.   Naikan therapy suggests that psychological problems are due to self-centeredness; self-observation is taught as a treatment

        d.   Morita therapy used to treat anxiety disorders to clear one's mind of perfectionism and to once again want practical activity

III. A Multiperspective Approach

    A.   Human behavior can be studied scientifically

    B.   Most abnormal behavior is the product of both psychological and biological processes

    C.   Each human being is unique

    D.   A comprehensive view of abnormal behavior is accomplished by examining different perspectives

Chapter Boxes

- The Mental Health Professions
  - A. There are four mental health professions each with its own training and theoretical perspectives
  - B. **Psychiatrists, clinical psychologists, psychiatric social worker**, and **psychoanalyst.**

- Western and Non-Western Culture-Bound Syndromes
  - A. Many psychopathologies occur across cultures
  - B. Some disturbances are specific to certain culture and societies
    - a. Non-Western syndromes are important to consider when evaluating individuals from other cultures
    - b. Some disturbances are Western culture-bound syndromes

- The Homeless and Mentally Ill
  - A. About one-third of the homeless are thought to be suffering from mental disorders
  - B. Some live in inexpensive single-room-occupancy "hotels"
  - C. Homeless individuals often had normal lives

Learning Objectives (LO)

By the time you are finished studying this chapter, you should be able to do the following:

1. List and describe four criteria for defining abnormality and list four categories of behavior that most societies consider indicative of mental disorder (4-7).

2. Describe how cultural and gender differences complicate the task of defining normal and abnormal behavior (7-8).

3. List and describe the essential features of the medical model of abnormal behavior, and list the advantages and criticisms of the medical model as presented in your text (9-11).

4. List and define six perspectives that the text cites as alternatives to the medical model, and describe the kinds of mental health professionals employed within them (11-12).

5. Cite the contributions of Hippocrates, Galen and Ascleplades to the study of abnormal behavior, and contrast their views to those that prevailed in more ancient societies (11-14).

6. Discuss how the cultural atmosphere of the Middle Ages influenced attitudes and actions toward the mentally ill during that period (14).

7. Discuss the degree to which witch hunting during the Renaissance was related to prevailing attitudes toward the mentally ill (14).

8. List the contributions of Pussin, Pinel, Esquirol, Tuke, Rush, and Dix to the reform of mental health care in the eighteenth and nineteenth centuries (15-17).

9. Define moral therapy and discuss its place in the development of modern psychotherapy (17).

10. Describe the social and historical factors that led to the rise and decline of large mental hospitals from the late nineteenth to the mid-twentieth centuries (18-19).

11. Describe how the work of Wundt, Kraepelin, Kraffi-Ebing, and Mesmer laid the foundation for the development of modem abnormal psychology (19-2 1).

12. Cite the contributions of Liebeault, Bernheim, Charcot, Breuer, and Freud to the development of modern psychotherapy (21-22).

9

13.   Describe how African and Asian cultures differ from Western cultures in their understanding and treatment of mental disorders (23-24).

14.   List three assumptions your text uses in constructing a multiperspective approach to abnormal behavior, and discuss the benefits of such an orientation (24).

Lecture Leads (LL)

Norms influencing behavior and perception (LL 1-1
Consider sharing the following quote to illustrate the extent to which norms affect nearly every aspect of our lives: "Culture not only helps to determine what foods we eat, but it also influences when we eat (for example, one, three, or five meals and at what time of the day); with whom we eat (that is, only with the same sex, with children or with the extended family); how we eat (for example, at a table or on the floor; with chopsticks, silverware, or the fingers); and the ritual of eating (for example, in which hand the fork is held, asking for or being offered seconds, and belching to show appreciation of a good meal), These eating patterns are habits of culture." (Gollnick & Chin, 1986, pp. 6-7) Before you read this quote to students, ask them to describe how their culture affects eating habits. Hupka et al. (1997) found cross-cultural differences in the extent to which different colors are associated with emotions. For example, Russians associated envy with black, purple, and yellow.

Resources:
Gollnick, D., & Chin, P. (1986). Multicultural education in a pluralistic society (2d ed.). New York: Merrill/Macmillan.

Hupka, R. B. et al. (1997). The colors of anger, envy, fear, and jealousy: A cross-cultural study. Journal of Cross-Cultural Psychology, 28, 156-171.

Cultural differences in nonverbal communication (LL 1-2)
You can underscore the importance of culture by extending the discussion of culture to other forms of nonverbal communication. The textbook focuses on proxemics, that is the study of how space communicates meaning. There are other areas of interest where intercultural differences emerge such as vocal behavior, eye contact, and touch. A good addition of this lecture is to bring in how mental health professionals need to be sensitive to these differences especially in diagnosis and therapeutic relationships. Tie in the lecture to any experiences of students who have interacted in other cultures that have different nonverbal cues and norms.

Resources:
Hickson, M. L., & Stacks, D. W. (1989). Nonverbal communication: Studies and applications (2d ed.). Dubuque, IA: Brown.

Richmond, V. P., McCroskey, J. C., & Payne, S. K. (1987). Nonverbal behavior in interpersonal relations. Englewood Cliffs, NJ: Prentice-Hall.

Sue, S., Zane, N., & Young, K. (1994). Research on psychotherapy with culturally diverse populations. In A. E. Bergin & S. L. Garfield (Eds.), Handbook of psychotherapy and behavior change (4th ed., pp. 783-817). New York: John Wiley.

Taijin kyofusho (LL 1-3)
As the textbook points out, abnormality and our perception of it is influenced by cultural factors. Taijin kyofusho is a social phobia that is common in Japan, but nearly nonexistent in the United States and other western cultures. This social phobia-like disorder consists of an irrational fear of offending others by one's awkward social or physical behavior. For example, a Japanese individual would be overly concerned if their eye contact, body odor, trembling hands, or unpleasant facial expression offended another. The etiology of taijin kyofusho is probably based on the Asian culture's social customs emphasizing modesty and proper public behavior.

Resources:
Friedmann, C. T. H., & Faguest, R. A. (1982). Extraordinary disorders of human behavior. New York: Plenum Press.

Kirmayer, L. J. (1991). The place of culture in psychiatric nosology: Taijin kyofusho and DSM-III-R. Journal of Nervous and Mental Disease, 179, 19-28.

Kleinknecht, R. A., Dinnel, D. L., Kleinknecht, E. E., Hiruma, N., & Harada, N. (1997). Cultural factors in social anxiety: A comparison of social phobia symptoms and taijin kyofusho. Journal of Anxiety Disorders, 11, 157-177.

Lebra, W. P. (1976). Culture-bound syndromes, ethnopsychiatry, and alternate therapies. Honolulu: University of Hawaii

Abnormal behavior and treatment in art (LL 1-4)
An effective way to start the class is to show slides illustrating how abnormal behavior and its treatment were reflected in the art of the Middle Ages. For example, show Hogarth's Rake's Progress (illustrating conditions at Bethlehem Hospital), van Hemessen's Stone of Folly (showing brain surgery to treat madness), and Examination of a Witch. Consider other sources of art, such as galleries, libraries, and if you have one, an art history department. The Bettmann Archive and Granger Collections, and the Archives of the History of American Psychology (University of Akron) are excellent sources as well. You could also include more contemporary works that convey different aspects of abnormal behavior.

Resource:
Cohen, B. M., & Cox, C. T. (1995). Telling without talking: Art as a window into the world of multiple personality. New York: W.W. Norton.

Careers in mental health (LL 1-5)
Some of your students may be interested in pursing a career in one of the areas of mental health. Develop a lecture that explains the differences with regard to education, training, and orientation. A guest speaker from any of the mental health professions would be a very good addition. You may also want to mention the current controversy regarding

12

allowing clinical psychologists' prescription privileges. Perhaps students can brainstorm and identify pros and cons allowing these psychologists to prescribe certain drugs. An extension is to provide students with a perspective on where psychologists are employed. Bring in a recent copy of the APA Monitor and show students the want ads focusing on the different types of settings where psychologists and other mental health workers are employed.

Resources:

DeLeon, P. H., Sammons, M. T., & Sexton, J. L. (1995). Focusing on society's real needs. American Psychologist, 50, 1022-1032.

Kilburg, R. R. (1991). How to manage your career in psychology. Washington, DC: American Psychological Association.

Tyler, L. E. (1992). Counseling psychology: Why? Professional Psychology: Research & Practice, 23, 342-344.

http://www.apa.org/students/ (American Psychological Association's web site provides students with information regarding career options.)

Medical student syndrome (LL 1-6)
Early on in the course is a good time to introduce the concept of the Medical Student Syndrome. A brief discussion of it can serve as a caution. You may want to consider saying that throughout the class, students will be exposed to many different disorders. It is somewhat typical for students to think that they suffer from the disorder. Remind students of the criteria for abnormality as discussed in the textbook. In most cases, those students who believe they have a particular disorder do not. However, inform your students of the services available on campus and community that they may wish to consult. Hardy (1997) reported students majoring in psychology to be more worried about their psychological health than those majoring in other fields. She also found that learning about psychological disorders was helpful in reducing students' fears about their own psychological status. However, these same students reported an increase in fear about their families' mental health.

Resource:

Hardy, M. S. (1997). Psychological distress and the "medical student syndrome" in abnormal psychology students. Teaching of Psychology, 24, 192-193.

Talking Points (TP)

Student-generated examples (TP 1-1)

To increase participation, have students generate examples for each of the definitions of abnormality as they are presented in class. Ask for personal and cultural examples to illustrate each definition's strengths and weaknesses.

Culture-specific abnormalities: Fact or Fiction? (TP 1-2)

Before you lecture on Chapter 1 or before students read it, present to them a number of the culture-specific disorders. Use the disorders presented on page xx. Throw in some disorders that students are familiar with, such as depression and anxiety. For each disorder, ask your students if they think the disorder is real or if you've just made it up.

Eating a bug and other things (TP 1-3)

To illustrate the importance of context in abnormality, ask your students if they would be willing to eat a bug? Tell them that wherever they are in the afternoon, they should take a nap. In some cultures, it is perfectly acceptable to eat bugs and to take a siesta. Take a quick look at your female students in class and identify those who are wearing jeans by saying "Shame on you" to each. In a different place and time, it would be considered unacceptable for women to be in public with pants. You might also want to commend women wearing dresses, but only if their ankles are not showing!

Statistical rarity (TP 1-4)

Remind students that abnormal is to normal as infrequent (or uncommon, atypical) is to frequent (or common, typical). To outline the limitations of the statistical definition of abnormality, ask your students if they would like to win a multimillion-dollar lottery, but add that only one student can. Who would like to be abnormal? Or use a full-ride scholarship or a sports record as further examples.

Group differences (TP 1-5)

It is a good idea to talk about within group variation in the section on group differences. Often times there is more variation within a group than between two groups. Also, it is worth mentioning that in any between group differences, there will be overlap.

Relating etiology to treatment (TP 1-6)

An important theme that you will want to stress to students is the relationship between etiology and treatment. How one explains abnormality will shape how it is treated. To drive home the point, query students.

What is normal and abnormal here? (TP 1-7)

Ask your students to think of behaviors, traditions, customs, and mores that would be considered normal in their neighborhood or community, but abnormal in others areas or regions of the country. Ask students to share experiences where they live (e.g., wearing a cowboy hat for senior pictures in high school, the opening of deer hunting season as a holiday, kissing in public).

Real people (TP 1-8)
It is critical to convey to students that even though we talk about people with psychiatric disorders in somewhat detached clinical ways, they still are people who are more similar to us than different. One way to convey this is to tell about the rich and famous with psychological disorders. Here is a sampling: Howard Hughes (obsessive-compulsive disorders), NFL Announcer John Madden (fear of flying), Karen Carpenter (eating disorders), The Doors' Jim Morrison (substance abuse), and 60 Minutes' Mike Wallace (depression). Ask students for other examples. Augment this talking point with the activity that involves a survey to illustrate that all of us are directly or indirectly touched by psychological disorders.

Scientific journals in abnormal psychology (TP 1-9)
Bring some relevant scientific journals (e.g., Journal of Clinical Psychology, Behavior Therapy, Journal of Consulting and Clinical Psychology; Psychosomatic Medicine, Journal of Abnormal Psychology, Journal of Behavioral Medicine, Archives of General Psychiatry) to class. Suggest to students that publishing research is critical in the scientific process to disseminate information. Briefly summarize the type of research reported in the journals by reading the titles of articles. For other journal ideas, check the reference section of the textbook.

Help with terms (TP 1-10)
One way to help students understand a vocabulary term is to break the term down. For example, "genic" as in psychogenic and biogenic refers to "beginning" or "of." (e.g., The Book of Genesis). Therefore, in the biogenic model, abnormal behavior has its causes in the biology of the body.

Bedlam (TP 1-11)
Bethlehem Hospital in London is described in the textbook as an early mental asylum. The hospital also became a popular tourist attraction where a cent was charged for admission. Tours were also given of Lunatics' Tower in Vienna in the late 1700s for the price of a ticket. Help students put this into perspective by asking for their reactions to charging admission to tour a prison, women's shelter, or AIDS clinic.

Cross-Cultural Teaching

People who stand too close to us may seem **pushy**...	p. 4
There is a more **liberal** approach than the two we just discussed...	p. 6
is able to meet the demands of his or her life--**hold down a job**, deal with friends and family, **pay the bills on time**, and the like.	p. 6
Mr. Sinha...tried to avoid having sex with wife, though he often **slipped** and felt guilty about this.	p. 8
This controversy is not as heated today as it was in the **sixties** and **seventies**...	p. 10
Biological researchers do not claim that organic changes are the **root cause**...	p. 11
They are the result of centuries of **trial and error**.	p. 11
The wise and **mild-mannered** Sir Thomas Moore...	p. 13
Benjamin Rush...known as the "**father** of American psychiatry."	p. 17
Dix took a job teaching **Sunday school** in a prison.	p. 17
there were simply not enough advocates of moral therapy to **staff** them.	p. 18
the mentally disturbed were once again seen as **freakish** and dangerous.	p. 18
Many people emerged from their lobotomies in a permanent **vegetative** state.	p. 18
A number of so-called halfway houses, however, are merely **seedy** hotels...	p. 19
a situation called "**revolving door** syndrome"...	p. 19
since they lack the money even for the cheapest **flophouse**.	p. 20
Many ... are dependent on city shelters and **soup kitchens**.	p. 20
end up on the street **penniless** and in desperate need of care.	p. 21
he asked patients to relax on a couch and simply to **pour out** whatever came to mind.	p. 22
Other techniques shared by Western and African psychotherapy are emotional **venting** and group treatment.	p. 23
they are allowed to take up tasks and **mix with people** again.	p. 23

Activities and Demonstrations (ACT/DEMO)

Background knowledge probe (ACT/DEMO 1-1)
Objective: To assess the breadth and depth of knowledge that your students bring to your course
Materials: Background Knowledge Probe Handout
Procedure: Before you begin presenting material, ask your students to take this brief assessment. The probe will help students measure their own background knowledge of abnormal psychology as well as providing you with valuable information.
Discussion: Briefly review the terms presented on the handout. Point out what chapters the terms will appear in. Ask students who claim to have an understanding of a term to discuss it. At the end of the semester, administer the probe again to determine gains in understanding.

Defining abnormal behavior (ACT/DEMO 1-2)
Objective: To demonstrate the difficulty in making judgments about what is abnormal
Materials: none
Procedure: Students should be divided into groups of about four or five. Each group should be given two different cases of someone suffering from a severe psychological disorder. These cases should be short and can be condensed from the ancillary case book or from the textbook. Have half of the groups make a case for one individual to be judged "normal" and the other to be "abnormal." The remaining groups do the opposite. The students should use the textbook or any other personal information they may have.
Discussion: Ask the students to develop a diagnosis based on stereotypes they have brought to the class.

Survey of psychological disorders (ACT/DEMO 1-3)
Objective: To demonstrate how abnormality has affected all and to document the most prevalent disorders
Materials: Survey of Psychological Disorders Handout
Procedure: Students should anonymously fill out the survey indicating if family members or friends suffer from any other disorders.
Discussion: Collect the surveys and rank the disorders with regard to frequency. Emphasize how these disorders affect not only the individual but also family and friends. Keep the data that you collect to identify any trends.

Role playing (ACT/DEMO 1-4)
Objective: To learn about the historical perspectives of abnormality
Materials: Role Playing Handout
Procedure: Put students into groups of six and assign a historical role to each. Instruct them that prior to the next class meeting, they must review the material related to their role and be prepared to role play their part. On the following class day, have all of those students with same role meet to compare notes and to discuss the role and its perspectives. Then regroup the students into their original groups. Each student should

be given a chance to role play their assigned part. Encourage your students to "debate" and rebut each other's perspectives.

Discussion: Follow-up with students writing a paper summarizing their part's perspective, as well as the perspective of the other roles in their group.

Do something abnormal (ACT/DEMO 1-5)
Objective: To illustrate the social and personal consequences of abnormal behavior
Materials: None
Procedure: Ask your students to do something abnormal. It must not be illegal, immoral, or dangerous. While this activity can be very effective, you want to approach it with some caution. A good idea is for the students to tell you what they plan to do.
Discussion: Require students to write a short paper describing why the behavior they performed is abnormal according to the textbook as well, as to discuss any contexts in which the behavior is not abnormal.

Films and Videos

Abnormal Behavior. CRM. A general overview of abnormal behavior. This film emphasizes the childhood antecedents for various disorders and includes views of individuals manifesting severe psychopathology as well as some controversial treatment procedures, including ECT.

Abnormal Behavior.- A Mental Hospital. MCG. A documentary about treatment in a mental hospital. Gives students an overview of treatment concerns and diagnostic issues.

An Ounce of Prevention. ANN/CPB. *The World of Abnormal Psychology.* Discusses prevention in abnormal psychology.

Brainwaves. PBS. Explores the physical explanations and treatments for mental illness from late eighteenth-century Europe to the present.

Committed in Error: The Mental Health System Gone Mad. FHS. This is the story of a man who spent 66 years incarcerated and forgotten in mental health institutions, although there was never anything wrong with him. This story takes place in Britain, but it could as easily have happened in the U.S., where similar errors have occurred.

King of Hearts. UA. This classic film depicts the experiences of a English soldier who is sent to scout out a German-occupied French village inhabited solely by members of the local insane asylum. This is a moving portrayal of both normal and abnormal behavior.

Looking at Abnormal Behavior. ANN/CPB. *The World of Abnormal Psychology.* Defines abnormal behavior.

Madness. ANN/CPB. The Brain. Compelling human portraits of schizophrenics and their families are featured, dramatically illustrating the effects of a split between the thinking and feeling parts of the brain. Scientists' efforts to pinpoint the brain's anatomical changes are chronicled.

Mistreating the Mentally Ill. FHS. This program focuses on the U.S., Japan, India, and Egypt, examining how each culture sees mental illness and treats the less accepted members of society. It concludes that the problem is not merely due to a shortage of funds, but can be attributed to the indifference of society to the mentally ill.

New Race and Psychiatry. FHS. The issue of race within psychiatry is at its most apparent in the psychiatric hospitals and institutions where, as one doctor who appears in this program puts it, "there is an over-representation of black people." There is also a problem of misdiagnosis and mistreatment because some medical staff don't understand why people from different cultures behave contrary to their expectations. This program looks at the issues of racism in mental health care, and at some black self-help groups that offer alternatives to the conventional psychiatric practices that have failed to meet the needs of the black community.

Out of Sight, Out of Mind. PBS. Episode two traces the rise and fall of the asylum, from the establishment of asylums during the Enlightenment, through the high point of Victorian reformist optimism, to the decline of the asylum in the 20th century. The hour concludes by raising the impact of the pharmacological revolution of the 1950s and 1960s and civil rights reforms of the 1960s as reasons for the current policy of deinstitutionalization.

The Enlightened Machine. ANN/CPB. The Brain. Beginning with the 19th century experiments of Viennese physician Franz Joseph Gall, the creator of the pseudo-science of phrenology, this episode moves rapidly to the forefront of 20th-century science, using microphotography to show how the brain organizes its "electrical symphony"-- neurotransmitters crossing synaptic gaps.

The Scandal of Psychiatric Hospitals: When the Goal Is Insurance Reimbursement. FHS. While mentally ill patients are being discharged because their insurance benefits have expired, perfectly healthy Americans are being locked up in mental hospitals while the hospital draws their insurance. This program shows how one group of hospitals herded up patients and held healthy Americans unnecessarily hostage.

To Define True Madness. PBS. This first episode examines past misconceptions and modern myths: how mental illness has been confused with neurological disease, moral judgments, deceptive appearances, and cultural stereotypes. The program discusses how mental illness looks to others now and in the past, how it has been misrepresented in art and literature, how it feels to those who experience it, and how it is diagnosed by doctors and psychiatrists.

19

Using Movies and Mental Illness as a Teaching Tool

The first class can be used to introduce the ways in which the instructor plans to incorporate films in the class. Students will be enthusiastic about using movies to supplement the text, and will want to volunteer examples of films they have seen that address mental illness, substance abuse, or developmental disabilities. It may be useful to have students generate a list of films relevant to the class; of course, almost every film on the list will be discussed in *Movies and Mental Illness*.

Films like *Snake Pit* and *Chattahoochee* will be useful to get students thinking about how treatments for people with mental illness has changed – and not changed – over the past few decades. However, these films are not as widely available as some others.

Having your students watch *The Madness of King George*, an award winning film that should be available in every corner video store, will set the stage for a provocative discussion of differential diagnosis. King George suffered from porphyria, a genetically transmitted metabolic disorder that produces psychiatric symptoms. The film is an excellent springboard for discussions of the limits of psychiatric diagnosis; the ways in which the King would have been treated differently today; and the historical tendency to assume that physical disorders we don't understand are psychiatric in nature. This may also be a good time to initiate a discussion of the mind/body problem and the ways in which *psyche* and *soma* interact. A quotation from Lord Chesterfield may serve to get the discussion started: "Psyche and soma are inextricably linked, and one can't suffer without the other sympathizing."

Movie	Link to Chapter	Page Reference to Wedding and Boyd
• Psycho series • Halloween series	perceptions of abnormality (p. 4)	p. 5
• Snake Pit • Chattahoochee	historical perspective on treatment (p. 12)	p.163 p. 163
• One Flew Over the Cuckoo's Nest • Frances • Angel at My Table	treatment (p. 11)	p. 7, 163 p. 163 p. 163

Classroom Assessment Techniques (CAT)

Muddiest Point (CAT 1-1)
Instruct students to write about an issue, concept, or definition presented in Chapter 1 that they find most confusing or difficult to understand.

Directed Paraphrasing (CAT 1-2)
In two or three sentences, students should paraphrase some important idea, concept, or definition presented in Chapter 1. Consider paraphrasing the medical model, the biogenic theory, the relationship between cause and treatment, Pinel's contribution to moral therapy, or deinstitutionalization..

Definition Matrix (CAT 1-3)
Using the handout, students should identify each definition of abnormality presented in the textbook. For each criterion, students should provide a definition, an example, and advantages and disadvantages of the criterion. Students should attempt to write only a few words or phrases.

Suggestions for Essay Questions

- ❑ Why should clinicians be aware of a patient's cultural and ethnic background?
- ❑ Explain the relationship between explaining abnormal behavior and treating abnormal behavior.
- ❑ As you consider the historical conceptions of abnormal, what themes do you see that emerge and then reemerge later?

Background Knowledge Probe
Handout

For each term, indicate your degree of understanding using the following scale:

1 - I have heard of this
2 - I have heard of this, but can't really say what it means
3 - I have heard of this and have some general idea of what it means
4 - I have heard of this and could explain it to someone

medical model	1	2	3	4
psychiatrist	1	2	3	4
norms	1	2	3	4
deinstitutionalization	1	2	3	4
DSM-IV	1	2	3	4
test-retest reliability	1	2	3	4
comorbidity	1	2	3	4
mental status exam	1	2	3	4
medical model	1	2	3	4
ABAB design	1	2	3	4
incidence	1	2	3	4
defense mechanism	1	2	3	4
id	1	2	3	4
diathesis	1	2	3	4
genotype	1	2	3	4
monozygotic twins	1	2	3	4
panic disorder	1	2	3	4
generalized anxiety disorder	1	2	3	4
dissociative amnesia	1	2	3	4
migraine headache	1	2	3	4
premorbid adjustment	1	2	3	4
mania	1	2	3	4
antisocial personality disorder	1	2	3	4
detoxification	1	2	3	4
paraphilia	1	2	3	4
positive symptoms	1	2	3	4
flat affect	1	2	3	4
clanging	1	2	3	4
expressed emotions	1	2	3	4
Alzheimer's disease	1	2	3	4
might terrors	1	2	3	4
PKU	1	2	3	4

Survey of Psychological Disorders
Handout

Please indicate if a family member or a friend has or had any of the following disorders or problems. Do not put your name on this survey.

	Family member	Friend
phobia (objects, animals, places, insects)		
panic disorder		
generalized anxiety (anxious all the time)		
mental retardation		
learning disability (reading, mathematics)		
stuttering		
attention-deficit/hyperactivity disorders		
Alzheimer's disease		
Parkinson's disease		
head trauma (brain injury)		
alcoholism		
dependency on caffeine		
dependency on nicotine		
dependency on pain killers		
dependency on tranquilizers		
schizophrenia		
depression		
bipolar disorder (manic-depressive)		
eating disorders (anorexia nervosa, bulimia)		
chronic insomnia		
narcolepsy (attack of sleep)		
sleep apnea (breathing stops in sleep)		
stress-related (ulcer, asthma, high blood pressure)		
tension or migraine headaches		
antisocial behavior (chronic fighting, lying, stealing)		
pathological gambling		
anger/impulse control problems		
exhibitionism (exposing one's genitals)		
voyeurism (Peeping Tom)		
transexualism		
transvestisms (cross dressing)		
victim/perpetrator of child abuse, incest, rape		
victim/perpetrator of domestic violence		

Role Playing
Handout

In this activity, you are to adopt a historical or cultural role and to assess a case study. Make sure you have reviewed the material related to your role in the textbook. Your interpretation of the case study ought to reflect the era in which you lived and the prevailing theories of that era. Specifically, your task is to identify the nature of the disorder, suspected cause, and a recommendation for treatment. You should prepare to defend your conclusions.

Case Study:

Kevin is a 33 year old male. Kevin is an only child from an upper class family. His parents pay all of his bills and provide him with a monthly stipend. His father and mother describe Kevin as "odd, but harmless." He lives alone in a three-bedroom apartment. For the past few years, Kevin has collected and stored in his apartment piles and piles of newspapers and magazines. The piles are so high that they touch the ceiling in some places in the apartment. Sometimes his apartment is so filled with newspapers and magazines that he cannot open the front door. Whenever he goes outside, he will check wastebaskets and dumps for newspapers and magazines. In the basement of the apartment building, he keeps a second cache of newspapers and magazines for, as he says, "Just in case." When asked to explain his collection, he claims that he might need the newspapers and magazines sometime. He claims that the moment he starts tossing out the newspapers and magazines, he might need to read a specific article or story. In addition, Kevin cannot understand why other people are so willing to dispose of their newspapers and magazines; he says, "They'll be sorry one day."

1.   You are an ancient Hebrew priest.
2.   Hippocrates
3.   Plato
4.   Galen
5.   You are a practitioner of Naiken
6.   You are a practitioner of Moriata

Definition Matrix
Classroom Assessment Technique

Term	Definition	Example	Advantage	Disadvantage
Norm violation				
Statistical rarity				
Personal discomfort				
Maladaptive behavior				

Chapter 2

Diagnosis and Assessment

Chapter Map

Section	Instructor Manual Components
Diagnosis and Assessment: The Issues • Why Assessment? • The Diagnosis of Mental Disorders • Assessing the Assessment: Reliability and Validity • Problems in Assessment	*History of testing (LL 2-1)* *Clinical biases (LL 2-2)* *Assessment (TP 2-1)* *Examples of description and prediction (TP 2-2)* *ICD and culture (TP 2-3)* *Labels students apply to themselves (TP 2-4)* *DSM-IV (TP 2-51)* *Validity and reliability of a calculator (TP 2-6)* *Dimensional classification (ACT/DEMO 2-1)* *Axes and case study (ACT/DEMO 2-2)*
Methods of Assessment • The Interview • Psychological Tests • Laboratory Tests • Observation in Natural Settings	*The Interview (LL 2-3)* *Using clock drawing as neuropsychological assessment (LL 2-4)* *Child behavioral assessment (LI 2-5)* *Joe and methods of assessment (TP 2-7)* *Students' personal experiences with testing (TP 2-8)* *Gardner and multiple intelligences (TP 2-9)* *"Projecting" in projective tests (TP 2-10)* *Testing materials and reports (TP 2-11)* *Response set/Social desirability set (ACT/DEMO 2-3)* *Neurological assessment (ACT/DEMO 2-4)*
Cultural Bias in Assessment	

Chapter Outline

I. Introduction
    A. **Psychological assessment** is the collection, organization, and interpretation of information about a person and his or her situation
    B. Ancient societies sorted people for prediction
    C. Ancient societies practiced psychiatric classification

II. Assessment: The Issues
    A. Why Assessment?
        1. Assessment has two goals
            a. Description of personality, cognitive functioning, mood, and behavior
            b. Prediction and its values relate to practical applications
        2. Reassessment of patients is important in managed health care
    B. The Diagnosis of Mental Disorders
        1. **Diagnosis** occurs when a problem is classified within a set of categories and labeled accordingly
        2. The Classification of Abnormal Behavior
            a. Several classification systems have been used; the first comprehensive one was developed by Kraepelin
            b. American Psychiatric Association published its first classification system in 1952
            c. DSM-IV was published in 1994
        3. The Practice of Diagnosis
            a. Each category has a description and set of specific criteria
            b. Diagnosis supplies description of patient's problem and **prognosis** or prediction of its future course
            c. A common vocabulary is important and diagnostic labeling is required
        4. Criticisms of Diagnosis
            a. Diagnosis tied to medical model
            b. Diagnosis falsifies reality
            c. Diagnosis may discount gradations between forms of abnormality
            d. Diagnosis gives illusion of explanation
            e. Diagnostic labeling may be harmful
    C. Categorical vs. Dimensional Classification
        1. Categorical classification places patients into diagnostic dimensions of pathology
        2. Dimensional classification could offer more information
        3. Defending diagnosis
            a. Research depends on diagnosis
            b. Research requires consistent and meaningful diagnosis

4. DSM-IV
    a. Specific diagnostic criteria
        i. essential features
        ii. associated features
        iii. diagnostic criteria
        iv. differential diagnosis
    b. Five axes of diagnosis
        i. Axis I - Clinical syndrome
        ii. Axis II - Personality disorders or mental retardation
        iii. Axis III - General medical disorders
        iv. Axis IV - Psychosocial and environmental disorders
        v. Axis V - Global assessment of functioning
    c. Unspecified etiology

D. Assessing the Assessment: Reliability and Validity
    1. Reliability
        a. **Reliability** is a measure of consistency
        b. Three criteria of reliability
            i. internal consistency
            ii. test-retest reliability
            iii. interjudge reliability
        c. Reliability of psychiatric diagnosis is low
        d. Specific diagnostic criteria increases reliability
        e. Low coverage results in higher reliability
        f. More patients are put into residual categories
        g. More diagnostic categories have been added
    2. Validity
        a. **Validity** refers to extent to which test measures what it is suppose to measure
        b. **Descriptive validity** is extent to which it provides significant information
            i. Pattern of symptoms is important
            ii. Most patients show **cormorbidity** by meeting diagnostic criteria for more than one Axis I disorder
        c. **Predictive validity** refers to degree to which questions of cause, prognosis, and treatment are answered
            i. High predictive validity requires high reliability
            ii. Changes in DSM may result in improved validity

E. Problems in Assessment
    1. Assessor's behavior, physical appearance, race, and sex can influence assessment
    2. Practical reasons, such as financial circumstance, can influence assessment
    3. Specific diagnosis criteria and decision rules minimize problems
    4. Assessment should rely more on actuarial judgment
    5. Some assessors do not follow diagnostic rules

III. Methods of Assessment
    A. The Interview
        1. The **interview** consists of a face-to-face conversation
        2. Can vary from structured to unstructured and will depend on purpose of interview
        3. Can introduce interview's subjectivity and biases
        4. Diagnostic interviews are highly structured
            a. Mental status exam is a broad exam
            b. Purpose of MSE is to detect dementia and other organic brain disorders
    B. Psychological Tests
        1. **Psychological test** is a standard procedure in which patient responds to series of stimuli; scoring is more objective
        2. **Psychometric approach** identifies stable personality **traits**
        3. Intelligence tests
            a. First psychological assessment techniques were **intelligence tests** used in French school system by Binet
            b. Final score on the test presented as **intelligence quotient (IQ)**
            c. Wechler tests yield general IQ, performance IQ, and verbal IQ
            d. Intelligence tests are carefully designed and have high internal consistency, test-retest reliability, and predictive validity
            e. Intelligence tests may be culturally biased
            f. Intelligence testing may reflect a too narrow view of mental abilities
        4. Projective Personality Tests
            a. **Projective personality tests** based on assumption of psychodynamic in drawing out people's real motives by responding to ambiguous stimuli
            b. The Rorshach
                i. **Rorshach Psychodiagnostic Inkblot Test** consists of cards with inkblots to which the subject must react
                ii. Has a free-association phase and inquiry phase
                iii. Highly structured scoring methods using a detailed manual
            c. The TAT
                i. **Thematic Apperception Test (TAT)** is series of pictures
                ii. Subject asked to describe picture, story, and character(s)
                iii. Is used to detect specific kinds of information

        d.   Evaluation of projective tests
             i.   Poor interjudge reliability
             ii.   Supporters claim that projective tests are only method that is open and flexible enough to provide information about unconscious processes

5.   Self-Report Personality Inventories
        a.   **Self-report personality inventories** ask subjects about themselves
        b.   The MMPI
             i.   **Minnesota Multiphasic Personality Inventory-2** compares subject responses to those with psychiatric diagnoses
             ii.   Test items that differentiate between normal and abnormal groups comprise the MMPI
             iii.   Test results in scores on ten clinical scales
             iv.   MMPI-2 consists of control scales to determine validity of responses and can be used to assist interpretation
             v.   Pattern of scores is used for interpretation and indicating the degree of overall disturbance
             vi.   Some concern regarding **response set** such as social desirability and acquiescence
             vii.   Can be scored by computer
        c.   The MCMI-III
             i.   Intended to assist in diagnosis of personality disorders
             ii.   Yields ratings on DSM personality disorders

6.   Psychological Tests of Organic Impairment
        a.   Diagnosis must distinguish between psychogenic causes and biogenic causes
        b.   Tests can determine the type of neurological problem
        c.   Paper and pencil tests are valid measures
             i.   Bender Visual-Motor Gestalt Test requires subjects to reproduce designs
             ii.   Halstead-Reitan Neuropsychological Battery assesses functioning of specific areas of brain

C.   Laboratory Tests
     1.   Direct testing of structure and function of nervous system
     2.   **Electroencephalogram (EEG)** measures electrical activity of brain cells
     3.   Sophisticated measures have been developed
         a.   Computerized tomography (CT) uses a series of x-rays
        b.   Positron emission tomography (PET) traces radioactive particles
        c.   Magnetic resonance imaging (MRI) uses magnetic fields

4. Using the relationship between emotion and physiology, psychogenic disorders may be detected
    a. **Polygraph** includes a number of sensors that pick up physiological changes
    b. **Galvanic skin response (GSR)** detects sweat gland activity
    c. **Electromyogram (EMG)** senses electrical activity of muscles
5. **Polysomnography** uses several measures and can identify nature of subject's problem
6. Physiological tests have several advantages
    a. Processes measured are those that subject cannot report
    b. More precision with good reliability and validity
    c. A problem is interpreting the psychological significance of results

    D. Observation in Natural Settings
1. **Situational variables** influence behavior
2. **Person variables** influence behavior
3. To assess behavior accurately, assessment must occur in natural settings
4. Direct observation has several advantages
    a. It does not depend on self-report
    b. Reduces assessment errors
    c. Observation provides workable answers
5. Direct observation has several disadvantages
    a. It requires much time
    b. Presence of observer may be reactive
    c. Behavior being studied may change due to observation
6. Use of recording devices raises some ethical problems

IV. Cultural Bias in Assessment
    A. Cultural bias exists in assessment such as use of second language in interview
    B. DSM-IV includes caution about misapplying diagnosis without considering cultural and ethnic differences
    C. Correcting bias may actually increase bias in diagnosis

Chapter Boxes

- On Being Sane in Insane Places
  - A. Rosenhan used eight pseudopatients, who presented themselves at mental hospitals
  - B. Pseudopatients diagnosed as schizophrenic and admitted; thereafter, made no complaints
  - C. Normal behaviors were seen as consistent with original diagnosis
  - D. Upon discharge, they were classified as in remission
  - E. Study was widely debated and gave support to the diagnostic system

- Comorbidity: Disturbance as a Package
  - A. Comorbidity occurs when two or more disorders occur simultaneously
  - B. Comorbidity is more common than having just one disorder
  - C. Questions regarding the existence of comorbidity have been raised versus just one disorder (e.g., antisocial personality disorder and substance dependence)
  - D. Answers influence theories of causation and treatment

Learning Objectives (LO)

By the time you are finished studying this chapter, you should be able to do the following:

1.   Define psychological assessment and list two goals of the assessment process (28-29).

2.   Define psychiatric diagnosis, list four criticisms of diagnosis, and explain why diagnosis is used in spite of these criticisms (29-31).

3.   List and describe the five axes of diagnosis used in DSM-I`V, and compare this approach to diagnosis to the dimensional system of classifying mental disorders (32-33).

4.   Define the concept of reliability in assessment and describe three kinds of reliability discussed in the text (33-34).

5.   Define the concept of validity in assessment and describe two types of validity mentioned in the text (34-37).

6.   Summarize the text's discussion of problems in assessment and what can be done about them (37 38).

7.   Discuss how the interview is used as an assessment tool, and summarize its advantages and disadvantages (38-39).

8.   List four currently used intelligence tests and review the controversial aspects of using intelligence scores in psychological assessment (40-42).

9.   List and briefly describe four personality tests (two projective and two self-report) discussed in the text and discuss the pros and cons associated with each (43-48).

10.   List and describe two psychological tests for the detection of organic impairment (48-49).

11.   Describe five types of physiological lab tests highlighted in your text that are used in connection with psychological assessment (49-50).

12.   Discuss the advantages and disadvantages of using observation 'in natural settings as an assessment tool (50-52).

13.   Explain how cultural bias can make accurate assessment and diagnosis difficult (52).

Lecture Leads (LL)

History of testing (LL 2-1)
As early as 2200 B.C., China was conducting psychological testing. Every three years, the Chinese Emperor would test his officials. Assessment was an important part of China's civil service, which existed for three thousand years. Applicants for civil service would be assessed in several areas such as writing, arithmetic, and music. Those wanting a civil appointment had to pass successfully through three levels of assessment. The first level required candidates to write a poem and thematic narrative. Their writing skill and penmanship were used to weed out unsuitable applicants. The second level and third level consisted of more rigorous testing that lasted three days and nights. Contemporary psychometric intelligence testing can be traced back to Galton. He measured intelligence by assessing such things as reaction time. He also studied the heritability of intelligence by analyzing twins and eminent families.

Resources:
Cohen, R. J., Swerdlik, M. E., & Smith, D. K. (1992). Psychological testing and assessment: An introduction to tests and measurement. Mountain View, CA: Mayfield.

Pressley, M., & McCormick, C. B. (1995). Advanced educational psychology for educators, researchers, and policymakers. New York: Harper Collins.

Clinical biases (LL 2-2)
One bias that clinicians, and for that matter all of us, are susceptible to is the confirmation bias. We actively seek out information that confirms our expectations and ignore or discount information that disconfirms them. The clinician who experiences the confirmation bias becomes even more confident of the validity of clinical judgment. The hindsight bias is another error that can cloud clinical judgment. The hindsight bias, or the I-knew-it-all-along phenomenon, is the tendency to have known an outcome after the outcome occurs. These after-the-fact explanations and confirmation bias were believed to have played a role in Rosenhan's classic study involving normal individuals complaining of hearing voices, who were later admitted and diagnosed as schizophrenic. Once admitted, they stopped the psychiatric complaints. However, the staff interpreted normal behavior and life histories in the context of their diagnoses. The textbook describes the actuarial approach to assessment. Actuarial interpretation is based on statistical methods and empirical evidence. In forming a judgment, the actuarial prediction uses formal rules while clinical judgment uses less formal rule and therefore, is more susceptible to the biases of the clinician.

Resource:
Myers, D. (1993). Social psychology. New York: McGraw-Hill.

The Interview (LL 2-3)

Expand the coverage of the interview method by focusing on issues of ethics and matching interviewers to respondents. In framing the latter issue, Weiss writes, "to what extent it is necessary for the interviewer to be an insider in the respondent's world in order to be effective as an interviewer" is an important consideration in interviewing. Observable characteristics such as ethnicity, gender, age, dress, physical appearance, and socioeconomic status do influence both respondent and interviewer. Weiss suggests that for the most part it is best to be "an insider," which allows a relationship to develop. However, he describes situations where he as an outsider had to be instructed regarding the respondent's social, economic, and cultural world. In some circumstances, being an outsider to the respondent's world may be an advantage; for instance, one might be more willing to open up to an outsider who is less likely to be critical.

Resource:

Weiss, R. S. (1994). Learning from strangers: The art and method of qualitative interview studies. New York: Free Press.

Using clock drawing as neuropsychological assessment (LL 2-4)

Patients have been assessed using clock drawing for many years where they are asked to draw and copy clock faces. Freedman et al. suggest that these tasks require visuospatial and visuomotor processes requiring contributions from a number of brain regions. In addition, clock drawing requires auditory language skills, attention, and motor output. Patients must have adequate executive functions of "planning, organizing, and simultaneous processing…to coordinate the multiple steps." For example, while drawing the numbers of a clock, one must keep intact their spatial layout following the curve of the clock. Clock drawing analysis can be used as a screening tool and in diagnosis. Clinicians using this tool pay particular attention to such characteristics as placing clock hands in the center, providing enough space for numbers, no omission of numbers, correct order of numbers, and the contour of the clock. Freedman et al. provide examples of clocks drawn by patients with brain lesions, brain injury, dementia, and disconnection syndrome as well as normative data.

Resource:

Freedman, M., Leach, L., Kaplan, E., Winocur, G., Shulman, K. I., & Delis, D. C. (1994). Clock drawing: A neuropsychological analysis. New York: Oxford University.

Child behavioral assessment (LL 2-5)

When assessing children, the clinician is faced with some unique challenges. If there is concern for the child's social development, a number of sociometric techniques have been developed. These techniques assess peer relationships. For instance, to determine peer status, peer ratings are sometimes used. Children are given a list of classmates and asked to indicate on a 1 to 5 Likert-scale how much they enjoy playing with each child. Sometimes, the Likert-scale includes a series of faces showing different degrees of frowning and smiling. In addition, instead of using the DSM-IV, which is a clinically derived classification system, clinicians may opt for empirical approaches to assess children. These approaches use statistics to identify interrelationships between behavior. Typically, the child's behavior is assessed by identifying the extent to which a particular characteristic is present. Using sophisticated statistical tools and large samples, relationships between behaviors are determined, thus producing syndromes. Research has identified two general clusters of behavior. The first cluster is typically called externalizing and includes specific behaviors such as destructiveness and disobedience. The second cluster, internalizing, may consist of anxiety and shyness. The empirical approach uses correlations as the basis of assessment and diagnosis. Several instruments have been developed to identify syndromes such as The Child Behavior Checklist and Child Behavior Profile. A child receives a score for each general cluster and can be compared to norms of both referred and nonreferred children.

Resources:
Ollendick, T. H., & Hersen, M. (1984). Child behavioral assessment: Principles and procedures. New York: Pergamon Press.

Wicks-Nelson, R., & Israel, A. C. (1997). Behavior disorders of children (3d ed.). Upper Saddle River, NJ: Prentice-Hall.

Talking Points (TP)

Assessment (TP 2-1)
Make sure you stress the idea that the manner in which behavior is assessed is based on how human behavior is conceptualized and understood, which is shaped by one's own culture and experiences.

Examples of description and prediction (TP 2-2)
To illustrate the goals of assessment in a different way, ask students for examples of the last time *they* described behavior (e.g., "Wow, that guy really made a fool of himself," "My roommate never picks up her stuff") and predicted behavior (e.g., "I bet she'll go out with him,""He'll probably register for another class"). Remind them that like clinicians, we also attempt to describe and predict behavior, though using different methods and approaches.

ICD and culture (TP 2-3)
Knowing what your students know about culture-bound syndromes, ask them for pros and cons of an international classification system (i.e., International Classification of Diseases).

Labels students apply to themselves (TP 2-4)
The textbook presents an argument that labels can be harmful to people. Ask your students to come up with pejorative labels that they apply to themselves and to others (e.g., nerd, jock, blonde, geek, ped). If they have trouble, instruct them to think back to high school for examples. Your discussion should focus on how we interpret and react to people solely based on labels. You may also want to share how labels have changed over the years. For example, in the early days of intelligence testing, the labels used were idiot, imbecile, and moron and these were accepted clinical terms. How about now?

DSM IV (TP 2-5)
Bring a copy of the DSM-IV and share with your students a few specific examples of the elements of specific diagnostic criteria. Also show the various committees and subcommittees that worked on this most recent revision. Even though the fourth edition is more research-based and involved field trials, with any project of this magnitude and number of participants, there is also compromise.

Validity and reliability of a computer keyboard (TP 2-6)
To illustrate the concepts of validity and reliability, students should think of a computer keyboard. For example, if you type a ten-page research paper, does the "t" key always type a "t"? If your friend uses the same keyboard, will she get a "t" when using the same key? If you must type an article summary, does the "t" key type a "t"? Does the label on the key accurately describe what you get when you hit it? Ask your students for other examples.

Joe and methods of assessment (TP 2-7)

As you discuss the various methods of assessment, try to integrate the textbook's running presentation of Joe and his responses to the various tests. As you travel through this section and share Joe's responses, get a few students to evaluate his responses after each method is presented. When you conclude this section, place students in groups of 3 to 4 to share their evaluation of Joe and to offer a diagnosis. Alternatively, ask students to write about their evaluation and diagnosis.

Students' personal experiences with testing (TP 2-8)

This idea should be approached with appropriate sensitivity. Ask students for volunteers to share their own experiences with psychological and laboratory testing. For example, a student who has had an MRI scan can relate aspects of the experience that are not covered in the textbook.

Gardner and multiple intellgiences (TP 2-9)

Howard Gardner has added an eighth intelligence to his theory of multiple intelligence-- naturalist, which is the ability to recognize animals and plants.

"Projecting" in projective tests (TP 2-10)

To put it differently, the premise behind projective measures is that when we are confronted with vague or ambiguous stimuli (e.g., incomplete sentence, inkblot), we will "project" our unconscious motives, desires, and conflicts into our responses.

Testing materials and reports (TP 2-11

The textbook presents a number of tests. Students will really appreciate it if you bring these tests or parts of the tests to class for their review. Bringing in the WAIS-R or WISC-III will make these tests more real. In addition, bring in a copy of a MMPI-2 or California Personality Inventory (CPI) profile and case summary, and actual scans from MRI, PET, and EEG tracings. If your department has a biofeedback unit with galvanic skin response or electromyograph, consider a demonstration for your students.

astrology was also being used as the basis of **personal horoscopes**...	p. 28
in the **cost-conscious** atmosphere of **managed health care**...	p. 29
such as impulsiveness and **fits of anger.**	p. 29
in some cases depriving them of their **civil rights.**	p. 29
and a **homemaker**...	p. 31
all the pseudopatients spent a **good part of the day**...	p .31
the only things standing in the way of conversion to this system are tradition and **professional vanity.**	p. 32
Experienced diagnosticians harbor no hops that DSM-IV is **foolproof**...	p. 32
whether the disorder tends to **run in families**...	p. 33
some writers call them **"wastebasket categories"**...	p. 34
If a diagnosticians tends to be formal and **businesslike**...	p. 37
The **Veterans Administration**, for example, pays higher benefits to veterans...	p. 38
handsome people and **plain people**...	p. 38
he skills of **Michelle Kwan** and **Michael Jordan**...	p. 42
on a projective test it is hard for subjects to **"fake"** their responses...	p. 46
they were involved in a **child-custody case**...	p. 47
for the sake of a **lawsuit** claiming psychological injury...	p. 47
certain **pencil-and-paper tests** have proved valid measures...	p. 48
into receptacles of the same shapes while **blindfolded**...	p. 49
children who are coddled by their parents after **temper tantrums**...	p. 50
they are being watching by a person with a **clipboard.**	p. 51
gang members in **ghetto neighborhoods** may have...	p. 52

Activities and Demonstrations (ACT/DEMO)

Dimensional classification (ACT/DEMO 2-1)
Objective: To engage students in creating their own dimensional classification
Materials: Case studies
Procedure: Select several case studies from the textbook or other source. Place the students in small groups and assign each group a case study. Their task is to create a dimensional classification for their assigned case. Specifically, the groups will identify dimensions that provide more information than categorical classification. Dimensions might include interpersonal relationships, sleep quality, mood, activity level, self-defeating thoughts, severity, anxiety in social situations, identity formation, memory functioning, and communication ability. Each dimension will yield a score.
Discussion: Compare the dimensions that are created by students and the scores they assigned to each case.

Axes and case study (ACT/DEMO 2-2)
Objective: To demonstrate the use of the axes in the DSM-IV
Materials: None
Procedure: There are two parts to this activity. In the first part, students should create a fictitious person complete with a brief life history, demographical information (e.g., age, gender, marital status, SES), and some presenting psychological disorder. This can be done in groups or individually. (Alternatively, you could supply the cases.) In the second part, after the student-created cases are exchanged, students are to evaluate the case using the five axes of the DSM-IV, which is discussed on page 33 of the textbook. The students ought to focus primarily on Axes IV and V. You may wish to continue this activity by having students exchange their cases one more time
Discussion: Preface your discussion with the students with an acknowledgment that they are not familiar enough with DSM-IV nor qualified to make diagnosis, nor have they been presented with enough information in the cases. Go through at least several cases sharing how you would evaluate the information in the context of the axes.

Response set/Social desirability set (ACT/DEMO 2-3)
Objective: To demonstrate the effects of response set/social desirability set
Materials: Student Survey of Behaviors (Form A) (anonymously completed); Student Survey of Behaviors (Form B) (with student name)
Procedure: Give half of your students Form A and the other half Form B. Tell your students that you've been asked to give this survey to students. Tell your students to read carefully the instructions on the survey. When completed, the surveys should be brought up to the front. As students hand-in Form B (with student name), ask each to obliterate their names, indicating that a mistake was made in writing the instructions. Obviously, your request is to protect confidentiality.
Discussion: First, debrief your students by indicating that this is not a bona fide attitudinal measure and that you were not asked to give it to students. Second, explain that the purpose of the activity was to demonstrate response set. Engage the students in a

40

discussion of how they felt as they were completing the survey. Did those completing Form B feel as if their privacy was being invaded? Extend the discussion to interviews and surveys, and how the nature of certain question and response sets may create bias. Another option is to analyze the data and see if there are differences between the two sets of surveys, which could be attributable to response set.

Neurological assessment (ACT/DEMO 2-4)
Objective: To demonstrate the methods and principles of neuropsychological tests
Materials: Several neuropsychological tests that your department or other psychologists in your community have available
Procedure: Select and bring several examples of neuropsychological tests into class. (Consider the Bender Visual-Motor Gestalt Test, Halstead-Reitan Battery, or the Luria-Nebraska Neuropsychological Battery). Administer parts of these tests such as the Trial Making exam. If you do not have the expertise necessary to conduct this demonstration, a guest speaker could provide assistance.
Discussion: Discuss how neuropsychologists identify deficits by using these tests that are able to relate the deficit to specific areas of the brain. Your guest speaker can be a valuable resource with the interpretation of these tests if you are not qualified.

Films and Videos

Personality. MGH. A college student agrees to undergo a formal psychological assessment. His reactions to the test results as well as the reactions of others are highlighted.

Simulated Psychiatric Patient Interview. USC. This series of six cassettes covers methods of interviewing and introduces students to the clinical presentations of more common psychiatric disturbances, including schizophrenia, organic brain syndrome, and phobias.

Using Movies and Mental Illness as a Teaching Tool

This is the logical class in which to introduce the Mental Status Examination. A standardized and widely used Mental Status Examination is included as Appendix A of *Movies and Mental Illness*. Your students will appreciate it if you will take time to walk through the examination, answering any questions they might have. The instructor may want to actually administer the examination to a student to illustrate how the test might be used in clinical practice, and students can be encouraged to give the examination to family members or friends outside of class, with the caveat that they have not received sufficient training to interpret the examination or to draw clinical inferences from the results.

There is a brief scene in the movie *Powder* in which a psychologist is reporting the results of a series of psychological tests given to the film's protagonist. The psychologist states "All the tests indicate you have the most advanced intellect in the history of mankind. Do you understand what that means?" This vignette might serve as a vehicle for a class discussion of the limits of psychological testing, and the reasons the psychologist's statement simply doesn't make any sense.

Movie	Link to Chapter	Page Reference to Wedding and Boyd
• Born on the Fourth of July	assessment (p. 28)	p. 9
• Mr. Jones		p. 49
• Clean Shaven		p. 117
• One Flew Over the Cuckoo's Nest		p. 161

Classroom Assessment Techniques (CAT)

One-Sentence Summary (CAT 2-1)
Ask students to summarize a specific piece of information in this chapter by responding to the question, "Who does/did what to whom, when, where, how, and why?"

Focused Listing (CAT 2-2)
Select an important point from this chapter (e.g., DSM-IV; reliability; MMPI-2; cultural bias) and ask students to write five words or phrases that describe the point.

Learning Review (CAT 2-3)
Students are to write in order five of the most important ideas they learned in this chapter.

Suggestions for Essay Questions

- ❑ If you are a clinical psychologist diagnosing various mental disorders, how might your diagnoses lead to harmful effects?
- ❑ Why are reliability and validity important characteristics in assessment and diagnosis?
- ❑ Contrast categorical and dimensional classification.
- ❑ What types of assessment would be appropriate to administer if a clinician suspected depression in a patient?

Student Survey of Behaviors
Form A

Please answer the questions presented below. Do not put your name on the survey.

What is your major? _____

How old are you? _____

What was the income of your parents last year? _____

At what age did you have your first sexual experience? _____

When was your last sexual experience? _____

Have you ever had inappropriate sexual desires or thoughts?   YES   NO

Have you ever cheated on your partner (e.g., boyfriend, girlfriend, spouse)?   YES   NO

Have you ever considered cheating on your partner?   YES   NO

Have you ever been sexually attracted to any of your college professors?   YES   NO

Are you a good person?   YES   NO

If an elderly person needed help with her groceries, would you help? YES   NO

Have you ever shoplifted?   YES   NO

Have you ever cheated on a college test?   YES   NO

Have you ever committed plagiarism on a paper?   YES   NO

Have you ever ignored a stranded motorist who was in obvious need of help? YES   NO

WHEN YOU HAVE COMPLETED THE SURVEY, PLEASE BRING IT TO THE
FRONT OF THE ROOM WHERE IT WILL BE COLLECTED

Student Survey of Behaviors
Form B

Please answer the questions presented below. Please put your name where indicated so that you may be contacted for future research.

Name _____

What is your major? _____

How old are you? _____

What was the income of your parents last year? _____

At what age did you have your first sexual experience? _____

When was your last sexual experience? _____

Have you ever had inappropriate sexual desires or thoughts? YES   NO

Have you ever cheated on your partner (e.g., boyfriend, girlfriend, spouse)? YES   NO

Have you ever considered cheating on your partner? YES   NO

Have you ever been sexually attracted to any of your college professors? YES   NO

Are you a good person? YES   NO

If an elderly person needed help with her groceries, would you help? YES   NO

Have you ever shoplifted? YES   NO

Have you ever cheated on a college test? YES   NO

Have you ever committed plagiarism on a paper? YES   NO

Have you ever ignored a stranded motorist who was in obvious need of help? YES   NO

WHEN YOU HAVE COMPLETED THE SURVEY, PLEASE BRING IT TO THE FRONT OF THE ROOM WHERE IT WILL BE COLLECTED

Chapter 3

Research Methods in Abnormal Psychology

Chapter Map

Section	Instructor Manual Components
Characteristics of the Scientific Method • Skeptical Attitude • Objectives • Scientific Procedures	*The nature of science (LL 3-1)* *Predicting violent crimes (LL 3-2)* *How to think (LL 3-3)* *Ethics in research (LL 3-4)* *Skeptical attitude (TP 3-1)* *Objectives (TP 3-2)* *Case studies (TP 3-3)* *Independent and dependent variable (TP 3-4)* *The null hypothesis (TP 3-5)* *The data are…(TP 3-6)* *Placebo effects (TP 3-7)* *Ethics of double blind studies (TP 3-8)* *Research in the popular media (ACT/DEMO 3-1)* *Placebo effect (ACT/DEMO 3-2)*
Research Designs • Correlational Research • Epidemiological Studies • Experimental Designs • The Single-Case Experiment	*Importance of research methods (TP 3-9)* *Single-case experiment (TP 3-10)* *Identifying research designs (ACT/DEMO 3-3)* *Correlation coefficient (ACT/DEMO 3-4)* *Field trip (ACT/DEMO 3-5*

Chapter Outline

I. Characteristics of the Scientific Method
    A. Skeptical Attitude
        1. Skepticism is necessary because behavior is complex
            a. Many factors are needed to explain behavior
            b. It is difficult to identify these factors
        2. Skepticism is necessary because science is a human endeavor
            a. Scientists are not passive observers
            b. Many decisions made in science are subjective
    B. Objectives
        1. Four objectives are met through the scientific method
            a. Description is defining and classifying events and their relationships
                i. Descriptions must have reliability
                ii. Descriptions must have validity
            b. Prediction is based on description
            c. Control involves development of treatment and preventive strategies
            d. Understanding of behavior consists of identify cause(s)
                i. **Covariation** of events refers to two events varying together
                ii. **Time-order relationship** where cause must occur before effect
                iii. **Elimination of plausible alternative causes** rules out other likely causes
        2. Internal and External Validity
            a. **Confounding** often arises when eliminating plausible alternative explanations
            b. Studies free of confounding have **internal validity**
            c. **External validity** refers to degree to which results can be generalized
            d. **Generalizability** is ability of a finding to be applied to different populations, settings, and conditions
            e. **Representativeness** determines generalizability and refers to degree to which sample matches population
            f. Random sampling achieves representativeness; a **random sample** is where everyone in population has equal chance of being included
            g. Many studies use samples of convenience
            h. To **replicate** a study tests its generalizability
    C. Scientific Procedures
        1. The Hypothesis
            a. A **hypothesis** is a tentative explanation for behavior

b. Intuition and hunches often play roles in developing a hypothesis

c. **Clinicians** develop hypotheses by observing their patients' reactions to treatment

2. Operational Definitions

a. Hypotheses must be **falsifiable**, that is stated in a way that it can be proven untrue

b. Terms in hypothesis must have **operational definitions** with regard to operations that can be measured or observed

3. Methods of Control

a. **Independent variable** is factor that is manipulated to measure its effects

b. **Dependent variable** is factor that may be affected and whose changes will be measured

c. **Internal validity** when control techniques are properly used

i. Independent variable is manipulated at two levels-- experimental group and control group

ii. Other variables are held constant to prevent confounding

iii. Balancing is used to control factors that cannot be held constant--**random assignment** is most important balancing technique

d. Minimizing the effects of expectations

i. **Demand characteristics** are expectations that the subject has

ii. **Experimenter effects** are biases from experimenter expectations

iii. **Placebo** and placebo subject groups are procedures to control for demand characteristics and experimenter effect

iv. **Double-blind** procedure is when subject and experimenter are unaware of which treatment is given

e. **Statistical inference** is used to conclude that results are real and not due to chance

i. Assumption of **null hypothesis**

ii. Use of probability theory to determine odds of obtaining results if null hypothesis were correct

iii. Statistically significant leads to rejection of null hypothesis

f. Problems with statistical inference

i. Statistical significance does not necessarily mean finding is important

          ii.   Statistical significance does not necessarily mean **clinical significance**

II.   Research Designs
- A.   Correlational Research
  1. **Correlational research** examines relationships
  2. In **case-control designs**, cases (those with mental disorder) are compared with controls (those who do not)
  3. Correlation does not show causal relationships
  4. Relationships between variables may be due to **third-variable problem**
  5. Matching may solve third-variable problem
  6. **Longitudinal studies** involve examining same subjects over period of time
     - a. **High risk designs** involve examining subjects who have high likelihood of developing a disorder
     - b. Genetic high risk designs include subjects who are genetically predisposed to disorder
     - c. Behavioral high risk designs include subjects who have some behavioral characteristic that makes them at-risk
     - d. Caution is needed when inferring causation
- B.   Epidemiological Studies
  1. **Epidemiology** studies frequency and distribution of disorders within specific populations
     - a. **Incidence** is number of new cases within given time period
     - b. **Prevalence** is percentage of population that has disorder
     - c. **Duration** is average length of disorder
  2. Epidemiological studies are prone to pitfalls such as unrepresentative samples
- C.   Experimental Designs
  1. Clinical Trials
     - a. **Clinical trials** test effectiveness of treatments
     - b. Empirically supported treatments are those that pass the test of controlled experimental research, but may not be clinically significant
  2. Analogue Experiments
     - a. **Analogue experiments** are experiments that serve as models of real life
     - b. A high degree of internal validity is possible due to types of control necessary to identify causal relationships
     - c. Allows testing of variables that otherwise could not be manipulated
     - d. The more ethical an analogue experiment is, the less analogous it is likely to be

        e.   Animal models can be used to address problems of analogue experiments
- i. Animal models allow variables to be held constant
- ii. Some procedures are too intrusive to be used with humans
- iii. Long-term consequences of treatment and disorder can be assessed

        f.   Threats to external validity exist in analogue experiments

D. The Single-Case Experiment
1. Multiple groups of subject pose problems
2. **Single-case experiment** focuses on one person
3. First stage is baseline where behavior before treatment is assessed
4. Treatment is introduced; comparison is made
5. Common design is ABAB--baseline, treatment, baseline, treatment
6. Multiple-baseline design does not involve an interruption of treatment
7. Limitation of single-case design is weak external validity

Chapter Boxes

- The Case Study
    - A.   Detailed description of the subject
    - B.   Case study helpful to describe rare phenomena such as Tourette's disorder
    - C.   Case studies can provide counterinstance that violates widely accepted principle
    - D.   Limitations include problems with cause and effect relationships and generalizability
    - E.   Case studies most valuable as a complement to other methods

- The Correlation Coefficient: A Measure of Predictive Strength
    - A.   Correlation coefficient indicates how well one variable can predict another variable
    - B.   Direction can be positive or negative
    - C.   Magnitude ranges from 0 to 1.00
    - D.   Correlation coefficient represents only linear relationship, not curvilinear

- Treatment Development: An Example of Hypothesis Generation
    - A.   Hypothesis generation is a legitimate phase of research design
    - B.   Research conducted by Kohlenberg examined Functional Analytic Psychotherapy
    - C.   Treatment development is example of pilot testing

Learning Objectives (LO)

By the time you are finished studying this chapter, you should be able to do the following:
:

1. List and define four objectives of the scientific method (58-59).

2. List three conditions that must be met before cause and effect are established (59).

3. Distinguish between internal and external validity and describe the means by which each is obtained (59-60).

4. Describe the case study method of research and discuss its advantages and limitations (61).

5. Describe the process of designing an experiment, from hypothesis formation through the development of operational definitions and the establishment of independent and dependent variables (60-6 1).

6. Distinguish between experimental and control groups, and describe three kinds of control techniques that are applied to factors influencing the outcome of an experiment (61-63).

7. Explain how expectations on the part of experimenters and subjects can influence the outcome of an experiment, and describe measures that are commonly taken to minimize these expectations (63-64).

8. Discuss the role of statistical analysis and inference in scientific research (64-65).

9. Describe correlational research designs, tell what one can and cannot conclude from correlations, and why (65-67).

10. Define longitudinal studies, including high-risk designs, and discuss their advantages and shortcomings (67).

11. Define epidemiological studies and describe the difference between incidence and prevalence (68).

12. Define clinical trials and analogue experiments and give example of each (68-70).

13. Describe single case experimentation, give examples of two variations of this research design, and tell how it differs from a traditional case study (70-72).

Lecture Leads (LL)

The nature of science (LL 3-1)

The assumption and characteristics of science is an important topic for students to understand because they differentiate science from religion, philosophy, and pseudosciences such as astrology. For example, science assumes that events in nature are governed by predictable sequences of cause and effect (i.e., lawful) and that these sequences are observable and understandable. Behavioral sciences assume that behavior is determined by natural, external forces. Science is based on careful observations, which yields empirical evidence.

Resource:

Heiman, G. W. (1998). Understanding research methods and statistics: An integrated introduction for psychology. Boston: Houghton Mifflin.

Predicting violent crimes (LL 3-2)

A good example of an attempt to predict future behavior is Teplin, Abram, and McClelland's investigation of the relationship of mental disorder to violent crimes. A large sample of male jail detainees were interviewed using the National Institute of Mental Health Diagnostic Interview Schedule. Arrest records were evaluated for six years. Mental disorder and substance abuse did not predict the number of arrests for violent crimes. The study did reveal a slightly higher rate of arrest for those individuals with delusional and hallucinatory symptoms. You could use this study to illustrate how researchers go about attempting to make predictions and the importance of controlling for the effects of variables such as age.

Resource:

Teplin, L. A., Abram, K. M., McClelland, G. M. (1994). Does psychiatric disorder predict violent crime among released jail disorders? A six-year longitudinal study. American Psychologist, 49, 335-342

How to think (LL 3-3)

There are a number of very good sources dealing with critical thinking and statistics. Consider developing a lecture that describes some of the characteristics of uncritical thinking and how we can be misled by statistics. For example, testimonials and evidence persuade many people. Correlation among the general public is assumed to show causation. Graphs when inappropriately constructed and labeled can be quite misleading. Finally, we are likely to experience the hindsight bias and illusory correlation. These shortcomings make necessary the scientific method.

Resources:

Huff, D. (1954). How to lie with statistics. New York: Norton.

Smith, R. A. (1995). Challenging your preconceptions: Thinking critically about psychology. Pacific Grove, CA: Brooks/Cole.

Stanovich, K. E. (1996). <u>How to think straight about psychology</u> (4th ed.). New York: Harper Collins.

Ethics in research (LL 3-4)
Many of your students will have participated as subjects for experiments while in introductory psychology courses. Develop a presentation that summarizes research ethics and subjects' rights (e.g., informed consent, deception). Detail the obligations of the experimenters and the steps necessary for an experiment to be conducted on your campus, such as an institutional review committee.

Resource:
American Psychological Association. (1992). Ethical principles of psychologists and code of conduct. <u>American Psychologist, 47</u>, 1597-1611.

Talking Points (TP)

Skeptical attitude (TP 3-1)
To illustrate the importance of a skeptical attitude, bring in a tabloid magazine with particularly unbelievable stories. Select a couple of these articles and ask some students to read them. Ask them if they believe the article. Is it important to be skeptical. David Hume, the Scottish philosopher, argued that extraordinary claims, like many of those in the popular media, require extraordinary evidence. Ask your students what type of extraordinary evidence they would need before accepting the validity of these articles.

Objectives (TP 3-2)
As you discuss the objectives of the scientific method, point out that most people attempt to do the same. They describe behavior, they predict behavior, they control behavior, and they attempt to understand. Discuss with your students what separates "most people" as they attempt these objectives from scientists as they attempt the same objectives.

Case studies (TP 3-3)
To illustrate case studies, point out to students that they are the subjects of many case studies, such as medical records, school records, military records, IRS records, and baby books.

Independent and dependent variable (TP 3-4)
Here's a mnemonic device to help students with independent and dependent variables: ICED--"*independent* variable is the *cause* and the *effect* is the *dependent* variables."

The null hypothesis (TP 3-5)
One of the more interesting things about behavioral science is that it is not set up to prove or disprove hypothesis, but merely to fail to support a hypothesis or support a hypothesis. Many people assume that science provides proof for a hypothesis. The nature of probability shows that we can only be 99% sure of something.

The data are...(TP 3-6)
It is a good thing to remind students that the word "data" is plural. "The data are..." and "The data do..." are grammatically correct. It is also worth noting that "datum" is singular.

Placebo effects (TP 3-7)
Students are often exposed to placebo effects in their college life. This exposure can come in the form of alcohol; the alcohol content of many drinks can vary from very high to very low (e.g., near beer). Many college students can relate stories and you could ask them for examples when they thought they were consuming real beer but only drinking nonalcoholic beer. Another idea is to bring a package insert for medication. The insert will present what effects subjects experienced when given a placebo. Considered using ACT/DEMO 3-2 as a follow-up.

Ethics of double blind studies (TP 3-8)
Discuss with your students the ethics of. Should researchers be allowed to give a drug that save the lives of those in the experimental group, while giving a placebo to the control group? Should a person's life be left to a table of random numbers? How should researchers balance the need for well-controlled studies with the withholding of a potentially life-saving treatment? Use the pointed examples of treatments for AIDS and cancer.

Importance of research methods (TP 3-9)
Many students say that they just want to help people or perhaps they have no desire to become mental health professionals. Often they see no connection between their career goals and the usefulness of research methods. There are a couple of good strategies to convince them. First, our knowledge of psychopathology is based upon research methods. Point out that the validity of the material presented in the textbook is based upon somebody's faithful and appropriate use of research methods. Second, nearly everyone has or will be prescribed medication for a large number of disorders ranging from strep throat to high blood pressure to diabetes to bipolar disorder. We trust that those who developed these drugs carefully followed the scientific method. Third, as future mental health professionals, students will be in a position to evaluate the efficacy of various treatments for their clients. What better way is there to evaluate treatments than to apply one's knowledge of research methods?

Single-case experiment (TP 3-10)
Other terms for a single-case experiment that students might find useful are small-N research and N-of-one.

The earliest antipsychotic drug, for example, was developed by **accident**.	p. 58
More than anything else, scientists are **skeptical.**	p. 58
there is a **body of research** show that certain types of poor communication...	p.59
A good example is the infamous **"executive monkey"** study...	p. 59
The second monkey in each pair, called the **"yoked"** monkey...	p. 59
constituted a **"marker"** for the most severe types of **wife-beaters**	p.60
It took a **sharp-eyed** clinician to notice that the drug...	p. 60
If a hypothesis is to receive a **fair trial**...	p. 61
If, however, the subjects were assigned randomly--by **drawing lots,** for example...	p. 63
they will feel relaxed, **giddy,** and so on.	p. 63
and you always **toss a coin** to see who will pay the bill.	p. 64
is like a carpenter whether **a screwdriver is better than a hammer.**	p. 65
we could predict students' success in college on the basis of their **SAT scores.**	p. 66
such as age, gender, and **life circumstances.**	p. 68
When animal subjects are sued, a **nagging** question is always present...	p. 70
The single-case experiment resembles its **cousin,** the case study...	p. 70
whether children suffering from autism could be taught to **"look before they leaped."**	p. 71

Activities and Demonstrations (ACT/DEMO)

Research in the popular media (ACT/DEMO 3-1)
Objective: To demonstrate the amount of misleading and incomplete information presented in the popular media
Materials: Popular magazines and tabloid newspaper if an in-class activity
Procedure: After students are placed in groups of three or four, they should select several articles to analyze. The articles should be evaluated with regard to research design, method of data collection, and the quality of interpretation. Of particular interest is the misinterpretation of statistical evidence, such as presenting correlation as causation. An excellent modification of this activity is to instruct students to find the original source of the study. Students then compare the article in the popular media with the original article.
Discussion: Each group should present the articles and their evaluation. Point out common shortcomings and why misinterpretations are so common in the popular media.

Placebo effect (ACT/DEMO 3-2)
Objective: To demonstrate the effects of placebo on drinking behavior
Materials: Nonalcoholic beer
Procedure: Approach this activity with appropriate caution, reminding students of the legal drinking age and the importance of responsible drinking. Have a club or other student organization (e.g., fraternity, dorm house) that is noted for its parties with alcohol. join you as you plan this demonstration. At one of their parties, alcoholic beer should be substituted with nonalcoholic beer. Ask students to act as casual observers and collect data on the placebo effects of the nonalcoholic beer. In particular, these observers should describe the behavior of the participants. If the behaviors change, what are the changes. Observers may wish to interview some of the participants to see if they knew that a placebo had been provided.
Discussion: Lead a discussion on the power of placebo effects and the need to control for expectancy effects and demand characteristics.

Identifying research designs (ACT/DEMO 3-3)
Objective: To identify research designs in a literature search
Materials: Research article from journal
Procedure: This activity can be done individually or in groups. Students are asked to select one disorder presented in the textbook and to locate a related research article in the literature. The task is to analyze the research methodology used in the article.
Discussion: Not only is this an effective activity to preview the course topics, but it also involves exposure to scientific journals and methodology. This activity also familiarizes students with library resources. If you require a research paper in the course, this activity can act as a good starting point.

Correlation coefficient (ACT/DEMO 3-4)
Objective: To demonstrate correlation coefficient
Materials: None
Procedure: Select two pairs of variables that you can readily measure in class. The first pair of variables ought to be logically related to each other (e.g., height and shoe size), while the other variables pairing should not (e.g., height and number of siblings). Using students as subjects, collect and plot the data. Calculate the correlation coefficients.
Discussion: Students should attempt to interpret the coefficient with regard to direction and magnitude of relationships. It is also a good idea to reiterate that correlation does not indicate cause and effect relationships. Are there third variables that account for the relationships you analyzed?

Field trip (ACT/DEMO 3-5)
Objective: To introduce students to research methodology and your institution's research facilities
Materials: None
Procedure: Arrange for a tour of your institution's and department's research facilities. Your institution may have a center or institute conducting survey research, a physiology laboratory, a rat lab, or lab school. Ask colleagues who are currently conducting research in the facilities to briefly describe their projects. If possible, students may be able to observe subjects being tested. Instruct your students to develop a list of questions prior to the field trip.
Discussion: Students should be asked to describe the type of research conducted.

Films and Videos

Methodology.- The Psychologist and the Experiment. CRM. Demonstrations of the experimental methods using the work of Stanley and Schacter and Austin Riesen as examples. Research terms and concepts are used throughout.

New Directions. WGBH. Discussion of the future of psychology and new directions in research, theory, and application.

Scientific Approach. PSU. Outlines the scientific method as it applies to psychology.

Search for Solutions: Investigation. UM. This film focuses on the way progress is made in science.

Using Movies and Mental Illness as a Teaching Tool

It may not be necessary to assign a film to accompany this chapter. However, if a film is desired, the 1997 HBO movie *Miss Evers' Boys* is highly recommended as a way to trigger a classroom discussion of research ethics. This compelling film is an accurate historical account of the Tuskegee experiment, a study of the natural history of syphilis in untreated Black men.

It is shocking to realize that this experiment was continued long after efficacious treatments for syphilis had been developed. President Clinton publicly apologized to the survivors and families of the Tuskegee experiment in 1997, and the federal government paid reparations and committed public funds to sensitize researchers to ethical issues.

The film illustrates why human subjects committees are so vitally important. It may be useful to review some of the experiments conducted by Nazi physicians during the Second World War, and to debate whether or not deception is every justified in research. It will be interesting to discuss whether vulnerable people (e.g., prisoners, convicts, and people coping with mental retardation, mental illness, or addictions) can ever give meaningful informed consent. Finally, this discussion can lead naturally into a discussion of (a) eugenics and (b) the ethical use of animals in research.

Classroom Assessment Techniques (CAT)

Minute Paper (CAT 3-1)
Ask your students to write about unanswered questions they have concerning Chapter 3.

Minute Paper (CAT 3-2)
Students should describe what concept in Chapter 3 would be the most important to know for a layperson.

Focused Listing (CAT 3-4)
Select an important point from this chapter (e.g., ABAB design; dependent variable; placebo; internal validity) and ask students to write five words or phrases that describe the point.

Memory Matrix (CAT 3-5)
Students should use the handout provided to review the purposes, functions, and importance of key terms.

Suggestions for Essay Questions

- ❑ Why should mental health professionals such as clinical psychologists be aware of research methods in abnormal psychology?
- ❑ Describe some pitfalls, such as the effects of expectations, researchers face as they test hypotheses.
- ❑ Contrast the experimental designs of clinical trials, analogue experiments, and single case experiments. When are these types of designs most appropriate?

Identifying research designs
Handout

APA Citation of article:

Psychological disorder:

Type of research method:

Hypothesis:

Operational definitions:

Independent variable (s):

Dependent variable (s):

Subject groups:
        Experimental group:

        Control group:

Results:

Memory Matrix
Classroom Assessment Technique

Key Terms	**Function/Purpose/Importance**
confounding	
internal validity	
random sampling	
hypothesis	
operational definition	
independent variable	
dependent variable	
clinical significance	
correlational research	
longitudinal study	
epidemiology	
clinical trials	
analogue experiment	
single-case experiment	
ABAB design	
multiple-baseline design	

Chapter 4

The Biological, Psychodynamic, and Cognitive Perspectives

Chapter Map

Section	Instructor Manual Components
The Biological Perspective • Behavior Genetics • The Central Nervous System • The Peripheral Nervous System: Somatic and Autonomic • The Endocrine System • Evaluating the Biological Perspective	*Case studies: Biological and hereditary influences on behavior (LL 4-1)* *Early history of psychosurgery (LL 4-2)* *Nature and nurture (TP 4-1)* *Types of genetic studies (TP 4-2)* *Twin studies (TP 4-3)* *Biology as the basis for affect, behavior, and cognitions) (TP 4-4)* *Brain imaging (TP 4-5)* *Sympathetic division (TP 4-6)* *Brain used in performing tasks (ACT/DEMO 4-1)* *Field trip (ACT/DEMO 4-2)* *In-class twin study (ACT/DEMO 4-3)*
The Psychodynamic Perspective • The Basic Concepts of Freudian Theory • The Descendants of Freud • The Psychodynamic Approach to Therapy • Evaluating the Psychodynamic Perspective	*Jung's collective unconscious and archetype (LL 4-3)* *Freud as a neurologist) (TP 4-7)* *Personalizing id, ego, and superego (TP 4-8)* *Influence of pain and pleasure in behavior (TP 4-9)* *Dream diary (TP 4-10)* *Freud vs Erikson (TP 4-11)* *Examples of defense mechanism (TP 4-12)* *Freud's couch (TP 4-13)* *Countertransference (TP 4-14)* *Guest speakers (ACT/DEMO 4-4)* *Freud's influence (ACT/DEMO 4-5)* *Dream interpretation (ACT/DEMO 4-6)*

The Cognitive Perspective	Social cognitive theory (LL 4-4)
• The Background of the Cognitive Perspective • Cognitive Behaviorism • Cognitive Appraisal • Self-Reinforcement • Information Processing • The Cognitive Approach to Therapy • Evaluating the Cognitive Perspective	Effects of self-efficacy (LL 4-5) Sources of efficacy expectancies (LL 4-6) Formula (TP 4-15) Summarizing perspectives (ACT/DEMO 4-7)

Chapter Outline

I. The Biological Perspective
    A. Introduction
        1. Focus on interaction between behavior and organic functions
        2. Mind-body problem--relationship between physical and psychological aspects
    B. Behavior Genetics
        1. **Chromosomes** contain genetic instructions
        2. More than 2,000 **genes** are on a single chromosome
        3. **Behavior genetics** examines genetic influence on behavior
        4. **Diathesis-stress model** helpful in explaining most genetically influenced disorders
            a. Diathesis refers to constitutional predisposition
            b. Stress combined with diathesis results in abnormal behavior
        5. Clinical Genetic Studies
            a. **Genotype** is individual combination of genes; **phenotype** is individual combination of observable characteristics
            b. Family studies used to examine genetic influences
                i.   **Index case** is identified; examine other members of family to determine if they have same disorder
                ii. Evidence is only suggestive of genetic transmission since family members share environments
            c. Twin studies compare twins
                i.   **Monozygotic (MZ) twins** develop from single fertilized egg and have same genotype
                ii. **Dizygotic (DZ) twins** develop from two eggs fertilized by two sperm and have half of their genes in common
                iii. **Co-twins** examined to determine how many are **concordant**
                iv. Environment is still an important influence since MZ twins are raised more alike than DZ twins
            d. Adoption studies
                i.   Attempt to separate the effects of genetics and environmental influences
                ii. Mother-child adoption studies are easier to conduct
        6. Molecular Genetic Studies
            a. Molecular genetic studies identify which genes are involved in behavioral disorders
            b. Linkage analysis uses genetic markers as clue in locating gene controlling disorder

C. The Central Nervous System
1. **Nervous system** is vast network extending from brain to body
2. **Central nervous system (CNS)** consists of brain and spinal cord
   a. Primarily responsible for storing and transmitting information
   b. If problem in CNS, then problem in behavior
3. **Neurons** made upon several characteristics structural features (i.e., cell body, dendrites, axon, axon terminals, and myelin sheath)
   a. Impulse from one neuron to the next neuron continues by **neurotransmitter**
   b. Firing is all-or-none response
   c. Some impulses stimulate the nerve to fire, some inhibit firing
3. Neurotransmitters
   a. Neurotransmitters are chemicals stored in vesicles
   b. After release, it travels across gap and contacts **receptors** like key in lock
   c. **Reuptake** breaks down neurotransmitters and transported back to axon terminal
   d. Receptors can change
      i. Decrease in number or sensitivity is called down-regulation
      ii. Increase in number or sensitivity is called up-regulation
   e. Several neurotransmitters have been studied
      i. Acetycholine--body muscles, sleep disorders, and Alzheimer's disease
      ii. Dopamine--motor behavior, reward, schizophrenia
      iii. Enkephalins--act on opiate receptors
      iv. GABA--inhibitory effect
      v. Norepinephrine--fight or flight response, alertness
      vi. Serotonin--role in constraint, depression
   f. Drug treatment
      i. Psychopharmacology studies drug treatment of psychological disorders
      ii. Many drugs target neurotransmitters by increasing or suppressing action of neurotransmitter
4. The Anatomy of the Brain
   a. Cerebral cortex, sulci, gyri, longitudinal fissure, corpus callosum, central sulcus, lateral sulcus; lobes - parietal, frontal, temporal, occipital thought to have differing functions
   b. Cross section of brain reveals hypothalamus, limbic structures (e.g., amygdala, hippocampus), thalamus, basal

ganglia, cerebellum, pons, medulla, brain stem, reticular activating system, and ventricles

    c. Structures associated with abnormal behaviors

5. Measuring the Brain

    a. Electroencephalography (EEG) measures general brain activity by giving picture of brain's response to external stimuli

    b. **Positron emission tomography (PET)** and single photon emission computer tomography (SPECT) measure brain metabolism and function

    c. **Computerized tomography (CT)** and **Magnetic resonance imaging (MRI)** measure brain structure

    d. Each technique has advantages and disadvantages

6. Psychosurgery

    a. Surgery designed to reduce abnormal behavior is called **psychosurgery**

    b. Psychosurgical techniques have been refined, for example cingulotomy and stereotactic subcaudate tractotomy

    c. Psychosurgery has been used in treating severe obsessive-compulsive, depression and pain

    d. Psychosurgery is very controversial and is usually the last treatment resort

7. Lateralization: Effects of Language and Emotion

    a. **Lateralization** refers to differences between the two hemispheres

    b. Complex cognitive processes involve both hemispheres, yet different aspects are localized

D. The Peripheral Nervous System: Somatic and Autonomic

1. Peripheral nervous system is a network leading from CNS to body

    a. **Somatic nervous system** senses and acts on external world

    b. Autonomic nervous system of special interest to abnormal psychology

2. **Autonomic nervous system** controls smooth muscles, glands, and internal organs

    a. **Sympathetic division** mobilizes body to meet emergencies

    b. **Parasympathetic division** slows down metabolism and regulates organs so that they can rebuild energy supply

    c. Relationship between divisions is complex and they work together

E. The Endocrine System

1. **Endocrine system** produces **hormones** and is involved in many functions

2. Hypothalamus controls endocrine system

       3.   Hormones may be involved in specific psychological disorders such as depression, bipolar disorder, eating disorders, and stress-related disorders

  F.   Evaluating the Biological Perspective
      1.   Biochemical abnormality may be result not cause of disorder
      2.   Not all biological treatments are effective
      3.   Ethical issues are raised such as treatment, symptom reduction and its consequences
      4. ·   Cannot consider biogenic and psychogenic causation as either-or

II.   The Psychodynamic Perspective
  A.   Introduction
      1.   **Psychodynamic perspective** focuses on interaction of forces deep in the mind
      2.   Three basic principles
          a.   Psychic determinism refers to belief that behavior is determined by intrapsychic forces
          b.   True motives of behavior are unconscious
          c.   Forces are deeply affected by childhood experiences
      3.   Sigmund Freud founding father of psychodynamic perspective
          a.   Neurologist with practice in Vienna
          b.   No physical cause could be found for many of his patients' complaints
          c.   Developed **psychoanalysis**
          d.   Freud's theory has been revised
  B.   Basic Concepts of Freudian Theory
      1.   The Depth Hypothesis
          a.   Idea that nearly all mental activity occurs unconscious is **depth hypothesis**
              i.   Conscious consists of what person is aware of any given instant
              ii.   **Unconscious** consists of all materials that mind is not attending to
          b.   Disturbing material is forced out on consciousness in process called repression and
              i.   Material may erupt later into consciousness
              ii.   Material plays role in behavior
      2.   The Necessity of Interpretation
          a.   Revealing hidden, intrapsychic motives requires **interpretation**
          b.   Two layers of meaning in behavior
              i.   **Manifest content** or surface meaning
              ii.   **Latent content** or true, unconscious meaning
      3.   The Structural Hypothesis: Id, Ego, and Superego
          a.   **Structural hypothesis** describes interaction of forces

b. **Id** refers to primitive biological drives
    i. Aggression is drive
    ii. **Libido** is the sexual drive and major source of psychic energy
    iii. Id operates on pleasure principle
c. **Ego** mediates between id and forces that restrict id's satisfactions
    i. Ego operates on the reality principle.
    ii. Because of reality principle, higher functions, such as language, perception, and memory, develop
d. **Superego** represents moral standards of society and the parents

4. The Dynamics of the Mind
 a. When ego is overwhelmed by demands of id and superego, **anxiety** is experienced
 b. Anxiety signals ego that danger is at hand
 c. Anxiety can be managed in several ways
 d. **Defense mechanisms** distort or deny reality and are adaptive up to a point
    i. **Repression**--pushing down into unconscious unacceptable id impulses; most fundamental defense mechanism
    ii. **Projection**--unacceptable impulses are attributed to others
    iii. **Displacement**--transferring of emotion from one object to another
    iv. **Rationalization**--offering socially acceptable reasons for behavior done for unconscious and unacceptable motives
    v. **Isolation**--avoiding unacceptable feelings by cutting them off from events to which they are attached and reacting to events emotionlessly
    vi. **Intellectualization**--using smokescreen of abstract intellectual analysis of emotion
    vii. **Denial**--refusing to acknowledge external source of anxiety
    viii. **Reaction formation**--repressing anxiety-arousing feelings and expressing the exact opposite
    ix. **Regression**--returning to a earlier developmental stage
    x. **Undoing**--engaging in a ritual behavior or thought to cancel an unacceptable impulse
    xi. **Sublimation**--transforming and expressing sexual or aggressive energy into more socially acceptable forms

70

5. The Stages of Psychosexual Development
   a. **Psychosexual development** refers to series of stages in which child is motivated to gratify sexual and aggressive drives in body zones
   b. Ways in which id strivings are handled in these stages has consequences for adult personality
   c. The **oral stage**
      i. Mouth is focus of id
      ii. Search for oral stimulation
   d. The **anal stage**
      i. Anus is focus
      ii. Gratification gotten from retaining and expelling feces
      iii. Toilet training seen as crucial event since it is first difficult demand on ego
   e. The **phallic stage**
      i. Genitals is focus
      ii. Gratification gotten from masturbation
      iii. **Oedipus complex** is experienced
      iv. Boys experience **castration anxiety**
      v. Girls experience Electra complex and penis envy
      vi. Both boys and girls later identify with same-sex parent incorporating values from which superego develops
   f. Latency and genital stage
      i. **Latency stage** characterized by dormant sexual impulses
      ii. **Genital stage** is final phase of development and when sexual impulses reawaken
6. Normal and Abnormal Behavior
   a. Normal personality functioning motivated by irrational id
   b. Abnormal personality motivated by irrational drives and childhood experiences
   c. **Neuroses** are conditions of abnormal personality functioning involving ever-increasing anxiety, defenses, and maladaptive functioning
   d. **Psychosis** occurs when the ego collapses and involves a flood of id impulses and anxiety
C. The Descendants of Freud
   1. Revisions of Freud's theory involve three trends
      a. Pronounced emphasis on ego, less on sex
      b. Child's social relationships as central determinant of behavior
      c. Extended period of critical developmental influences

2.   Carl Gustav Jung--mind contains personal unconscious and also collective unconscious; goal in therapy is integration to become whole
3.   Alfred Adler--primary motivator is striving to attain goals and overcome handicaps; relationships with others are important; inferiority complex
4.   Harry Stack Sullivan--abnormality rooted in poor parent-child relationships; developed milieu therapy for treatment of psychoses
5.   Karen Horney--psychological disturbance result of basic anxiety, and a pervasive view of world as impersonal and cold; placed emphasis on men's greater prestige and opportunities
6.   Heniz Hartmann--ego develops independently of id and has its own functions; conflict-free expressions of ego are mind's cognitive process; developed **ego psychology**
7.   Erik Erikson--**ego identity** product of psychosocial development; personality affected by family and others; developmental stages occur throughout the life span characterized by challenges to ego
8.   Margaret Mahler--developed object relations; child's interaction with mother most important in psychological development; process of **separation-individuation** is greater and greater independence
9.   Heniz Kohut--developed **self psychology**; development of self dependent on vigor and calmness
10.   John Bowlby and Mary Ainsworth--developed attachment theory; basic determinant of adult personality is attachment; conducted studies of infant-mother pairs using Strange Situation paradigm

D.   The Psychodynamic Approach to Therapy
    1.   **Psychoanalysis** is foundation of psychodynamic therapies
    2.   Freudian Psychoanalysis
        a.   Source of neurosis was anxiety experienced by ego
        b.   Bring unconscious material out into consciousness
        c.   Analyst interprets client's remarks using four techniques
            i.   In **free association**, client verbalizes whatever thoughts come to mind without censoring them
            ii.   **Dream interpretation** allows identification of manifest content and latent content
            iii.   Client may show **resistance** to avoid painful material; analyst interprets resistance
            iv.   In analysis of **transference**, analyst assesses transfer of emotion from important people in client's life to analyst
    3.   Modern Psychodynamic Therapy
        a.   A modified form of psychoanalysis is practiced today
        b.   Therapists take a more active role in therapy session
        c.   Pay more attention to client's current life
        d.   Most therapy is briefer and less intensive

E.	Evaluating the Psychodynamic Perspective
	1.	Psychodynamic Theory versus the Medical Model
		a.	Was first purely psychological approach to abnormal behavior
		b.	Saw abnormal behavior to be problem in individual's emotional life
	2.	Criticisms of Psychodynamic Theory
		a.	Lack of experimental support
			i.	Claims have never been tested in scientifically controlled experiments
			ii.	Case studies open to bias
			iii.	Clinical evidence used since phenomena is too complex
			iv.	Some evidence support and some evidence contradicts Freudian theory
		b.	Dependence on inference
			i.	Assumption is mental processes are unconscious and therefore must rely on inference
			ii.	Inference subject to bias
		c.	Unrepresentative sampling and cultural bias
			i.	Theory based on limited sample of middle-class Viennese women between 20 and 45 years old
			ii.	Freud lived in society that emphasized social-class distinctions
		d.	Reductiveness
			i.	Dismal view of human life
			ii.	Humans driven by instincts beyond conscious control
	3.	The Contributions of Psychodynamic Theory
		a.	Theory helped to demythologize mental disorders
		b.	Mentally disturbed have no monopoly on irrationality
		c.	Importance of increasing client's self-knowledge underlies most forms of psychotherapy
		d.	Influenced art, literature, history, and education

III.	The Cognitive Perspective
	A.	Introduction
		1.	**Cognitive perspective** argues that abnormal is product of mental processing
		2.	Many psychological disturbances involve serious cognitive disturbances
		3.	Certain cognitive patterns may be actual causes of disorders
	B.	The Background of the Cognitive Perspective
		1.	Cognitive perspective grew out of behavioral perspective
		2.	**Cognition** is the mental processing of stimuli

C. Cognitive Behaviorism
    1. An alliance between cognitive view and behavior view is **cognitive behaviorism**
    2. Mental processing of environmental stimuli influences behavior
    3. Albert Ellis: Irrational Beliefs
        a. Rational emotive therapy developed by Ellis
        b. Based on idea that psychological problems caused by people's reactions to events and not events themselves
            i. A is for activating experience
            ii. B is for beliefs that irrationally follow
            iii. C is for consequences
        c. Problems stem from irrational beliefs that need to be confronted and disputed
    4. Aaron T. Beck: Cognitive Distortions
        a. Psychological disorders often associated with specific patterns of distorted thinking
        b. Distorted thoughts centered on triad--self, world, and future
        c. Distortions become automatic and need to be replaced with more reasonable thoughts
D. Cognitive Appraisal
    1. Evaluating stimuli is called **cognitive appraisal** and involves using one's memories, beliefs, and expectations
    2. Person's interpretation of stimulus determines response to it
    3. **Attribution** is one form of cognitive appraisal and includes three dimensions
    4. Dimensions influence feelings of hopelessness and helplessness
    5. Cognitive Variables Affecting Behavior
        a. Competencies--unique set of skills acquired through past learning
        b. Encoding strategies--special way of perceiving and categorizing experience
        c. Expectancies--develop sense of what is likely to lead to rewards and punishments
        d. Values--we place different meaning on different stimuli
        e. Plans and goals--behavior is guided by plans and goals
        f. Bandura's expectancies
            i. Outcome expectancies--expectation that a behavior will lead to a certain result
            ii. Efficacy expectancies--expectation that one will be able to execute a behavior successfully; believed to be determinant of coping behavior
E. Self-Reinforcement
    1. Behavior is molded by reinforcement from environment
    2. Most potent reinforcement and punishment comes from the mind

F.   Information-Processing
        1.   Information processing refers to how the mind takes in, stores, interprets, and uses information from environment
                a.   Automatic processing operates without conscious awareness and may be part of many abnormal behavior patterns
                b.   Controlled processing requires logic and consideration
        2.   Computer as model of human mind
        3.   Taking in certain information and filtering out the rest is called **selective attention** and may play a role in some abnormal behaviors
        4.   Organizing structures
                a.   A **schema** is an organized structure of information about a particular domain of life
                        i.   Schemas influence how we select and process new information
                        ii.   Self-schemas are schemas that refer to our self-concept and identity
                b.   Irrational beliefs can cause anxiety and depression
G.   The Cognitive Approach to Therapy
        1.   **Cognitive restructuring** attempts to help clients change the ways they perceive and interpret events
        2.   Self-instructional training emphasizes modifying self talk--the things people say to themselves before, during, and after actions
        3.   Ellis' and Beck's Cognitive Therapies
                a.   In **rational-emotive therapy**, client's irrationality is pointed out
                b.   Irrational beliefs are disputed and questioned, and more rational beliefs are modeled and rehearsed
        4.   Constructivist Cognitive Therapy
                a.   **Constructivist cognitive therapy** emphasizes construction of new patterns
                b.   Self-exploration through writing is important process
        5.   Common Strategies in Cognitive Therapy
                a.   **Hypothesis testing** involves clients testing their assumptions in real world
                b.   In **Reattribution training**, client's distorted attributions are changed
                c.   **Decatastrophizing** is a technique where client considers what would happen if worst fear were realized
H.   Evaluating the Cognitive Perspective
        1.   Criticisms of Cognitive Psychology
                a.   It is unscientific since theory is based on inferring forces that cannot be observed

        b.   Recognizing that life is not rational may not be enough to produce therapeutic change

        c.   Changing thinking may not be appropriate or right

        d.   Basis of how cognitive therapy works is unknown

2.   The Contributions of Cognitive Theory

        a.   Focuses on specific, operationalized variables

        b.   Insists on empirical evidence

        c.   Techniques can be easily applied

        d.   Cognitive therapy most successful with depression, substance dependence, and some personality disorders

        e.   There are manuals available describing how to administer and evaluate cognitive therapy

Chapter Boxes

- The Minnesota Study of Twins Reared Apart
    - A.   Study began in 1979 and has examined more than 100 sets of MZ and DZ twins
    - B.   Information is collected on each twin and then any differences or similarities are compared
    - C.   Genetic factors account for large part of behavioral variability
    - D.   Being reared in same environment has small effect on development of similar traits
    - E.   Genetic influences have been found for drug abuse and antisocial behavior, but not for alcohol abuse

- Psychodynamic Theory and Female Development
    - A.   Freud's ideas based on girls not having a penis
    - B.   Girls, according to Freud, consider themselves already castrated, resulting in inferior superego
    - C.   Opposition has come from Horney, Chodorow, and Gilligan
    - D.   Girls' task is to internalize feminine role
    - E.   Boys' task is to renounce feminine role and separate from their mothers

- A Cognitive Approach to Transference
    - A.   Experimental study of transference from the cognitive perspective
    - B.   Schemas hold memories about and feelings toward significant others
    - C.   Results produced transference

Learning Objectives (LO)

By the time you have finished studying this chapter, you should be able to do the following:

1. Define and briefly describe the field of behavior genetics, and explain the diathesis-stress model of mental disorder (78-79).

2. Briefly explain how family studies, twin studies, adoption studies, and molecular genetics studies are conducted and list the advantages and shortcomings of each (79-82).

3. Describe the functions of the cell body, dendrites, axon, axon terminals, myelin sheath, and synapse in connection with the neuron (82-83).

4. List six neurotransmitters important in the study of abnormal behavior, and describe their major functions as currently understood (83-85).

5. Name and describe the functions of the four lobes of the cerebral cortex and of the brain structures noted in italics in your text (85-87).

6. Briefly describe the EEG, CT, PET, and MRI as tools for investigating the brain (88-89).

7. Describe the major functional differences between the right and left hemispheres of the cortex (89-90).

8. Describe the functions of the somatic and autonomic divisions of the peripheral nervous system, and further distinguish between the functions of the sympathetic and parasympathetic divisions of the autonomic system (90-92).

9. Describe what hormones are and summarize their role in the functioning of the endocrine system (92).

10. List pros and cons of the biological perspective and compare it to the medical model (92-93).

11. List three basic principles held in common by almost all psychodynamic theorists (93).

12. Describe the three levels of consciousness proposed by Freud, and explain why Freud believed that behavior and experience need to be interpreted and not merely taken at face value (94).

13. Describe the functions and characteristics of the id, ego, and superego (94-95).

14. Define anxiety as Freud viewed it, and list and describe eleven defense mechanisms against anxiety. (95-97).

15. List and describe four stages of personality development in Freudian theory (97-99).

16. Summarize Freud's view of normal and abnormal personality functions (99-100).

17. Name ten psychodynamic-descendants of Freud and describe the contributions of each that distinguish them from Freud and from each other (100-105).

18. Describe the essential elements of psychoanalysis and tell how modem psychodynamic therapy differs from Freud's original method (105-106).
    □
19. List four criticisms of psychodynamic theory as well as three contributions made by this perspective (106-108).

20. Summarize the essential position of the cognitive perspective, and describe the historical factors which gave rise to this point of view (109-110).

21. Describe the contributions of Ellis, Beck, Mischel, and Bandura to the cognitive perspective (110-112).

22. Discuss the role of selective attention, schemas, and beliefs in information processing (112-113.

23. List and discuss the major approaches and strategies used in cognitive therapies and summarize the pros and cons of the cognitive perspective (113-116).

Lecture Leads (LL)

Case studies: Biological and hereditary influences on behavior (LL 4-1)
Students might appreciate a brief lecture on famous cases in abnormal psychology.
These cases would illustrate the relationship between brain and behavior and in a sense
further justify the biological perspective. Among the most well-known are Phineas Gage
and H.M. Phineas Gage suffered an accident involving a 13-pound rod traveling through
his head. Most introductory texts describe his case. H.M. suffered from global amnesia
following a neurosurgergy to treat epileptic seizures. There are several excellent case
books that provide more detailed summaries of these and other cases. Another excellent
approach is to summarize how various drugs affect the structures and fucntions of the
neuron and neurotransmitters.

Resources:

Diaz, J. (1997). How drugs influence behavior: Neuro-behavioral approach. Upper
    Saddle River, NJ: Prentice Hall.

Ogden, J. A. (1996). Fractured minds: A case-study approach to clinical
    neuropsychology. New York: Oxford University Press.

Sacks, O. (1985). The man who mistook his wife for a hat and other clinical tales. New
    York: Harper Perennial.

Early history of psychosurgery (LL 4-2)
The first widespread use of psychosurgery was the prefrontal lobotomy, developed in the
1930s by a Portuguese physician, Egas Moniz. Moniz found that cutting the connections
between the frontal lobe and the emotional areas found deep inside the brain calmed
uncontrollably violent patients by reducing the spread of neural activity. The procedure
involved inserting an instrument resembling an ice-pick up through each eye socket to the
frontal lobe severing the targeted connections. Originally Moniz injected alcohol into the
frontal lobe to destroy the frontal lobe. Many patients did become more placid with
many patients becoming very sluggish and in some cases vegetative.. Prefrontal
lobotomy was considered the panacea and during the heyday of the procedure about
50,000 procedures were conducted between 1939 and 1960. Moniz won the 1949 Nobel
prize in medicine for his procedure This procedure declined in the mid 1950s, as drug
therapies became the preferred method of treatment. Ironically, one of Moniz's
lobotomized patients shot Moniz, leaving him paralyzed. Valenstein has argued that the
tragedy was the result of several factors. For example, psychiatry was attempting to
become more "scientific" and this procedure was seen as a medical procedure. In
addition, violent, uncontrollable patients became more controllable and manageable; this
increased the staff's ability to maintain control. Since then psychosurgery has undergone
a kind of transformation as less brain tissue is destroyed. Instead of large brain areas
being ablated, clusters or pathways of cells are now destroyed. In the early 1960s it was
noted that for epileptic patients, bursts of electrical activity would often spread from one

hemisphere to the other, resulting in brain damage and, at times, death. For patients who had not responded to drug treatment, they severed the corpus callosum in a procedure known as spilt-brain operation of a commissurotomy. This procedure continues to be performed today, although surgeons are localizing seizure activity as much as possible and removing parts of the brain, as opposed to severing the connections between the two hemispheres. However, ethical issues still abound. It is easy to question the ethics of Moniz performing thousands of lobotomies as an outpatient surgery by inserting an ice pick in the corner of the eye. A valuable discussion with the students is to ask "How might people view the psychosurgeries of today 50 years from now." Will ECT be perceived tomorrow as we now perceive prefrontal lobotomy?

Resources:

Freeman, W. (1959). Psychosurgery. In S. Arieti (Ed.). American handbook of psychiatry (Vol. 2, pp. 1521-1540). New York: Basic Books.

Rodgers, J. E. (March/April 1992). Psychosurgery: Damaging the brain to save the mind. Psychology Today, 35-39, 78, 84, 86.

Valenstein, E. S. (I 986). Great and desperate cures.. New York: Basic Books.

Jung's collective unconscious and archetype (LL 4-3)
Carl Jung was one of Freud's favorite pupils and was significantly influenced by Freud. Freud once called Jung his "crown prince" and expected him to his successor. The relationship soured when their views became more divergent and soon deteriorated to the point of never again speaking to each other. One of these differing views was Jung's collective unconscious, which he argued was the basic force in personality. In this collective unconscious are archetypes, or the universal symbols. According to Jung these symbols are common to all people regardless of culture. For example two important archetypes are the anima (i.e., female) and animus (i.e., male). There may be some differences in the actual symbols used by a particular culture and there may be some slight variation in how the symbol is interpreted. Jung viewed the mandala, a concentrically arranged symbol, denoting unity and wholeness, as a symbol of the emerging self. The exact symbol varies. For instance, western mandalas take the form of the cross, fleur-de-lis, and the sun or the sun-wheel. Eastern mandalas take the form of the well-known Yin/Yang symbol, the Sricakra of Tibet, and the ankh. It is also interesting to note that certain symbols have similar meaning in a variety of cultures. Many symbols are actually interpreted in different cultures in very similar ways. To Christians the cross symbolizes humanity's connection to heaven through Jesus Christ. In China, the cross is often depicted in a square, symbolizing earth, with a circle over it, symbolizing the heavens. The Egyptian version of the cross, the ankh, symbolizes immortality; some African tribes view the cross as a symbol of divinity; the Hindu version of the cross, depicts the expansion of being.

Resources:

Carver, C. S., & Scheier, M. F. (1996). <u>Perspectives on personality</u> (3d ed.). Needham Heights, MA: Allyn & Bacon.

Cooper, J. C. (I 978). <u>An illustrated encyclopaedia of traditional symbols</u>. New York: Thames and Hudson.

Social cognitive theory (LL 4-4)

Social cognitive theory was created in response to the inadequacies of models that stress environmental determinants of behavior. There are several important core principles in social cognitive theory. Bandura (1977) acknowledged the role of the environment in behavior, for example, as when a person is directly reinforced for appropriate behavior. Behavior may also be acquired from the direct observation of others who are reinforced or punished (i.e., vicarious modeling). Moreover, Bandura introduced cognitive elements into this conceptual framework by emphasizing the individual's capacity to process information to regulate behavior. Self-regulation is therefore an important tenet of social cognitive theory. Bandura argued that individuals can exercise control over their thoughts, emotions, and behaviors. For instance, in the case of observational learning, individuals must attend to the model, remember what was seen, and be capable and motivated to repeat the observed behavior (Bandura, 1977). In each of these elements, self-regulation occurs as cognitive processes take place.

Resource:

Bandura, A. (1977). <u>Social learning theory.</u> Englewood Cliffs, NJ: Prentice-Hall.

Effects of self-efficacy (LL 4-5)

As the textbook describes, there are two type of expectancies. Self-efficacy refers to an individual's subjective belief that one can successfulyl carry out a behavior (Bandura, 1977, 1986). The difference between outcome expectancies and efficacy expectancies is important: "individuals can come to believe that a particular course of action will produce certain outcomes, but question whether they can perform those actions" (Bandura, 1977, p. 79). An individual wanting to diet, for instance, may expect to lose weight if an exercise regime is consistently followed (i.e., outcome expectancy), but questions his ability to adhere to such a regime (i.e., self-efficacy). Behavior, motivation, and emotions can be affected by one's sense of efficacy. An individual's level of self-efficacy can determine the types of situations and tasks that are selected (Bandura, 1977). An individual who possesses low self-efficacy regarding success in college will not likely pursue college courses; high self-efficacy is likely to lead one to accept and work towards such a goal. Individuals who find themselves in circumstances where they encounter obstacles are likely to persist if they have high self-efficacy. In other situations where there is low self-efficacy, obstacles are likely to lead to retreat (Bandura, 1977).

Resources:

Bandura, A. (1977). Social learning theory. Englewood Cliffs, NJ: Prentice-Hall.

Bandura, A. (1986). Social foundation of thought and action. Englewood Cliffs, NJ: Prentice-Hall.

Sources of efficacy expectancies (LL 4-6)
According to the cognitive perspective, changes in behavior are likely to be based upon changes in the individual's self-efficacy (Bandura, 1977, 1997). The effectiveness of many therapeutic techniques is believed to be due to their effect on clients' personal efficacy. In a review of the research, Bandura (1992) found strong support for the idea that improvements in self-efficacy are associated with performance enhancements. Therefore, a desire to change individual behavior should be considered in the context of changing self-efficacy. Self-efficacy, as a psychological construct underlying behavioral change, has received much attention, especially in health psychology where high levels are found to be related to positive health behaviors such as stress management, smoking cessation, and weight control. The most powerful source of efficacy is past success since these are experiences of personal mastery. Self-efficacy is heighten following success and declines when there is failure. However, a series of strong accomplishments may serve to lessen the impact of subsequent failures. Effective modes of induction include participant modeling and practice. Observing others succeeding is also very powerful in creating personal efficacy. Modeling is the main mode of induction. Self-efficacy is developed as people are spoken to in a way that persuades them of their capacities. Suggestion, exhortation, and self-instruction are modes of induction. Individuals use this source as they monitor their arousal to determine their level of anxiety. Modes include relaxation and attribution training.

Resources:

Bandura, A. (1977). Social learning theory. Englewood Cliffs, NJ: Prentice-Hall.

Bandura, A. (1992). Exercise of personal agency through the self-efficacy mechanism. In Ralf Schwarzer (Ed.), Self-efficacy: Thought control of action (pp. 3-38). Washington, DC: Hemisphere Publishing Company.

Bandura, A. (1997). Self-efficacy: The exercise of control. Englewood Cliffs, NJ: Prentice-Hall.

Talking Points (TP)

Nature and nurture (TP 4-1)
Often times the issue of what determines behavior--one's genetic makeup or environment--is phrased as nature versus nurture. What the research on behavior genetics tells us is that there is a dynamic interaction between the two. Therefore, the more appropriate choice of worlds would be nature and nurture since the research has revealed less-than-perfect concordance rates

Types of genetic studies (TP 4-2)
Discuss the rationale for the various types of genetic studies that are conducted in psychology and psychiatry. Emphasize the differences in interpretation of twin studies, adoption studies, and sibling studies. Discuss the importance of understanding the genetic mechanisms that underlie many psychological disorders. Ask: What should society do when we find a gene for schizophrenia? Do we prevent these individuals from reproducing and thus eliminate the disorder?

Twin studies (TP 4-3)
We are often amazed at the similarities between twins who are raised apart. For example, one particular striking twin pair had the same name, same job, same vacation spot and drove the same model car.

Biology as the basis for affect, behavior, and cognitions) (TP 4-4)
Stress this tightly knit relationship by informing students that changes in the nervous system will affect us in profound ways. Be prepared to give examples such as Phineas Gage. Moreover, an understanding of how pharmacological agents affect the disorders presented in the textbook is dependent on understanding neurons and neurotransmitters. In fact, refer your students to Table 4.1 (Major Psychotherapeutic Drugs) pointing out that these drugs affect the very structures and processes described in this chapter.

Brain imaging (TP 4-5)
Locate some examples of EEG, PET scans, CT scans, and MRI scans to bring to class. Present them in the context of how they revolutionized our understanding of the brain.

Sympathetic division (TP 4-6)
An often used mnemonic to remind students of the difference of the actions of the sympathetic and parasympathetic divisions is that sympathetic begins with an "s" and so does "stress."

Freud as a neurologist) (TP 4-7)
Many students are under the assumption that Freud was a psychologist. He was an MD specializing in neurology with private practice. He founded his psychodynamic ideas on his clinical observations of his patients.

Personalizing id, ego, and superego (TP 4-8)
Ask students for examples of fictional and nonfictional individuals who embody these three forces.

Influence of pain and pleasure in behavior (TP 4-9)
Are sexuality, pleasures, and the avoidance of pain really primary motives in human life and behavior?

Dream diary (TP 4-10)
Have students keep a dream diary for a week. Ask them to record their impressions of what their dreams might mean on both the conscious and unconscious levels.

Freud vs Erikson (TP 4-11)
As the textbook presents, Freud believed that personality was formed by the age of six or seven. On the other hand, Erikson suggests that personality development is lifelong, as his psychosocial theory reflects. Have students discuss these two differing viewpoints. Ask students to give examples, albeit anecdotal, of personality formed by an early age and personality being formed throughout one's life.

Examples of defense mechanism (TP 4-12)
Solicit the help of students in developing relevant examples of the defense mechanisms presented in this chapter.

Freud's couch (TP 4-13)
Some researchers have argued that the real reason Freud used a couch was that eye contact made him feel uncomfortable. Students should enjoy "analyzing" that!

Countertransference (TP 4-14)
The textbook describes transference where the patients "transfer" their feelings for significant others to the psychotherapists. In countertransference, the therapist projects feelings to the patient. One way that the therapist can understand and control countertransference is to undergo psychoanalysis as part of the training.

Formula (TP 4-15)
To better understand the historical relationship among the various perspectives is to present "mathematical formula" to illustrate the cause(s) of behavior. For instance, traditional behaviorism explains the origin of behavior to be a simple function of the environment $[B = f(e)]$ which led to $[B = f(p \bullet e)]$. In this modification, behavior is believed to be the result of an interaction between the person and the environment, but maintains that behavior is a product of an interaction. Social cognitive theory asserts a triadic reciprocal causation among behavior, internal cognitive variables, and the environment as all are interactive or "interlocking determinants of each other." Reciprocal determinism, all fashioned as a triangle, allows a better understanding of the continuous interaction of behavior, environment, and cognitions.

85

With the help of advanced technology, research can now **flip a switch**...	p. 78
But establishing the degree of genetic influence is a much **thornier** issue.	p. 78
If a sufficient amount of neurotransmitter crosses the synapse, the receiving neuron will "**fire**"...	p. 83
in loss of control over **gross-motor behavior**...	p. 85
the cerebellum, which in involved in posture, physical balance, and **fine-motor** coordination...	p. 87
this can reveal tumors or lesions that may be the **root cause** of the problem.	p. 88
but the name was changed because the word **nuclear** frightened many patients.	p. 88
Their **great virtue** is their ability to reveal brain structure...	p. 89
This lateralization is most **pronounced**...	p. 90
Have drugs been used as a "**quick fix**"...	p. 92
From this **seed** grew his theory of psychoanalysis...	p. 93
the contents of the unconscious are kept **tightly sealed** from our awareness.	p. 94
as **handed down** from Freud...	p. 94
she can calm her fears by going to **childbirth classes**...	p. 96
to go on with the **business of living**.	p. 96
surrounding it with a **smokescreen** of abstract intellectual analysis...	p. 97
a regressed adult may be reduced to a **babbling**, helpless creature...	p. 97
both the sane and insane are motivated by the irrational id, with its **reckless** drives.	p. 99
the Oedipus/Electra complex is nothing if not a **social drama**.	p. 100
anxiety ...makes it almost impossible for the, as they grow up, to **weather** the threats to the self...	p. 101
the proper treatment for neurosis was to **coax** the unconscious material...	p. 105
They may change the subject, make jokes, or **pick a fight** with the analyst...	p. 106
We can never know to what degree psychodynamic therapists' expectations **color** the patient's responses...	p. 107
the **die is cast** in early childhood...	p. 108
person who becomes extremely depressed at not receiving a **birthday card**...	p. 110
these two people will react differently when someone **cuts in front** of them...	p. 111
the result that the **mind is flooded** with information.	p. 112
urged to call a few friends on the phone and suggest a **get-together**.	p. 114

Activities and Demonstrations (ACT/DEMO)

Brain used in performing tasks (ACT/DEMO 4-1)
Objective: To review the structures and functions of the brain
Materials: None
Procedure: This activity is best done in small groups. After students are placed in groups, ask each group to list three activities (e.g., playing the piano, watching a baseball game, reading a mystery novel, listening to music, hearing bad news, drinking a cool glass of water, using a word processor). Next, the group should describe the brain areas that are being used as the activity is performed. A fun addition is to bring to class a real brain and use it to point out the various structures.
Discussion: Following the group work, review the activities and brain areas involved. This is an excellent way to illustrate the interrelationships between brain and behavior.

Field trip (ACT/DEMO 4-2)
Objective: To introduce the students to brain imaging techniques
Materials: None
Procedure: Arrange with your local hospital or medical center for a tour of their brain imaging facilities. Instruct the students to meet at the local hospital or medical center. If the facility is a long distance away, suggest car pooling. Many students will have some knowledge of this type of equipment but will probably never have seen it in operation. Ask the students to develop a list of questions prior to attending this tour that they would like the personnel to answer.
Discussion: Either after the tour or during the next class period, ask for additional questions from the students. Ask what they thought was the most interesting aspect of the tour.

In-class twin study (ACT/DEMO 4-3)
Objective: To demonstrate the relationship between concordance rates and twin behavior
Materials: Twins
Procedure: You may have to locate a pair and invite them to your class. Twin studies are often used to provide support for the hereditary basis of mental illness. This relationship is becoming stronger as we discover more genetic relationships. A common misconception held by the general public is that twins think, act, and feel the same way most of the time. Develop a list of questions on attitudes and preferences. You can use this list to demonstrate that twins may show greater similarities than nontwins. Ask for two same-sex students who are not related to come to the front of the room. Keeping track on an overhead transparency ask the students-twins and nontwins-to write down their attitudes and preferences in response to your questions. Then summarize each pair's answers in terms of concordance on their attitude or preference.
Discussion: Your data are likely not to have very large concordance rates, especially for the nontwins. If the twins have higher concordance rates, you can discuss the implications of concordance rates and psychological disorders, such as schizophrenia.

Emphasize that higher concordance rates do not guarantee that one twin will suffer from the same disorder as the other but the probability is increased. If you do not get an effect, you can discuss why there appeared to be no effect. This could be due to your questions or the absence of an effect. What are some of the problems associated with twin research, particularly longitudinal studies?

Guest speakers (ACT/DEMO 4-4)
Objective: To illustrate the differences among the perspectives
Materials: None
Procedure: Invite speakers to your class to discuss how the different perspectives play out in professional practice. Specifically, invite a psychiatrist, neuropsychologist, psychoanalyst, and a cognitive-behaviorist to class. If at all possible, invite them to appear together to engage in a friendly, informal debate. Of particular interest is the degree to which they "use" tenets of other perspectives. Is eclecticism a characteristic of professional practice? Make sure you schedule this presentation early, since many mental health professionals are very busy.
Discussion: Beforehand, instruct students to review this chapter and be prepared to ask questions of their guest speakers. Afterwards, ask students to compare and contrast the speakers' presentations.

Freud's influence (ACT/DEMO 4-5)
Objective: To illustrate the influence of Freud's work on everyday life
Materials: Miserandino's 15-item questionnaire
Procedure: Students should fill out the 15-item questionnaire regarding their agreement with several statements used in everyday life that stem from Freudian constructs for example "People who chronically smoke, eat, or chew gum have some deep psychological problem."
Discussion: This lack of appreciation is due, perhaps, to a healthy degree of skepticism regarding Freud's work instilled by previous instructors. The range of student agreement with the 15 statements in Miserandino's classes was between 4 and 12 with a mean agreement of 6.5 indicating that, at some level, every student subscribed to a belief that was rooted in psychoanalytic concepts. Perhaps the most significant aspect to administration of this questionnaire is how it facilitates discussion of why students feel the way they do regarding the statements and where their beliefs originated. Miserandino also indicates that the questionnaire serves as a good swing point for discussing psychoanalytic theory.

Resource:
Miserandino, M. (1994). Freudian principles in everyday life. <u>Teaching of Psychology</u>, <u>21</u>, 93-95.

Dream interpretation (ACT/DEMO 4-6)
Objective: To demonstrate the Freudian dream interpretation techniques
Materials: None
Procedure: Have students write on a piece of paper one of their most recent vivid dreams. Do not have the students identify themselves on this project. Collect the papers and either start the discussion, if you are very well versed in this area, or study the papers overnight and select the best for a discussion the following class period.
Discussion: Read the dreams and after each reading, ask for student input into the interpretation of the meaning of the material contained in the dream from a psychodynamic perspective. Guide the discussion and correct any misinterpretation.

Summarizing perspectives (ACT/DEMO 4-7)
Objective: To summarize the perspectives of psychopathology
Materials: Handout
Procedure: Students are placed in groups of three to four and asked to fill in the handout. Specifically, they should describe how each perspective conceptualizes the cause of the abnormal behavior and treatment approaches. If you wish, you may give groups specific ideas within each perspective to focus on (e.g., genetics, neurotransmitters within biological perspective).
Discussion: Following the group work, form new larger groups to go over what they discovered as they summarized the perspectives.

Films and Videos

Biofeedback: Listening to Your Heart (Documented Associated). Explores the use of biofeedback- to control emotional problems and diseases.

C.G. Jung: A Matter of Heart (Insight Media). An in-depth biography of Jung that utilizes footage of home movies, some of his interviews, and interviews with some of his family, friends, and students. It is a very well made documentary.

Exploring the Human Brain. UM. Covers the scientific study of the brain, intelligence, emotion, and control of disease.

Freud Under Analysis. WGBH. Traces the development of Freud's major ideas.

Freud: The Hidden Nature of Man. IM. Examines Freud's theories of psychoanalysis: the Oedipus complex, the unconscious, infantile sexuality, and the relationship of the id, ego, and superego.

IQ. PSU. Is intelligence inherent or is it environmental?

Madness and Medicine, Parts 1 & 2 PSU. This is a must-see ABC News close-up film that presents a somewhat negatively-biased portrayal of psychiatry's impact on people with mental disorders. Negative side effects of drug treatment, ECT, and psychosurgery are highlighted.

Madness, .Brainwaves. ANN/CPB The third installment covers modern attempts to cure mental illness through physical treatment.

Mind and Matter. FHS. Examination of the work of Jung.

Mysteries of the Mind. FHS. This program explores neurochemical and genetic factors in manic-depressive and obsessive-compulsive disorders, alcoholism, and other mood disorders.

*Notable Contributions to the Psychology of Personality (*Macmillan Films) A series of a number of psychologists discussing their work. Includes B.F. Skinner, Carl Jung, Carl Rogers, Erich Fromm, and Erik Erikson.

Psychodynamic Considerations and Defense Mechanisms. KSU. This video provides an in-depth view of the unconscious and highlights how the unconscious operates both verbally and behaviorally.

Psychological Defenses. IM. Part 1 explains repression, denial, and regression. Part 2 distinguishes healthy and unhealthy uses of defense mechanisms, including projection, rationalization, identification, displacement, reaction formation, and sublimation.

Rational-Emotive Therapy. PSU. An overview of RET through interviews with Albert Ellis.

The Brain, Mind and Behavior, Program 1-8. ANN/CPB. Research techniques including nuclear medicine, genetics, and immunology that enable scientists to examine the basic neuroscientific basis of behavior.

The Man Who Mistook His Wife for a Hat. FHS. Interviews with Oliver Sacks investigating problems of perception and Alzheimer's disease.

The Mind. PBS. This PBS series focuses on mental development, both in normal and abnormal populations.

The Otto Series. IU. This classic series of five films introduces formulations and treatment plans for a middle-aged man from behavioral, phenomenological, psychoanalytic, and social perspectives.

The Talking Cure. PBS. Traces the development of Freud's therapy.

Using Movies and Mental Illness as a Teaching Tool

No single film effectively contrasts these three different perspectives; however, instructors should be able to show brief vignettes from several films to illustrate all three approaches to therapy. For example, there are scenes in *Mr. Jones* that document the extent to which Richard Gere's bipolar disorder is effectively controlled by Lithium (biological). *Ordinary People* presents compelling scenes in which Judd Hirsch, playing a psychiatrist, helps his patient confront repressed traumatic memories (psychodynamic). In *Good Will Hunting* Robin Williams plays a counseling psychologist who appears to operate out of a cognitive behavioral perspective (despite the frayed copy of *I'm OK; You're OK* sitting on his desk). It will be relatively easy to excerpt scenes from all three films to demonstrate the general differences in style and method that separate practitioners of each approach.

The poignant kitchen scene between the basketball coach's wife and her young lover in Peter Bogdanovich's *The Last Picture Show* offers an excellent example of some of the vegetative symptoms of depression and you may want to show this excerpt in the context of your discussion of biological theories of mental illness. Films like *The Hospital* and *Scent of a Woman* present numerous examples of the kinds of cognitive distortions so common in depressed and suicidal individuals. As a homework assignment, you may want to have your students view these films and write down every example they find of irrational thinking or cognitive distortions.

Movie	Link to Chapter	Page Reference to Wedding and Boyd
• Mr. Jones • Raging Bull • One Flew Over the Cuckoo's Nest • Regarding Harry • I'm Dancing as Fast as I Can • An Angel at My Table • Frances	biological perspective on cause and treatment (p. 78)	(p. 49) (p. 131) (p. 161) (p. 137) (p. 167) (p. 167) (p. 167)
• Prince of Tides	psychodynamic perspective on cause and treatment (p. 93)	(p. 6172
• Scent of a Woman • The Hospital	cognitive perspective on cause and treatment (p. 109)	(p. 53) (p. 54)

Classroom Assessment Techniques (CAT)

Focused Listing (CAT 4-1)
Select an important point from this chapter (e.g, concordant, free association, diathesis-stress model) and ask students to write five words or phrases that describe the point.

Muddiest Point (CAT 4-2)
Instruct students to write about an issue, concept, or definition presented in Chapter 4 that they find most confusing or difficult to understand.

Directed Paraphrasing (CAT 4-3)
In two or three sentences, students should paraphrase some important idea, concept, or definition presented in Chapter 4. Consider paraphrasing the biological perspective, cognitive appraisal, psychosexual development, transference, and rational-emotion therapy.

Suggestions for Essay Questions

- In what ways do genetic and environmental variables interact to influence behavior?
- Describe the brain imaging techniques of PET,CT, and MRI.
- How does the conflict between id, ego, and superego lead to mental disorders?
- If you were Sigmund Freud, how would you respond to critics who claim that psychodynamic thought lacks experimental support?
- Describe the underlying assumptions of the cognitive perspectives.

Summarizing perspectives

Perspective	Suspected Cause of Abnormality	Treatment
Biological		
Psychodynamic		
Cognitive		
Behavioral		
Family Systems		
Sociocultural		
Integrated Perspective		

Chapter 5

The Behavioral, Family Systems, and Sociocultural Perspectives

Chapter Map

Section	Instructor Manual Components
The Behavioral Perspective • The Background of Behaviorism • The Assumptions of Behavioral Psychology • The Basic Mechanisms of Learning • Other Mechanisms Associated with Learning • Abnormal Behavior as a Product of Learning • The Behavioral Approach to Therapy • Evaluating Behaviorism	*Common characteristics of therapists (LL 5-1)* *Little Albert: The rest of the story (LL 5-2)* *Relationship between perspective and treatment (TP 5-1)* *Pavlov and classical conditioning (TP 5-2)* *"Give me twelve..." (TP 5-3)* *Classical conditioning (TP 5-4)* *Learning in psychopathology (TP 5-5)* *Learning in everyday life (TP 5-6)* *Systematic desensitization (TP 5-7)* *Getting back on the horse (TP 5-8)* *Perceptions of behavior therapy (TP 5-9)* *Applying principles of behaviorism (ACT/DEMO 5-1)* *Illustrating principles of behaviorism (ACT/DEMO 5-2)*
The Family Systems Perspective • Family Systems Theories • Family Systems Theory and Abnormal Behavior • Family and Couple Therapy • Evaluating the Family Systems Perspective	*Using family drawings to assess relationships (LL 5-3)* *Couple therapy (LL 5-4)* *Satir's conjoint family therapy (LL 5-5)* *AVANTA (TP 5-10)* *Creating scripts (ACT/DEMO 5-3)*

The Sociocultural Perspective	Analyzing famous people (ACT/DEMO 5-4)
• Mental Illness and Social Ills • Mental Illness and Labeling • Prevention as a Social Issue • Evaluating the Sociocultural Perspective	
Integrating the Perspectives	Delivery of therapy through technology (LL 5-6) Diathesis-stress model (TP 5-11) Summarizing perspectives (ACT/DEMO 5-5)

I.   The Behavioral Perspective
    A.   **Behavioral perspective** views behavior as result of environmental experience or learning
        1.   Cause of behavior is in environment
        2.   Proximal focus in treating behaviors
    B.   The Background on Behaviorism
        1.   Behaviorism rose in reaction to subjective analysis of one's thought processes
        2.   **Learning** is explanation of behavior
        3.   Mechanisms of learning laid foundation for behaviorism
            a.   Pavlov: The Conditioned Reflex
                i.   **Conditioned reflex** is basic mechanism of learning
                ii.   Many responses were result of simple learning process
            b.   Watson: The Founding of Behaviorism
                i.   Believed psychology should focus on observable and measurable behavior
                ii.   Rejected introspection as method
                iii.   Found emotional responses to be conditioned
            c.   Thorndike: The Law of Effect
                i.   Studied relationship between behavior and its consequences
                ii.   Formulated **law of effect** describing how consequences can strengthen and weaken behavior
            d.   Skinner: Radical Behaviorism
                i.   Developed **radical behaviorism** - everything person does, says, or feels is behavior
                ii.   Focused on practical applications of experimental analysis
                iii.   Contingencies in environment could be altered to change behavior
    C.   The Assumptions of Behavioral Psychology
        1.   Study behavior by examining learning history
        2.   Stimuli and responses must be observed and measured
        3.   Goal of psychology is prediction and control of behavior
            a.   Laboratory settings provide easy prediction and control
            b.   Real-life settings add complexity
         4.   Focus on outside of organism to locate real causes of behavior
    D.   The Basic Mechanisms of Learning
        1.   Respondent conditioning
            a.   Pairing of stimuli leads to conditioning to what is initially a neutral stimulus

        b.   **Respondent conditioning** is learning of conditioned response
- i.   Unconditioned stimulus (UCS)
- ii.   Unconditioned response (UCR)
- iii.   Conditioned stimulus (CS)
- iv.   Conditioned response (CR)

2.   Operant conditioning

    a.   Operant behavior is associated with outcomes

    b.   **Operant conditioning** involves increasing or decreasing likelihood of behavior by its consequences

    c.   Association between behavior and consequence is a **contingency**

    d.   **Reinforcement** refers to process where events in environment that increase probability that behavior will be repeated
- i.   A **primary reinforcer** is one that we respond to instinctively
- ii.   **Conditioned reinforcers** are stimuli that we have learned to respond to through association to primary reinforcers
- iii.   **Positive reinforcement** strengthens response
- iv.   **Negative reinforcement** strengthens response by avoidance or removal of aversive stimulus

    e.   **Punishment** refers to process where behavior decreases in frequency

    f.   Negative reinforcement and punishment are often confused for several reasons
- i.   Similar consequences do not have similar effects on all people
- ii.   It is hard to think of reinforcement as negative

    g.   Functional analysis identifies variables controlling behavior

E.   Other Mechanisms Associated with Learning

    1.   **Extinction** is elimination of a response by withdrawing reinforcer that maintained it

    2.   **Generalization** occurs when organism responds to similar stimuli

    3.   **Discrimination** is learning to distinguish among similar stimuli

    4.   **Shaping** refers to reinforcement of successive approximations of desired response

    5.   Learning to follow rules: Instructions as discriminative stimuli

        a.   Behavior is acquired through modeling or imitation

        b.   Modeling can occur without verbal instruction or external reinforcement

F.   Abnormal Behavior as a Product of Learning

    1.   Normal behavior seen as due to genetics and experience

    2.   Abnormal behavior seen as due to genetics and experience

        a.   Explanations favor complexity over simplicity

        b.   Emphasis more on entire life history of individual

        c.   Behavior is defined within its context

    3.   Skeptical of usefulness of labeling people, which suggests medical model

    4.   Function of behavior not form is basis of prediction and influence

    5.   Learning may be an important variable in abnormal behavior

G.   The Behavioral Approach to Therapy

    1.   Using same mechanisms believed to produce normal behavior

    2.   Respondent Conditioning and Extinction

        a.   Maladaptive behavior can be unlearned

        b.   Systematic desensitization

            i.   **Systematic desensitization** based on weakening bond between stimuli and anxiety

            ii.   Client given relaxation training

            iii.   **Hierarchy of fears** developed

            iv.   Client practices relaxing while confronting fears in hierarchy either in vivo or through imagining

            v.   Effective for wide variety of problems

        c.   Exposure

            i.   Extinction as a clinical practice has replaced systematic desensitization

            ii.   Patients are confronted with experiences they fear without reinforcement

            iii.   Flooding involves prolonged confrontation

            iv.   In graded exposure, the confrontation is gradual

    3.   Operant Conditioning

        a.   **Contingency management** involves the manipulation of consequences of behavior

        b.   Behavior can be changed by managing its contingencies

    4.   Multicomponent Treatment

        a.   A disorder has many facets

        b.   Different treatments address various problems

    5.   The New Radical Behavioral Therapies: Integrating Acceptance with Change

        a.   Incorporates behavioral principles with acceptance

        b.   Dialectical behavior therapy emphasizes validation and skills training

    6.   Behavior Therapy: Pros and Cons

        a.   There are several criticisms of behavior therapy

            i.   It is superficial since it does not focus on patient's past or have insight as primary goal

            ii.   It addresses patient's symptoms and ignores underlying causes

            iii.   It denies individual freedom

        b.   Behavior therapy has been shown to be effective in treating wide variety of problems
              i.   It tends to be faster and less expensive than other treatments
              ii.   Paraprofessionals and nonprofessionals can use it
              iii.   It can be reported, discussed, and evaluated with precision

H.   Evaluating Behaviorism
    1.   Criticisms of behaviorism
        a.   Oversimplification
              i.   It reduces life to small measurable units of behavior
              ii.   Ignores deeper workings of the mind
        b.   Determinism
              i.   Argues that there is no free will
              ii.   Argues that whatever we do is due to learning history
        c.   The Issue of "Control"
              i.   Suggests that behavioral engineering could be used for totalitarian regime where people are coerced by reinforcement
              ii.   Control actually refers to predictability and using scientific laws
    2.   The Contributions of Behaviorism
        a.   Adherence to objectivity and precision in behavioral research
        b.   Behaviorists recognize broad range of responses as legitimate
        c.   Treatment methods are promising with wide range of disorders and are applied in many settings

II.   The Family Systems Perspective
    A.   Family Systems Theories
        1.   In **family systems theories,** abnormal behavior seen as product of habitual relationship patterns with family
        2.   The abnormal behavior is a reflection of poor family functioning
        3.   Communication theory suggests that faulty communication within family causes psychopathology
            a.   Double-bind communication consists of contradictory messages
            b.   Ambiguous messages is a demand without information how it is to be met
            c.   Hostile, runaway exchanges result in escalations to greater hostility
            d.   Silent schisms is where the family splits into factions
        4.   Structural theory argues that relationships as units and boundaries

5. Differentiation of self is key to healthy functioning
6. Overlap exists between family systems theories and behavioral approaches
    a. Balance theory describes the ratio of positive to negative behaviors as important
    b. Reactivity in a marriage is tendency to respond to immediate contingencies of situation rather than long-term contingencies

B. Family Systems Theory and Abnormal Behavior
1. Abnormal behavior may be due to individuals encouraging symptoms through complementary behaviors
2. Expressed emotion may play a role, where the more EE in a family, the higher the risk of relapse
3. Family is seen as "sick" rather than an individual in the family

C. Family and Couple Therapy
1. Family Therapy
    a. Popularity of **family therapy** increased in past 25 years
    b. Disturbance is seen as being in family unit
    c. **Strategic approach** is oldest and most influential and uses paradoxical intention as a technique
    d. In **structural family therapy** family is analyzed as set of interlocking roles
    e. Psychodynamic family therapy and behavioral family therapy have been developed
2. Couple Therapy
    a. **Couple therapy** attempts to alleviate relationship problems and abnormal behavior
    b. Different approaches emphasize different aspects of relationships
        i. Behavioral couple therapy focuses on increasing positive behaviors
        ii. Cognitive couple therapy helps couples to identify cognitive distortions in relationships
3. Family and Couple Therapies: Pros and Cons
    a. Appear to be more successful than individual therapy
    b. Scope of treatment now being broadened
    c. Research on outcomes of therapy is uneven, however

D. Evaluating the Family Systems Perspective
1. Perspective is consistent with psychodynamic, behavioral, and cognitive approaches
2. Analysis of patient-therapist relationship reveals importance of empathy and responsiveness
3. Some findings have not held up to research
4. Family systems theory limited in scope

5.   Most therapists have no interest in proving techniques scientifically

III.   The Sociocultural Perspective
    A.   **Sociocultural perspective** views abnormal behavior to be result of broad social forces
    B.   Mental Illness and Social Ills
        1.   Social ills cause psychological ills
        2.   Focus should be on social ills such as poverty
    C.   Mental Illness and Labeling
        1.   Sociocultural view suggests that labeling occurs because individuals violate social norms
        2.   Behavior consistent with role is reinforced; inconsistent behavior is punished-becoming a self-fulfilling prophecy
        3.   Class, Race, and Diagnosis
            a.   Psychological disturbances related to social class
            b.   Differences found between people of lower socioeconomic class and those of middle-class
                i.   People with lower socioeconomic backgrounds labeled psychotic and hospitalized
                ii.   People with higher socioeconomic backgrounds labeled neurotic and not hospitalized
            c.   Race affects diagnosis
                i.   Blacks more likely to be diagnosed as alcoholic or schizophrenic
                ii.   Whites more likely to be diagnosed as depressed
    D.   Prevention as a Social Issue
        1.   Approach to treatment involves community prevention programs
        2.   Three levels of prevention exist
    E.   Evaluating the Sociocultural Perspective
        1.   Conditions in society do contribute to psychological disturbances
            a.   Some argue that socially engendered stress is primary cause
            b.   Some argue that socially engendered stress is secondary cause
        2.   More controversy with notion that abnormality is a cultural artifact maintained through labeling

Chapter Boxes

- The Limitations of Change: An Acceptance-Based Approach to Couple Therapy
  A. Integrative Behavioral Couple Therapy is based on radical behavioral perspective
  B. Assumes couples have engaged in habitual, destructive patterns of interaction for many years
  C. Approach teaches partners to accept each other
  D. Techniques involve turning problems into strengths and tolerance
  E. Pilot study suggests IBCT to be effective

- African-American Protest and the Mental Health Establishment
  A. Historical examples of stresses affecting black people
  B. Protests seen as signs of psychological disturbance

Learning Objectives (LO)

By the time you have finished studying this chapter, you should be able to do the following:

1. Describe the major contributions of Pavlov, Watson, Thorndike and Skinner to behavioral psychology (122-124).

2. List and explain four fundamental assumptions of the behavioral approach (124-125).

3. Briefly summarize the basic processes of respondent and operant conditioning (125-126).

4. Define reinforcement and punishment, and distinguish among primary, secondary, positive, and negative reinforcement (125-126).

5. Define the concepts of extinction, generalization, discrimination, three-term contingency, rule governed behavior, shaping, and modeling (125-129).

6. Summarize the behavioral view of mental disorder (128-130).

7. Briefly describe systematic desensitization, exposure therapy, contingency management, multicomponent treatment, and recent radical behaviorist approaches to treatment involving integration and acceptance (130-132).

8. List and discuss the criticisms leveled at the behavioral perspective, as well as three contributions attributed to this point of view (133-135).

9. Summarize the essential concepts of the family systems perspective, making reference to communication theory structural theory, balance theory, and the work of Murray Bowen (135-136).

10. Summarize the family systems approach to disorder and therapy, using examples from family therapy and couples therapy (136-139).

11. List two contributions and three criticisms of the family systems perspective referred to in our text (139-141).

12. List and discuss two ways in which the sociocultural perspectives accounts for abnormal behavior (141-143).

13. Summarize the pros and cons of the sociocultural perspective (143-144).

Lecture Leads (LL)

Common characteristics of therapists (LL 5-1)

There are several characteristics that typify therapists of all perspectives. In terms of educational background, almost all psychotherapists hold masters' or doctoral degrees in clinical or counseling psychology. In most states, only professionals who have the appropriate educational background (usually a doctoral degree such as Ph.D.; Psy.D.; Ed.D.) and have passed a state exam may use the title "psychologist." Licensed therapists are able to practice more or less independently, whereas unlicensed therapists are supervised on a regular basis. These state licensing laws help to regulate who performs psychotherapy. The titles "counselor" and "therapist" often may be legally used without any special training or license. Psychiatrists are medical doctors (MDs) who specialize in psychiatry. Training and educational background will influence the therapist's approach to the etiology and treatment of abnormal behavior. For instance, psychiatrists tend to adhere to the biological perspective, and therefore, are likely to treat abnormality with medication. However, there are suggestions to grant some psychologists prescription privileges. Another common trait among therapists is their code of conduct regarding clients. For example, sexual contact between therapist and client is a prime example of the therapist violating ethical guidelines and not acting in the best interests of the client. Therapist-client communication is confidential. Unless clients provide written consent or are dangerous to themselves or others, all records and information regarding therapy sessions are held in confidence. When the client shares with the therapist an intent to attempt suicide or harm a third party, the therapist has a legal obligation to protect both the client and society. This may involve breaking confidentiality on a need-to-know basis. All therapists need to develop an atmosphere of rapport and trust with their clients for effective psychotherapy to occur. All forms of psychotherapy require some degree of client self-disclosure, and the extent to which the clients are at ease with their therapists often dictates the rate of progress in therapy. In addition to self-disclosure, the client must trust the therapist enough to follow the therapist's direction and interventions. In fact, trust can lead to the all-important belief that the therapist and therapy will help the client. Although rapport and trust are qualities that most of us desire in our personal relationships with others, the therapist-client relationship should not be misconstrued as a friendship. The relationship is strictly a professional one; it is time-limited and should not include socializing outside therapy sessions, because the therapist needs to maintain objectivity. Every so often, the American Psychological Association will publish a list of psychologists who have violated one of APA's ethical guidelines.

Resources:

Beutler, L. E., Machado, P. P., Neufeldt, S. A. (1994). Therapist variables. In A. E. Bergin and S. L. Garfield (Eds.). Handbook of psychotherapy and behavior change (4th ed.). New York: John Wiley.

Crits-Christoph, P., Baranackie, K.L., Kurcias, J. S., & Beck, A. T. (1991). Meta-analysis of therapists effects in psychotherapy outcome. Psychotherapy Research, 1, 81-91.

Engler, J., & Goleman, D. (1992). <u>The consumer's guide to psychotherapy</u>. New York: Simon & Schuster.

Lichtenstein, E. (1980). <u>Psychotherapy: Approaches and applications</u>. Monterey, CA: Brooks/Cole.

Little Albert: The rest of the story (LL 5-2)

 In 1916, John B. Watson began doing studies on babies at the Phipps Clinic of Johns Hopkins University in Baltimore. His particular area of research at this time was in the area of emotions. Watson felt that children did not have a natural fear of things such as furry animals but developed them through conditioning. Enter Albert B., alias Little Albert, a child of a wet nurse at the Phipps Clinic, upon whom Watson and a colleague, Rosalie Rayner (more about her later), set out to test whether emotional reactions could be classically conditioned. Little Albert was nine months old at the time of the experiment, which was carried out in 1919. Although Watson intended to recondition Albert not to fear the rat, he never got the chance because Albert was adopted by a family outside of Baltimore (Cohen, 1979). Albert's subsequent history is unknown, but somewhere there may be a 70-year-old man alive today who is scared to death of rats but can't figure out why! The Little Albert study was the last published academic work for Watson though he later went on to a successful career in advertising. His relationship with Rosalie Rayner was not just professional. They had met in 1919 when she, after graduating from Vassar College, came to Johns Hopkins to get a master's degree under Watson at the Phipps Clinic. Though he was 42 years old and married, Watson fell in love with the 19-year-old Rayner and they began a passionate love affair. After Watson's wife found out about the Watson-Rayner affair, so did the president of Johns Hopkins. He forced Watson to resign. The ensuing sensational divorce trial was front-page news in Baltimore and received national publicity. Watson eventually married Rosalie Rayner on January 3, 1921.

Resources:

Cohen, D. (1979). <u>J. B. Watson: The founder of behaviorism</u>. London: Routledge & Kegan Paul.

Duke, C., Fried, S., Pliley, W., & Walker, D. (1989). Contributions to the history of psychology: LIX. Rosalie Rayner Watson: The mother of a behaviorist's sons. <u>Psychological Reports, 65</u>, 163-169.

Harris, B. (1979). Whatever happened to Little Albert? <u>American Psychologist, 34</u>, 151-160.

Paul, D. B., & Blumenthal, A. L. (1989). On the trail of Little Albert<u>. Psychological Record, 39</u>, 547-553.

Using family drawings to assess relationships (LL 5-3)
Stein suggested that clinicians in pediatric practice can use the drawings of family members made by children. The drawings represent an alternative approach to assess development of the children and family dynamics. Drawings can be used longitudinally to evaluate how family relationships have changed. Family drawings can also be used as part of school readiness examination. Several examples of cases and family drawings are presented in the article.

Resource:
Stein, M. T. (1997). The use of family drawing by children in pediatrics practice. Journal of Developmental & Behavioral Pediatrics, 18, 334-339.

Couple therapy (LL 5-4)
Couple therapy is a form of family therapy and makes the assumption that relationships and communication patterns are related to maladaptive behavior. Therefore each spouse must participate in therapy since it is assumed that men and women have equal power, both social and economic, inside and outside of their marriage. For this reason, it should not be surprising that most couple therapists refrain from taking on cases of spouse abuse, and many couple therapists that do have been criticized as being insensitive to women's issues. Lipchik notes that there is considerable variance between spouse abuse cases, and in some instances the males involved are not the "psychopathic misogynistic killers" they are portrayed to be by the media. In many instances they want help to overcome their problems and are amenable to therapy. Lipchik argues that occasionally in these cases couple therapists need to look beyond the orthodox approach of helping the woman leave the violent partner and never return. A variation of couple therapy is behavioral couple therapy that teaches partners problem solving and communication skills. It also encourages couples to accept what they cannot change with regard to maladaptive behavior or situational variables.

Resources:
Cordova, J. B., & Jacobson, N. S. (1993). Couple distress. In D. H. Barlow (Ed.), Clinical handbook of psychological disorders. A step-by-step treatment manual (2d ed.). New York: Guilford

Epstein, N. Baucom, D. H., & Rankin, L. A. (1993). Treatment of marital conflict. A cognitive-behavioral approach. Clinical Psychology Review, 13, 45-57.

Kelly, J. B. (1982). Divorce: An adult perspective. In B. B. Wolman (Ed.), Handbook of developmental psychology. Englewood Cliffs, NJ: Prentice Hall.

Lipchik, E. (1991). Spouse abuse: Challenging the party line. The Family Therapy Networker, 15, 59-63.

Satir's conjoint family therapy (LL 5-5)
Another family therapy is that of Virginia Satir. In her model, there is a clear emphasis on personal growth and health, rather than on psychopathology. For growth to occur, the environment must be nurturing and supportive, and we as individuals must recognize our inner selves. From there, we can reach out from this center. Our communications must be clear and direct. For instance, family members are taught how to send intended messages and learn skills to receive messages.

Resources:
Satir, V. (1983). Conjoint family therapy. Palo Alto, CA: Science and Behavior Books.

Satir, V., Bamnen, J., Gerber, J., & Gomori, M. (1991). The Satir Model: Family Therapy and Beyond. Palo Alto, CA: Science and Behavior Books.

Delivery of therapy through technology (LL 5-6)
As technology advances, more and more venues to delivery therapy have emerged. Talk psychologists have long been a fixture on television and radio. In fact, the Dr. Laura Schlessinger Show is currently one of the most popular talk radio programs. Predictably, forms of therapy and related information are now offered on the Internet. Among the topics that can be researched is assistance for personal problems-it is possible to access a variety of web sites that are happy to help. However, as with the quality of any other available information, the American Psychological Association (1995) cautions that this profusion of therapeutic insights raises ethical questions. The APA has noted psychologists who offer services on-line are merely "offering guidance for people who seek help resolving crises or simple answers to everyday questions of living." New York City psychologist Dorothy Litwin argues that: "This is definitely not a substitute for face-to-face psychotherapy," and the APA has become concerned that "the emergence of cybertalk signals unfolding ethical questions in psychology." Despite the potential for ethical conundrums, many respected organizations provide help on-line.

Resources:
Ainsworth, M. (March 1997). The Metanoia guide to internet mental health services [On-line]. Available: WWW URL http://www.metanoia.org/imhs/.

American Psychological Association. (March 1996). APA's new help center providing consumer information via the world wide web. APA News Release [On-line]. Available: WWW URL http://www.apa.org/releases/helpcen.html.

Sleek, S. (November 1995). On-line therapy services raise ethical questions. APA Monitor [On-line]. Available: WWW URL htttp://www.cmhc.com/articles/apal.htm.

Wallace, P. M. (1997). Psych on-line 97: Abnormal, clinical and counseling. Madison, WI: Brown & Benchmark.

Talking Points (TP)

Relationship between perspective and treatment (TP 5-1)

Have students discuss the impact that identification with a particular paradigm has, both on the scientist and the practitioner. While most students concentrate on the negative aspects of such an adoption, try and elucidate some of the positive aspects. Bring up the fact that the type of treatment they would receive as a patient would differ radically depending on the paradigm the therapist followed. How could they discern whether such a strategy would be useful for them?

Pavlov and classical conditioning (TP 5-2)

It is important to point out to students that Pavlov was not a psychologist, but a neurophysiologist studying digestion. Yet he discovered classical conditioning by accident; in fact, he found the conditioning of the dogs to be a hindrance. Pavlov's accidental discovery is interesting because it says something about science and research. First, important findings are often made serendipitously. Second, many important discoveries for psychology are made by those not in the field (e.g., medicine), and that research in two fields can be combined. An article in a recent APA Monitor (May 1998) describes such a combination in the fields of virology and psychology than lead to the emergence of psychoneuroimmunology.

"Give me twelve..." (TP 5-3)

John B. Watson, the founder of behaviorism, has to be credited with a concept that can be used as a lecture starter. The concept was to give him a healthy baby and he could turn it into anything he wants--beggar, doctor, or even President of the United States-with behavioral principles. In other words, reinforcement is more dominant and influential than other predispositions. It does not matter what you start with because behavioral principles are more powerful. Ask the students if they believe this radical behaviorist perspective. Could all you are really be only your reinforcement history?

Classical conditioning (TP 5-4)

The terminology of classical conditioning gives many students trouble. An effective approach is to focus students' attention on the meaning behind the words. For example, what does "unconditioned" and "conditioned" mean? It is helpful to define "unconditioned" as "unlearned" and "conditioned" as "learned." Then proceed to define "stimulus" and "response" and put the translation together as in "unlearned behavior."

Learning in psychopathology (TP 5-5)

The behavioral perspective asserts that both abnormal and normal behavior are learned in much the same way. Develop a lecture on how a specific normal behavior and a parallel abnormal behavior could develop. Continue this discussion with the use of the techniques of classical conditioning, operant conditioning, and modeling. Compare and contrast the methods in developing your abnormal and normal behavior.

Learning in everyday life (TP 5-6)
Have students keep a log of behaviors they engage in everyday that they believe are learned and maintained by classical and operant conditioning.

Systematic desensitization (TP 5-7)
As you go through systematic desensitization, ask students to come up with their own hierarchy of fears. Some suggestions include asking someone out for a date, test taking, or preparing for a speech. Point out that what matters with regard to the hierarchy is that it is personalized or unique for each individual.

Getting back on the horse (TP 5-8)
One could argue that the old adage about getting back on the horse after being bucked off is based on the principle of exposure.

Perceptions of behavior therapy (TP 5-9)
There appears to be a negative labeling bias against behavioral techniques. Many individuals equate behavior therapy with brainwashing, involuntary behavior change, and indoctrination. Behavioral therapists have been increasingly concerned about consumer perceptions of these techniques. Make sure you disavow students of these misperceptions. In fact, point out that they themselves practice behavior therapy whenever they attempt to change environmental contingencies (e.g., using reinforcement).

AVANTA (TP 5-10)
Virginia Satir, a pioneer in family therapy, established an organization to teach her principles. The organization was named Avanta, which means "to move forward": in Latin. The name is apropos given Satir's philosophy on communication and personal growth. As a learning check, ask students to come up with fictitious names of organizations for the other perspectives presented in the textbook.

Diathesis-stress model (TP 5-11)
As you present the diathesis-stress model, ask students to give examples of factors from each perspective that increases a person's vulnerability. For instance, a person's vulnerability increases if they come from a family whose communication is ambiguous (family systems) or from a lower socioeconomic level (sociocultural).

Behavior is only the **surface** of mental functioning...	p. 122
Environmental experience...is the **sum of all** life experiences.	p. 122
made it the **battle cry** for a new school of psychology...	p. 123
a dog, a sealskin coat, and a bearded **Santa Claus mask**.	p. 123
when the behaviorist moves out of the laboratory into the **world at large**...	p. 125
This assumption is an **article of faith.**	p. 125
between a friendly smile and a **malicious grin**...	p. 127
Imagine a **child learning to dive.**	p. 127
at a **high school dance**...	p. 127
a list of anxiety-producing situations in order of their **increasing horror** to the client	p. 130
Most desensitization, however, takes place in the **consulting office**...	p. 131
The **hoped-for result** is that they will realize that the thing they fear.	p. 131
whereas the clear **spelling out** of treatment goals in behavior therapy.	p. 132
sacrifice the intangibles for the sake or rigor.	p. 133
has been the subject of **endless controversy.**	p. 134
To explain this...uses a **bank account metaphor.**	p. 136
lest the network **sabotage treatment**...	p. 137
discuss the **pros and cons** without **emotional overreaction**...	p. 139
the homework assignment of writing a **joint letter** to the third party...	p. 140
Therefore, the field remains dominated by charismatic lecturers.	p. 141
discrimination against minority groups and women, and **homophobia**...	p. 141
raised eyebrows from people who know about his "past"...	p. 142

Activities and Demonstrations (ACT/DEMO)

Applying principles of behaviorism (ACT/DEMO 5-1)
Objective: To demonstrate behavior techniques on changing behavior
Materials: None
Procedure: Divide students into groups of four to five each. Have the students discuss a common problem we all have, procrastination. Instruct the groups to develop a treatment plan using the principles of classical conditioning, operant conditioning, and modeling, to help them modify this problem. Ask for volunteers from each group to implement each of the plans for one week. At the end of the week, ask each student to be prepared to discuss his or her experience.
Discussion: Have each student report to the other students the relative efficacy of each plan. Summarize each plan on an overhead transparency, as the reports are made. Lead a discussion on the relative merits of each plan, what worked, and what did not and why.

Illustrating principles of behaviorism (ACT/DEMO 5-2)
Objective: To demonstrate the principles of behaviorism
Materials: Copy of selected articles
Procedure: There are several very effective ways to demonstrate the principles of behaviorism. You could lead each demonstration described in the resources presented below or assign groups of students to conduct the demonstrations. Consult the articles referenced.
Discussion: As each demonstration unfolds and following them, review the principles of classical and operant conditioning.

Resources:

Gibb, G. D. (1983). Making classical conditioning understandable through a
    demonstration technique. Teaching of Psychology, 10, 112-113.

Greenspoon, J. (1955). The reinforcing effect of two spoken sounds on the frequency of
    two responses. American Journal of Psychology, 58, 409-416.

Keith-Spiegel, P. (1988). Operant conditioning demonstrations. L. T. Benjamin, Jr. &
    K. D. Lowman (Eds.), Activities handbook for the teaching of psychology (Vol. 1).
    Washington, DC: American Psychological Association.

Morgan, W. (1974). The shaping game: A teaching technique. Behavior Therapy, 5,
    271-272.

Smith, R. A. (1987). Jaws: Demonstrating classical conditioning. In V. P. Makosky, L.
    G. Whittemore, & A. M. Rogers (Eds.), Activities handbook for the teaching of
    psychology (Vol. 2). Washington, DC: American Psychological Association.

Watson, D. (1981). Shaping by successive approximations. L. T. Benjamin, Jr. & K. D. Lowman (Eds.), <u>Activities handbook for the teaching of psychology</u> (Vol. 1). Washington, DC: American Psychological Association.

Creating scripts (ACT/DEMO 5-3)
Objective: To illustrate the approach of family systems perspective
Materials: None
Procedure: After students are placed in small groups, instruct them to develop written scripts of a therapist-client(s) dialogue. The therapist should subscribe to and use a family systems approach. The groups may select the particular problem but should revolve around communication difficulties within the family unit (e.g., double-bind communication; ambiguous messages).
Discussion: Have each group read the dialogue. The remaining students can point out specific techniques or themes used in the dialogue.

Analyzing famous people (ACT/DEMO 5-4)
Objective: To apply the perspective in analyzing a famous person
Materials: None
Procedure: This activity is best conducted in small groups. Ask the students to suggest candidates for the analysis; choose a person whose public image is complex enough to permit an interesting discussion (e.g., Dennis Rodman, Michael Jackson, Bill Clinton). The students are to perform an informal analysis of the individual from one of the perspectives described in the textbook.
Discussion: Students may complain that they don't really know how the person feels; that is a good place to point out the value of testing and personal interviewing in personality diagnosis. Ask each group to give a brief synopsis of their analysis.

Summarizing perspectives (ACT/DEMO 5-5)
Objective: To summarize the perspectives of psychopathology
Materials: Handout
Procedure: Students are placed in groups of three to four and asked to fill in the handout. Specifically, they should describe how each perspective conceptualizes the cause of the abnormal behavior and treatment approaches. If you wish, you may give groups specific ideas within each perspective to focus on (e.g., genetics, neurotransmitters within biological perspective).
Discussion: Following the group work, form new larger groups to go over what they discovered as they summarized the perspectives.

Films and Videos

A Conversation with B.F Skinner. CRM. Skinner presents his views on the potential for environmental control of behavior.

B. F Skinner and Behavior Change: Research, Practice, and Promise. PSU. Behavioral interventions in various settings, including a fear of dental procedures, learning social skills at a youth center, controlling epilepsy in a hospital, and working with a developmentally disabled child at home.

B.E Skinner Demonstrates Operant Conditioning. PSU. In a classroom setting, B. F. Skinner demonstrates, with pigeons, the application of Thorndike's Law of Effect in operant conditioning.

B.F. Skinner on Behaviorism. Insight Media. Skinner discusses positive reinforcement, behavior modification, and other operant conditioning principles.

Behavior Modification: Teaching Language to Psychotic Children. Appleton-Century-Crofts. Demonstrates how reinforcement has been applied to teach children with autism.

Behavior Therapy: An Introduction. UM. Demonstrates different approaches to behavior therapy, operant, classical, and observational.

Exploring the Human Brain. UM. Covers the scientific study of the brain, intelligence, emotion, and control of disease.

IQ. PSU. Is intelligence inherent or is it environmental?

Multimodal Marital Therapy (Arnold Lazarus). PSU. Arnold Lazarus conducts a therapy session with a distressed couple, using techniques from both cognitive and behavioral perspectives.

Notable Contributions to the Psychology of Personality. Macmillan Films. A series of a number of psychologists discussing their work. Includes B.F. Skinner, Carl Jung, Carl Rogers, Erich Fromm, and Erik Erikson.

One Step at a Time: An Introduction to Behavior Modification. CRM. The behavior of mental patients is modified using positive reinforcement.

The Mind. PBS. This PBS series focuses on mental development, both in normal and abnormal populations.

The Otto Series. IU. This classic series of five films introduces formulations and treatment plans for a middle-aged man from behavioral, phenomenological, psychoanalytic, and social perspectives.

Token Economy: Behaviorism Applied. Demonstrates the use of token economies with three different populations: psychotics, the retarded, and prisoners.

Using Movies and Mental Illness as a Teaching Tool

The scene in *A Clockwork Orange* in which Alex is being treated with behavioral methods is dramatic and a bit overdone, but it is guaranteed to generate a provocative class discussion about the appropriate limits of behavior therapy.

Films are replete with scenes demonstrating family pathology. For example, the interactions between mother and son in *Ordinary People* -- and between father and son in *Shine* or *Dead Poets' Society* -- will get your students thinking about how families affect the expression of mental illness. The suicide scene in *Dead Poets' Society* and the bathtub defecation scene in *Shine* are especially powerful trigger scenes for classroom discussion.

Benny and Joon presents a relatively positive portrayal of serious mental illness, and the scene in which Benny and his poker playing buddies appear to be oblivious to Joon's idiosyncratic behavior illustrates how context influences the interpretation of the significance of aberrant behavior. Similar points can be made with scenes from *The Gods Must be Crazy*, *Lord of the Flies*, and, especially, *King of Hearts*.

Movie	Link to Chapter	Page Reference to Wedding and Boyd
• A Clockwork Orange	behavioral perspective on cause and treatment (p. 122)	p. 169
• Scent of a Woman • Dead Poet's Society • Ordinary People • Shine • David and Lisa • On Golden Pond •	family relationships and cause and treatment (p. 135)	p. 57 p. 59 p. 61 p. 120 p. 121 p. 127
• The Fisher King • One Flew Over the Cuckoo's Nest	sociocultural themes (p. x)	(p. 121) (p. 161)

Classroom Assessment Techniques (CAT)

Sentence Summary (CAT 5-1)
Ask students to summarize a specific perspective in this chapter by responding to the question, "Who does/did what to whom, when, where, how and why?"

Muddiest Point (CAT 5-2)
Instruct students to write about an issue, concept, or definition presented in Chapter 5 that they find most confusing or difficult to understand.

Minute Paper (CAT 5-3)
Ask your students to write on what important question they have that remains unanswered.

Suggestions for Essay Questions

❑ Describe how the behavioral perspective explains abnormal behavior and how it is treated.
❑ React to the criticism that the principles of behaviorism could be used to coerce people. Support your view.
❑ Create a vignette describing a family conversation that illustrates the family systems perspective to abnormal behavior.
❑ What does the notion "social ills cause psychological ills" mean?

Summarizing perspectives
Handout

Perspective	Suspected Cause of Abnormality	Treatment
Biological		
Psychodynamic		
Cognitive		
Behavioral		
Family Systems		
Sociocultural		
Integrated Perspective		

Chapter 6

Anxiety Disorders

Chapter Map

Section	Instructor Manual Components
Anxiety Disorder Syndromes • Panic Disorder • Generalized Anxiety Disorder • Phobias • Obsessive-Compulsive Disorder • Posttraumatic Stress Disorder	*Famous people with anxiety disorders (LL 6-1)* *Trichotillomania: A hair-pulling obsession (LL 6-2)* *What is anxiety? (TP 6-1)* *Medical student syndrome (TP 6-2)* *Panic disorder with agoraphobia (TP 6-3)* *Phobos (TP 6-4)* *Are you phobic? (TP 6-5)* *Obsessions? (TP 6-6)* *Examples of posttraumatic stress disorder (TP 6-7)* *Survivor guilt (TP 6-8)* *What's the matter with me? (ACT/DEMO 6-1)* *Specific phobias (ACT/DEMO 6-2)* *Simulating panic attack (ACT/DEMO 6-3)* *Role playing anxiety disorders (ACT/DEMO 6-4)*
Anxiety Disorders: Theory and Therapy • The Psychodynamic Perspective: Neurosis • The Behavioral Perspective: Learning to Be Anxious • The Cognitive Perspective: Misperception of Threat • The Biological Perspective: Biochemistry and Medication	*Eye movement desensitization and reprocessing (LL 6-3)* *What happens to blood flow in the brain in anxiety disorders? (LL 6-4)* *What do agoraphobics think about during scary tasks? LL 6-5)* *Concordance rate for anxiety disorders (TP 6-9)* *Psychiatric journals (TP 6-10)*

Chapter Outline

I.   Introduction
    A.   **Anxiety**, a state of fear, has three basic components
        1.   Subjective reports of tension, apprehension, dread
        2.   Behavioral responses
        3.   Physiological responses
    B.   **Anxiety disorders** characterized by manifest anxiety or behavior aimed at warding off anxiety
    C.   Neurosis historically seen as related to anxiety
    D.   Anxiety disorders is single largest mental health problem in United States

II.   Anxiety Disorder Syndromes
    A.   Panic Disorder
        1.   **Panic attack** characterized by sudden and unexpected anxiety
        2.   Subjective report of derealization and depersonalization
        3.   Disorder often first recognized by complaints of having heart attack
        4.   Two kinds of panic attack
            a.   Uncued attacks come out of the blue
            b.   Cue attacks occur in response to situational trigger
        5.   Stressful events common
        6.   Complication is agoraphobia, which is fear of being in situation where escape is difficult
            a.   Often preceded by panic attacks
            b.   DSM-IV lists agoraphobia as complication of panic disorder
        7.   Panic attacks can be induced in lab using pharmacological agents
        8.   Groups at risk
            a.   Affects 3.5% of population; agoraphobia affects 5.3%
            b.   Gender, age, and marital status are risk factors
            c.   Similarity across ethnic groups and cultures, but symptoms vary
    B.   Generalized Anxiety Disorder
        1.   **Generalized anxiety disorder** is chronic state of diffuse anxiety
        2.   Common areas of worry include family, money, work, and health
        3.   Generalized anxiety disorder is distinct from panic disorder
            a.   Symptom profiles differ
            b.   Has more gradual onset than panic disorder
            c.   Run in families, but run separately
        4.   Groups at risk
            a.   Age at onset is early
            b.   Gender and marital status are risk factors
            c.   Similarity across cultures

C. Phobias
   1.   **Phobias** involve two factors
      a.   Intense and persistent fear of object or situation that poses no real threat
      b.   Avoidance of phobic situations
   2.   Specific phobia
      a.   **Specific phobias** involve **acrophobia, claustrophobia** and animal phobias
      b.   Most people can manage their specific phobia without much difficulty
   3.   Social phobia
      a.   **Social phobia** characterized by avoidance of performing certain actions in front of others for fear of embarrassing or humiliating themselves
      b.   Common social phobias include public speaking, eating in public, and using public bathrooms
      c.   Fears restrict choice; it may interfere with work
      d.   Social phobics have characteristics that make them prone to social rejection
      e.   Social phobia is not specific phobia for social situations
      f.   Distinguishing social phobia from other syndromes is difficult
      g.   Social phobics recall themselves as being shy in childhood
      h.   Groups at risk
          i.   Often begin in childhood
          ii.   Affects up to 11% of population
          iii.   Gender, ethnicity, and SES are risk factors

D. Obsessive-Compulsive Disorder
   1.   **Obsession** is thought or image that is intruding and irresistible
   2.   **Compulsion** is action that is repeated again and again
   3.   Obsessions are common in general populations, but pathological obsessions do not pass, but are recurrent and involve scandalous or violent themes
   4.   Compulsions generally related to duty and caution
      a.   Cleaning rituals
      b.   Checking rituals
   5.   Can be completely disabling
   6.   Individuals with obsessive-compulsive disorder generally do not show characteristics of obsessive-compulsive personality disorder
   7.   Not related to problems of excess that are seen as means to an end
   8.   Obsessive-compulsive disorder does overlap with depression
   9.   Groups at risk
      a.   Affects 2-3% of general population
      b.   Marital status is a risk factor
      c.   Females and males equally at risk

        d.   Usually appears in late adolescence or early adulthood

        e.   Onset may be related to stressful event

E.   Posttraumatic Stress Disorder

    1.   **Posttraumatic stress disorder** is severe psychological reaction to traumatic events

    2.   Source of stress is external event that is very traumatic

    3.   Symptoms consists of heightened arousal, reactions to reminders of trauma, and numbing to surroundings

    4.   Symptoms generally appear shortly after trauma, but there may be an extended time between event and onset of symptoms

    5.   Combat can trigger disorder but is typically preceded by accumulated stress

    6.   Victims of civilian catastrophes may also be related to posttraumatic stress disorder

    7.   Those that escape a disaster may experience survivor's guilt

    8.   Groups at risk

        a.   Affects 8% of population

        b.   Marital status, gender, ethnicity, and type of trauma are important

        c.   Not all people are disabled by traumatic experiences because severity of trauma is significant

        d.   Coping and attributional style related to reaction to trauma

        e.   Environment to which individual returns to following trauma important

        f.   Nature of trauma affects posttraumatic stress disorder and type of symptoms

    9.   Problems in the classification of posttraumatic stress disorder

        a.   In DSM-IV, reactions to ordinary trauma considered adjustment disorders

        b.   Most victims show symptoms of posttraumatic stress disorder

        c.   There is disagreement regarding classifying posttraumatic stress disorder as an anxiety disorder

III.   Anxiety Disorders: Theory and Therapy

    A.   The Psychodynamic Perspective: Neurosis

        1.   The Roots of Neurosis

            a.   Anxiety is viewed as coming from external danger and breakdowns of ego attempt to satisfy id without violating demands of reality and superego resulting in neurosis

            b.   Anxiety chronically experienced is generalized anxiety disorder

            c.   Anxiety builds up in panic disorder as id impulses move closer to the conscious mind

            d.   In phobia, ego defends against anxiety by displacing it

        e.   Symptoms of obsessive-compulsive disorder affect its explanation

        f.   Anxiety disorders differ in choice of defense and some research support it

        g.   Bowlby's attachment theory suggests that disturbances in parent-child relationship may lead to anxiety disorder

    2.   Treating Neurosis

        a.   Goal is to expose and neutral material ego is defending against

        b.   **Free association.** dream analysis, **resistance**, and **transference** used to reveal unconscious material

        c.   Therapy moving toward briefer, face-to-face therapies directed more to present and specific symptoms

B.   The Behavioral Perspective: Learning to Be Anxious

    1.   How We Learn Anxiety

        a.   Avoidance learning has two components

            i.   Respondent learning changing neutral stimulus to anxiety-arousing

            ii.   Avoidance of conditioned stimulus resulting in relief from anxiety

        b.   Disorders are variations on avoidance-reinforced anxiety

        c.   Research supports avoidance-learning theory, but has several problems

            i.   Some anxiety patients do report conditioning, some do not

            ii.   Traditional learning theory has difficulty explaining why very select, nonrandom types of stimuli become phobic objects

            iii.   Focus entirely on concrete stimuli and observable behaviors and not thoughts

        d.   Cognitive processes play important role in anxiety such as efficacy expectations and fear-of-fear

    2.   Unlearning Anxiety

        a.   Confrontation with feared stimulus

        b.   **Systematic desensitization** involves hierarchy of fears and relaxation

        c.   Systematic desensitization effective with specific phobias

            i.   Relaxation unnecessary

            ii.   **Exposure** with feared stimulus effective

            iii.   Imagined exposure with feared stimulus is **flooding**

            iv.   Exposure effective with anxiety disorders

        d.   More complex anxiety disorders may require combinations of different cognitive techniques

C.   The Cognitive Perspective: Misperception of Threat

    1.   Anxiety as Misperception

a. People with anxiety disorders misperceive or misinterpret stimuli, internal, and external

b. Panic disorder patients interpret bodily sensations as dangerous and continue to pay even closer attention to internal sensations

    i. Some research supports model

    ii. Model doesn't explain why panic attacks occurring during sleep are often not connected with dreams and some patients report catastrophic conditions after attack

c. Agoraphobia seen as extension of panic disorder where person appraises that they cannot cope with panic

d. Other anxiety disorders seen as variations on misinterpretation-of-threat theme

2. Reducing Perceptions of Threat

a. Focus is on panic attack itself rather than on avoidance behavior

b. Therapy involves three components

    i. Identify patient's negative interpretations of bodily sensations

    ii. Suggest alternative interpretations

    iii. Help patient test validity of alternative interpretation

c. Therapy has been successful at helping most patients to remain free of panic attacks

d. Questions remain on why therapy works; suggestions include exposure

e. Generalized anxiety disorder treated with combined cognitive and behavioral therapy

D. The Biological Perspective: Biochemistry and Medication

1. Genetic Research

a. Panic disorders has genetic basis; other disorders have weaker, but significant genetic bias; with generalized anxiety disorder having weakest evidence

b. A general vulnerability is inherited toward anxiety disorders in general rather than toward specific disorder

2. The Role of Neurotransmitters

a. Anxiety disorders involve GABA, which is an inhibitory neurotransmitter; it is affected by benzodiazepines

b. Panic disorder responsive to antidepressants suggesting another mechanism

    i. Chemical basis of panic disorder differs from generalized anxiety

    ii. Panic disorder may be closely related to depression

      c.   Panic attacks may be triggered by increased activity in locus ceruleus

      d.   Another model of panic disorder is called suffocation false alarm hypothesis; some individuals have hypersensitive monitors and produce false alarm

      e.   Obsessive-compulsive disorder related to serotonin abnormalities and the basal ganglia

      f.   Little is known about the biology of social phobia, but may involve serotonin abnormalities

      g.   Posttraumatic stress disorder may be explained by a hormonal theory suggesting hormones affect memory of trauma to the point that memory cannot fade

3.   Minor Tranquilizers

      a.   **Minor tranquilizers** are used to reduce anxiety

      b.   **Benzodiazepines** are very popular minor tranquilizers

           i.   Are CNS depressants

           ii.   Can lead to dose-dependent side effects such as daytime sedation, memory disturbances

           iii.   **Withdrawal** from benzodiazepines is a drawback and may be followed by rebound as is case of Xanax

           iv.   Short-acting and long-acting benzodiazepines have differing pattern of withdrawal

4.   Antidepressant Drugs

      a.   **Antidepressant drugs** used to elevate mood

      b.   Effective for panic disorder and obsessive-compulsive disorder

      c.   **MAO inhibitors** interfere with action of enzyme MAO

           i.   Effective treatment for anxiety disorders

           ii.   Can have adverse effects on brain, liver, and cardiovascular system

      d.   **Tricyclics** effective with panic disorder and obsessive-compulsive disorder, but with side effects

      e.   Selective serotonin reuptake inhibitors (SSRIs) block serotonin reuptake

           i.   Prozac is most widely prescribed antidepressant

           ii.   Prozac works well with social phobia and panic disorder, and obsessive-compulsive disorder

           iii.   SSRI can have side effects

      f.   Critics of antianxiety drugs suggest that drugs allow people to avoid their problems

           i.   Solution appears to be psychotherapy and drugs

           ii.   Some success with combined psychotherapy and drugs has been seen with panic disorder, but less clear with other anxiety disorders

Chapter Boxes

- Persian Gulf War Syndrome
    - A.   Gulf War was stressful for most participants
    - B.   Many veterans of Gulf War experienced symptoms of stress and anxiety after their return home
    - C.   Characteristics of Gulf War Syndrome mirror acute stress disorder and posttraumatic stress disorder
    - D.   Symptoms may be related to sources other than stress of combat
    - E.   Chemical weapons can produce long-lasting effects

- Anxiety and Selective Attention
    - A.   People with anxiety disorders pay more attention to threatening stimuli
    - B.   What patients attend to is influenced by type of anxiety disorder
    - C.   Stroop test revealed that anxious subjects pay more attention to color of threat words than color of nonthreat words

- Anxiety and the Middle-Aged Brain
    - A.   There is decreased incidence of anxiety disorders in middle-aged people
    - B.   Related to deterioration of locus ceruleus
    - C.   Locus ceruleus, part of brainstem that controls breathing and heart rate
    - D.   Changes in locus ceruleus slows the cells' functions
    - E.   Decrease in norepinephrine production

Learning Objectives (LO)

By the time you have finished studying this chapter, you should be able to do the following:

1. List three characteristics of anxiety and define the concept of anxiety disorder (150).

2. Define the Freudian concept of "neurosis" and explain why this concept is no longer used as a diagnostic category in *DSM-IV* (150).

3. Describe two varieties of panic disorder and explain its relationship to agoraphobia (151-152).

4. Describe generalized anxiety disorder and distinguish it from panic disorder (153).

5. Define phobia, and describe two categories of phobia mentioned in your text (153-155).

6. Define obsessive-compulsive disorder, distinguish between obsessions and compulsions, and distinguish between two varieties of compulsions (155-157).

7. Define posttraumatic stress disorder, list the factors associated with its occurrence, and discuss the problems associated with posttraumatic stress disorder as a diagnostic category (157-161).

8. Explain how the psychodynamic perspective views the causes of anxiety disorders and how such disorders should be treated (161-163).

9. Explain how the behavioral perspective accounts for and treats anxiety disorders, making specific reference to the two-process model and exposure therapy (163 - 165).

10. Explain the role of misperception in the cognitive perspective on anxiety disorders and describe cognitively based treatment techniques (165-168).

11. Describe the findings of genetic and biochemical research into anxiety disorders (168-171).

12. Describe biological treatments for anxiety disorders, making specific reference to the use of minor tranquilizers and antidepressant drugs (171-173).

Lecture Leads (LL)

Famous people with anxiety disorders (LL 6-1)
A memorable way to introduce this chapter is to talk about how anxiety disorders affect all people from all walks of life. In fact, there have been some rather famous people who have struggled with anxiety disorders such as Howard Hughes (the late billionaire-- OCD), John Madden (sportscaster--phobia), Mark Somers (game show host--OCD). Charles Darwin probably suffered from panic disorder with agoraphobia. This disorder caused Darwin impairment in nearly all areas of his life, and explains his reluctance to speak and meet with his colleagues. Figueroa argued that Sigmund Freud had symptoms that are consistent with panic disorder without agoraphobia and nicotine dependence. Ask students for more examples.

Resources:

Barloon, T. J., & Noyes, R. (1997). Charles Darwin and panic disorder. Journal of the American Medical Association, 277, 138-141.

Figueroa, G. (1997). Anxiety disorder and Freud's disease. Review of Medicine Chile, 125, 363-370.

Trichotillomania: A hair-pulling obsession (LL 6-2)
Spectrum disorders of obsessive-compulsive disorder are those disorders that resemble OCD in symptomlogy, family history, and treatment. One spectrum disorder that is related to or associated with OCD is trichotillomania, which is "an irresistible urge to pull one's hair out" *(Harvard Mental Health Letter,* 1990, p. 6). About half of the patients with trichotillomania (TM) experience heightened anxiety that produces the urge to pull out their hair from the scalp, eyebrows, and eyelashes. The other half of sufferers experiences a sense of pleasure from pulling out their hair. The primary symptom of this disorder is "recurrent pulling out of one's hair resulting in noticeable hair loss" (DSM-IV, 1994, p. 621). However, DSM-IV described associated features, which include hiding the disorder and thus avoiding social situations, examining and twirling off hair roots, pulling strands of hair between the teeth or eating them. While these symptoms may be done in private, "some individuals have urges to pull hairs from other people and may sometimes try to find opportunities to do so surreptitiously" (p. 619). They may also pull hairs from their pets, from dolls, or from fabrics. To treat TM, O'Sullivan (1993) suggested use of "competing responses"--that is, identify the situations or cues that trigger the behavior, then teach responses that make the hair pulling impossible, such as clenching the fist. Considering the number of people afflicted with this disorder, it seems surprising that we hear so little about it. Perhaps it is the secretive nature of trichotillomania that keeps it so well concealed.

Resources:

American Psychiatric Association. (1994*).* Diagnostic and statistical manual of mental disorders (4th ed.). Washington, DC: Author.

Neziroglu, F. (March, 1997). Obsessive-compulsive spectrum disorders: An overview. Mental Health Infosource [On-line]. Available: WWW URL www.mhsource.com/edu/psytimes/p970352.html.

O'Sullivan, R. L. (1993). What is trichotillomania and how is it treated? The Harvard Mental Health Letter, 10(5), 8.

Eye movement desensitization and reprocessing (LL 6-3)

In the last decade a new therapy has been developed that seems to be building a moderately strong research base. Eye movement desensitization and reprocessing (EMDR) involves recounting a traumatic, emotional memory while engaging in lateral eye movements. The client typically follows the finger or a pen as it is moved back and forth in front of the eyes. The back and forth motions are spaced about one second apart. A typical session lasts for about 90 minutes during which time these negative memories are replaced by positive ones. Scheck, Schaeffer, and Gillette used EMDR to treat a group of traumatized females between 16 and 25 years of age. They found that those who received EMDR experienced favorable and, in some cases, greater improvement than to a control group on measures of depression, anxiety, and stress. The underlying mechanism to account for EMDR's apparent effectiveness is not clear.

Resources:
Carlson , J. G., et al. (1998). Eye movement desensitization and reprocessing treatment for combat-related posttraumatic stress disorder. Journal of Trauma Stress, 11, 3-24.

Scheck, M., Schaeffer, J. A., & Gillette, C. (1998). Brief psychological intervention with traumatized young women: The efficacy of eye movement desensitization and reprocessing. Journal of Trauma Stress, 11, 25-44.

Shapiro, F. (1989). Eye movement desensitization: A new treatment for post-traumatic stress disorder. Journal of Behavior Therapy and Experimental Psychiatry, 20, 211-217.

What happens to blood flow in the brain in anxiety disorders? (LL 6-4)

Regional cerebral blood flow was measured in groups of patients with anxiety disorders. High-resolution single photon emission tomography was used to assess blood flow in patients with panic disorder with agoraphobia (n=15), obsessive-compulsive disorder (n=15), posttraumatic stress disorder (n=16), and health control group (n=15). Blood flow was positively correlated with anxiety. The level of anxiety experienced by subjects was positively correlated with whole brain blood flow. In addition, blood flow differed among the different anxiety diagnostic groups. The study also showed regional cerebral blood flow differences between obsessive-compulsive disorder and posttraumatic stress disorder compared to panic disorder and control group subjects. Specifically, the brain areas where different blood flow was observed were the bilateral superior frontal lobe and right caudate nuclei. The study also found a negative correlation between the severity of posttraumatic stress disorder and blood flow in both left and right caudate.

Resource:

Lucey, J. V. et al. (1997). Brain blood flow in anxiety disorders: OCD, panic disorders with agoraphobia, and post-traumatic stress disorder on single photon emission tomography. British Journal of Psychiatry, 171, 346-350.

What do agoraphobics think about during scary tasks? (LL 6-5)

Subjects with agoraphobia monitored their thinking as they drove alone or tolerated an enclosed place. A periodic beep signaled subjects to tape record what they there thinking. Over 1,800 tape-recorded statements were collected. The statements were analyzed and it was found that about 29% of the statements involved a preoccupation with their current level of anxiety. In about 15% of statements, subjects expressed skepticism that they could successfully complete the task of driving or tolerating an enclosure. The study also revealed that fewer than 1% of the statements contained references to danger or anticipatory anxiety or panic. The authors suggest that this rather low percentage presented a challenge to cognitive theories of phobia.

Resource:

Williams, S. L., Kinney, P. J., & Harap, S. T. (1997). Thoughts of agoraphobic people during scary tasks. Journal of Abnormal Psychology, 106, 511-520.

Talking Points (TP)

What is anxiety? (TP 6-1)
When you introduce this chapter, ask students to "free association" on the word anxiety. Point out that the word "anxiety" really is an abbreviation for a very complex list of components.

Medical student syndrome (TP 6-2)
Chances are pretty good that you will have some students who believe that they suffer from one of the anxiety disorders. Some will be experiencing abnormal psychology's version of the medical student syndrome; others will probably have what appears to be valid complaints. The critical questions are: Does the anxiety interfere with the individual's life? Does the anxiety prevent the fulfillment of roles and responsibilities? Of course, when in doubt refer them to the university counseling center or to a community service agency.

Panic disorder with agoraphobia (TP 6-3)
Here is a way to approach the topic of panic disorder with agoraphobia. After you have presented panic disorder, ask your students where they would rather be when having an attack? Most of them will respond with "at home." This gives a nice lead into agoraphobia.

Phobos (TP 6-4)
We get the word phobia from the Greek for fear, specifically the Greek god of fear, Phobos, who frightened his enemies.

Are you phobic? (TP 6-5)
The key thing for students to keep in mind about phobias is the irrationality of the fear. Pose this scenario to students: They are walking alone at night down a dark street. Suddenly a figure jumps out from the shadows showing a knife and demands their money. Are your students scared? Are they fearful? Do they have a phobia? Is it irrational to be fearful in that situation? Does the situation pose a real threat?

Obsessions? (TP 6-6)
As you start discussing OCD, differentiate obsessions of the innocent nature and those of a clinical nature. For instance, most of us have had a song or question like "Did I lock the door?" running through our minds. Contrast these types of obsessions with the type of obsessions characteristic of OCD. Ask the students to write on a piece of paper their most active obsession or compulsion. Do not have them identify themselves. After the students have turned in the papers, review and rank order them in terms of interest to the students. You can even reveal some of the not-too-dark secrets about your own obsessions and compulsions; this is especially relevant if you have some associated with the class or school. By revealing some of your obsessions and compulsions, the students will feel much more at ease when discussing many of the disorders later in the course.

Examples of posttraumatic stress disorder (TP 6-7)
Approach this suggestion with discretion. There are probably students in your class who have direct or indirect experience with PTSD. Perhaps they experienced a flood that destroyed their home or were assaulted. Maybe they have a relative who is a Vietnam veteran suffering from PTSD. If you wish, put out a request for examples of PTSD and then discuss it with those who come forward, but do so outside of class. If you and the student feel comfortable, have the student present the example in the next class meeting.

Survivor guilt (TP 6-8)
In the last several months there have been several school shootings in the United States. Two common questions asked by survivors of those shootings are "Why?" "I should have been the one shot or killed." Ask students for other examples of survivor guilt that they have seen in real-life events or fictitious examples from movies.

Concordance rate for anxiety disorders (TP 6-9)
It bears repeating that the concordance rate for panic disorder in MZ is 31 percent and not 100 percent. This suggests that there are environmental factors at work in the etiology of panic disorder. if not all anxiety disorders.

Psychiatric journals (TP 6-10)
Pharmacology manufacturers advertise their antianxiety drugs in several psychiatry journals. The advertisements often dramatically illustrate the type of symptoms and level of discomfort the anxiety disorders cause in people. Locate a couple of these advertisements and bring them to class. You can also develop an activity from this by either asking students to guess what anxiety disorder the particular ad is referring to or to get students to create their own advertisements for antianxiety drugs.

Cross-Cultural Teaching

A 27-year old married **electrician** complains of ...	p. 150
and a constant "**edgy**" and watchful feeling...	p. 150
whether his **wife will leave** him...	p. 150
Anxiety is **part and parcel** of human existence.	p. 150
Without it, we would probably all be **asleep at our desks**...	p. 150
People with panic disorder cannot go anywhere...to the **supermarket**	p. 151
it seems to descent "**out of nowhere**"...	p. 151
frequently shouting and **weeping**...	p. 152
Fear of air travel might be more debilitating to a **business executive**...	p. 153
a **city dweller** with a phobia for snakes need only avoid going to the zoo.	p. 153
to avoid encountering a stranger in the **lavatory**...	p. 154
as they generally have **overtones** of duty and caution.	p. 155
At the same time, they seem to **numb** themselves to their present surroundings.	p. 157
Some soldiers become depressed and **curl up in their bunks**...	p. 157
numerous **brushes with death**.	p. 158
Among the survivors of the **Mount St. Helens** eruption in 1980...	p. 158
volunteer **firefighters** who survived the huge wave of **brushfires**...	p. 159
since his father would sometimes play "**horsie**" with him...	p. 161
They change the subject, begin missing **appointments**...	p. 162
yet they still go onstage...	p. 164
panic attacks come "**out of the blue**."	p. 165
the disorder **runs in families**...	p. 168
rats can be bred for "**nervousness**"...	p. 169
often assumed to be a **plague of modern life**.	p. 171
simply going through a **hard time** in their lives.	p. 171
often cause headache, upset stomach, **jitteriness**, and sexual dysfunction.	p. 173
As a final **caveat**...	p. 173

Activities and Demonstrations (ACT/DEMO)

What's the matter with me? (ACT/DEMO 6-1)
Objective: To engage students in asking relevant questions about the anxiety disorders
Materials: a 3 x 5 index card for each student; masking tape
Procedure: Hand out one card per student. Ask them to write on the card one of the anxiety disorders. Collect the cards and then randomly distribute the cards, again one to each student. Ask the students to keep the cards face down. Next, students should help each other by taping the index card on their forehead with the disorder label face up. Students are now to walk around the classroom asking questions of others attempting to determine what disorder is taped to their head. Obviously, students cannot directly ask what disorder they have.
Discussion: Based on the answers they receive from their question, they should be able to identify which disorder has been assigned to them

Specific phobias (ACT/DEMO 6-2)
Objective: To illustrate the variety of specific phobias
Materials: Specific phobias handout
Procedure: There are two variations to this activity. Simply read the handout to the students, asking them what the specific phobia involves. Or, pass the handout to students with some terms and fears erased; ask students to supply the missing information.
Discussion: As students will see, almost anything can be the focus of a specific phobia. Everyone has some fears, spiders (Arachnaphobia), dirt (Mysophobia), or lightning (Astraphobia) are good examples. Ask the class to volunteer with a show of hands anyone who has a fear of spiders (Arachnaphobia). Several will raise their hands. Then ask the question, are these people phobic? Describe what a true spider phobic's behaviors might be like.

Simulating panic attack (ACT/DEMO 6-3)
Objective: To demonstrate a mild panic attack to the students
Materials: Pop quiz based on previously assigned (but rarely read) outside class readings
Procedure: Two words of caution--first, this activity will cause some amount of discomfort for students, therefore use your discretion. Second, if you do decide to use it, a critical element is your acting; be serious! Assign some outside reading and have it put on reserve in the library several weeks prior to this demonstration. Tell the students that they are to have these readings done by the date of this demonstration for discussion in class. These readings can be relevant to the material you are currently studying. The day of the demonstration come to class several minutes late and act very angry. Explain that you have learned from a student in the class that several students have cheated on the last formal examination and that you are very upset with students in general and the students in this class in particular. Explain that you have decided to invalidate the last examination and give everyone a zero on it since you cannot identify the specific students who have cheated. You have decided that the only "fair" thing to do is to give another examination and that the best method to assess the students' true knowledge of the subject

matter is to evaluate the outside readings. Distribute the pop quiz and explain that this will substitute for one-quarter or one-half of the course points. Be very stern and formal if any students question your authority. Tell the students that they have until the end of the class period to finish. Sit at the front of the classroom for about 5 minutes; this will allow most of the students to experience a mild panic attack, *but use your own judgment.* **Discussion**: Even the students who will have done the reading will not feel confident with this assignment. Make sure you debrief them following the experience. Ask students to describe the behavioral, cognitive, physiological, and affective dimensions of the experience. Remind them that many of us have experienced limited panic symptoms. Ask them to imagine how their lives would be disrupted if they experienced panic attacks on a regular basis.

Role playing anxiety disorders (ACT/DEMO 6-4)
Objective: To demonstrate the types of behaviors associated with anxiety disorders
Materials: Descriptions of anxiety disorders
Procedure: Have the students individually or in small groups select one of the anxiety disorders.. Their task is to develop a role play to illustrate the disorder as well as other information (e.g., effect on family, demographics, suspected etiology, treatment perspectives). Tell the students that they have at least overnight to prepare for their disorder and that they will be expected to role play the disorder in front of the class. If using groups, one person plays the role of the subject, and other group members can play family members, employers, friends, and clinician.
Discussion: Give feedback on the accuracy of the role play. Ask the students how they developed their role and who they used as a model. Was there any influence from the media? If so, what specific individuals did they use as models? You could show a video at this point that will reinforce the correct behaviors and change the incorrect ones.

Films and Videos

Anxiety: The Endless Crisis. IU. Discusses a wide range of anxiety-producing situations.

Anxiety: The Endless Crisis. PSU. This film explores anxiety from a range of situations and responses ranging from mild to potentially life-threatening.

Breathing Away Stress. FHS. Deep-breathing exercises designed to manage stress and promote relaxation.

Burnout. MTI. Discusses the danger signs of burnout and practical ways to deal with it.

Coping with Phobias. FHS. This program explains why people have phobias and how phobias can usually be overcome. It focuses on fear of flying. The program also visits a speech class to explain the dynamics of this phobia and provide specific suggestions on overcoming the fears involved.

Dealing with Stress. FHS. How to deal with stress without reducing job productivity, and how to change stress into motivation for positive achievement.

Fear Itself. FHS. Focuses on agoraphobia and the use of drug therapy, individual therapy, and support groups in treatment.

Getting a Handle on Stress. FHS. Examines risk for stress-related diseases, the effects of prolonged stress, and ways to reduce stress.

Interview with an Obsessive-Compulsive. PSU. This video is part of a continuing series of case interviews.

Male Stress Syndrome. FHS. Describes the ways men and women experience stress; discusses causes and cures of male stress syndrome.

Managing Stress. FHS. Distinguishes between positive stress, which can strengthen the immune system, and negative stress, which can increase the likelihood of illness. Describes how an individual can reduce stress.

Mysteries of the Mind. FSH. Discusses neurochemical and genetic components of manic depressive and obsessive-compulsive disorders, alcoholism, and mood disorders.

Obsessive-Compulsive Disorder. FHS. Once thought to be a psychological problem, obsessive-compulsive behavior may, in fact be rooted in chemical imbalances in the brain. Drug treatment now offers hope to. many whose lives have been dominated by the uncontrollable urges to perform and repeat actions as a ritualistic attempt to avoid anxiety.

Obsessive-Compulsive Disorder. The Boy Who Couldn't Stop Washing. FHS. Examines obsessive-compulsive behavior, by which individuals think they can keep something terrible from happening.

Panic! FHS. This program follows two agoraphobics through three years of treatment. A man discusses his phobia of poisoning himself, and a woman shows how she worked through a fear of flying. Researchers explain their evidence for a biological cause for anxiety disorders.

Post-Traumatic Stress Disorder. FHS. The term "post-traumatic stress disorder" (PTSD) was originally used to describe the symptoms of Vietnam veterans suffering from depression and rage. But PTSD is not limited to battlefield vets. Anyone who has had a deeply traumatic experience can develop PTSD and treatment techniques developed for

Vietnam veterans are now being used with other patients. Host Jamie Guth interviews a Vietnam veteran; she also spends time with an adult woman who is an incest survivor.

Posttraumatic Stress Disorder. FHS. Examines PTSD resulting from the Vietnam war and other traumas.

Progressive Relaxation Training. A Clinical Demonstration. PSU. Identifies the sixteen muscle groups involved in relaxation training and shows how the procedure is done.

Stress. FHS. Examines the many ways stress can affect people of all ages and demonstrates proven methods of coping with stress.

The Compulsive Mind. FHS. This program focuses on a woman with Obsessive Compulsive Disorder (OCD) who suffers from a fear of contamination. The woman describes her washing routines, explaining how she washes anywhere from eight to 200 times a day. A psychiatrist explains what OCD is and that these patients know their behavior is irrational. The program discusses the brain chemical serotonin and explains the role of medication and behavioral therapy in the treatment of OCD. Finally, the program observes the OCD patient as she works with her therapist.

The Psychobiology of Stress. IM. Investigates how the brain controls the stress response through regulation of the nervous system and of hormonal activity.

The Relaxation Response. FHS. Explains the relaxation response and discusses exercises designed to trigger it.

Treating Tourette's and Other Mental Illness. FHS. This program explains the imbalance in the brain chemical dopamine, which can cause Tourette's; how dopamine and other chemicals affect the brain; mental disorders and family history; diagnosis of Tourette's and other mental illness in children; medications and their side effects; psychotherapy and counseling; drug abuse and mental illness; and what imaging techniques reveal about mental illness.

Understanding Stress. IM. Explains stress and describes the key elements of an effective stress response.

When Panic Strikes. FHS. This program begins with a description of how it feels to have a panic attack. The victim found no physician who correctly diagnosed the condition. When she was finally diagnosed as agoraphobic, treatment included medication and exposure therapy. Panic attack patients can lead nearly normal lives with the proper combination of medication and behavioral therapy.

Women and Stress. FHS. Examines typical ways women deal with stress.

Using Movies and Mental Illness as a Teaching Tool

Most of your students will have seen and enjoyed *As Good As It Gets,* and they will appreciate getting a chance to review selected scenes from the film that illustrate the obsessive compulsive traits displayed by Jack Nicholson's character Melvin Udall (featured on the cover of *Movies and Mental Illness*).

It may be useful to have your students debate whether or not Nicholson's character presents a representative and realistic portrayal of the behavior of someone with an obsessive compulsive disorder. Your students will want to debate whether or not the therapist Robin Williams portrayed in *Good Will Hunting* could have helped Nicholson's character in *As Good As It Gets,* and students can be asked to research whether or not cognitive behavioral methods are superior to psychodynamic approaches in the treatment of OCD. (A compelling body of data suggests behavioral methods are the treatment of choice, and your students should be able to establish this fact with little difficulty.)

A lively discussion of the relationship between traumatic events and phobias can grow out of the opening scene from *Vertigo* in which Jimmy Stewart's plays a policeman who sees his partner fall to his death from the roof of a high building. Your students will be able to generate other examples of Hitchcock films in which trauma shapes the life of the protagonist.

Many of the films dealing with the adjustment of veterans returning home from war will illustrate post traumatic stress disorders, and it will be easy for professors to identify an appropriate stimulus film for class discussion (e.g., selected scenes from *The Deer Hunter, Platoon, Full Metal Jacket)*. Alternately, students can be assigned individual films from the Anxiety Disorders section of Appendix B of *Movies and Mental Illness* and charged with bringing the films to class, prepared to show brief vignettes illustrating the symptoms of PTSD. Instructors may want to introduce this chapter by briefly showing some of the group therapy scenes from *Fearless*, or Rod Steiger's concentration camp flashbacks from *The Pawnbroker*.

Movie	Link to Chapter	Page Reference to Wedding and Boyd
• Annie Hall • Manhattan	generalized anxiety disorder (p. 153)	p. 13 p. 13
• The Fisher King • Vertigo • Inside Out • Lonely Hearts • Rocky	phobias (p. 153)	p. 12 p. 13 p. 16 p. 19 p. 19
• As Good As It Gets	obsessive-compulsive disorders (p. 155)	p. 17
• Born on the Fourth of July • Fearless • Ironweed • The Pawnbroker • Coming Home	posttraumatic stress disorder (p. 157)	p. 9 p. 12 p. 13 p. 19 p. 19

Classroom Assessment Techniques (CAT)

Focused Listing (CAT 6-1)
Select an important point from this chapter (e.g., anxiety, survivor guilt, obsession, compulsion) and ask students to write five words or phrases that describe the point.

Learning Review (CAT 6-2)
Students are to write in order five of the most important ideas they learned in this chapter.

Muddiest Point (CAT 6-3)
Instruct students to write about an issue, concept, or definition presented in Chapter 6 that they find most confusing or difficult to understand.

Definition Matrix (CAT 6-4)
Using the handout, students should identify each anxiety disorder presented in the textbook. For each criterion, students should provide a definition, an example, and effective treatment options. Students should attempt to write only a few words or phrases.

Minute Paper (CAT 6-5)
Ask your students to write about an important question they have that remains unanswered.

Suggestions for Essay Questions

- What is anxiety and why is it sometimes harmful and at other times useful?
- Describe how anxiety is maladaptive in each of the anxiety disorders.
- You are a clinical psychologist treating a young woman with panic disorder. Using the cognitive perspective describe your approach in treating this patient.

Examples of Specific Phobia
Handout

Term	Object of fear
Acrophobia	Heights
Aerophobia	Flying
Anglophobia	England and things English
Anthropophobia	Human beings
Arachnophobia	Spiders
Arachibutyrophobia	Peanut butter sticking to the root of the mouth
Astraphobia	Storms; thunder and lightning
Bibliophobia	Books
Carnophobia	Meat
Claustrophobia	Closed spaces; confinement
Doraphobia	Fur
Gephyrophobia	Bridges
Hematophobia	Blood
Hydrophobia	Water
Kenophobia	Empty rooms
Logosphobia	Words
Mysophobia	Dirt
Nyctophobia	Darkness
Odontophobia	Teeth
Ophidiophobia	Snakes
Osphresiophobia	Body odors
Pogonophobia	Beards
Pyrophobia	Fire
Thanatophobia	Death
Dendrophobia	Trees
Xenophobia	Strangers

(taken from Melville, 1978)

Definition Matrix
Classroom Assessment Technique

Anxiety Disorder	Definition	Example	Treatment Options
Panic disorder			
Generalized anxiety disorder			
Phobias			
Obsessive-Compulsive disorder			
Posttraumatic Stress Disorder			

Chapter 7

Dissociative and Somatoform Disorders

Chapter Map

Section	Instructor Manual Components
Dissociative Disorders • Dissociative Amnesia • Dissociative Fugue • Dissociative Identify Disorder • Depersonalization Disorder • Groups at Risk for Dissociative Disorders	*Debating dissociative identity disorders (LL 7-1)* *Recovered memory of child abuse (LL 7-2)* *More information on dissociative identity disorder (LL 7-3)* *Case studies of dissociative and somatoform disorders (LL 7-4)* *Dissociative versus associative (TP 7-1)* *Dissociative disorders on soap operas (TP 7-2)* *Amnesia and fugue (TP 7-3)* *Dissociative identity disorder (TP 7-4)* *Sybil (TP 7-5)* *Role of childhood abuse in DID (TP 7-6)* *Prevalence of DID (TP 7-7)* *What's the matter with me? (ACT/DEMO 7-1)*
Dissociative Disorders: Theory and Therapy • The Psychodynamic Perspective: Defense Against Anxiety • The Behavioral Perspective: Dissociation as a Social Role • The Cognitive Perspective: Memory Dysfunction • The Biological Perspective: Brain Dysfunction	*Integrate alters? (TP 7-8)* *Guest speakers (ACT/DEMO 7-2)*

Somatoform Disorders • Body Dysmorphic Disorder • Hypochondriasis • Somatization Disorder • Pain Disorder • Conversion Disorder • Groups at Risk for Somatoform Disorders	*Case studies of dissociative and somatoform disorders (LL 7-4)* *Gender differences in body dysmorphic disorder (LL 7-5)* *Understanding origin of pain (LL 7-6)* *Pseudoseizure as conversion disorder (LL 7-7)* *Somatoform disorders (TP 7-9)* *A bad hair day (TP 7-10)* *Hypochondriasis (TP 7-11)* *Role playing somatoform disorders (ACT/DEMO 7-3)*
Somatoform Disorders: Theory and Therapy • The Psychodynamic Perspective: Defense Against Anxiety • The Behavioral Perspective: The Sick Role • The Cognitive Perspective: Misinterpreting Bodily Sensations • The Biological Perspective: Brain Dysfunction	*Somatoform and Dissociative disorders and the popular press (ACT/DEMO 7-4)*

Chapter Outline

I.   Introduction
      A.   **Hysteria** mimics a biogenic disorder
      B.   Dissociative disorders include disturbances of higher cognitive functions
      C.   Somatoform disorders are disorders that take physical form

II.   Dissociative Disorders
      A.   Dissociative disorders involve dissociation of personality components typically integrated
            a.   Psychological functions screened out of awareness
            b.   Dissociative disorders occur without demonstrable damage to brain
      B.   Dissociative Amnesia
            1.   Amnesia is partial or total forgetting of past experiences
                  a.   Can occur by head injury or brain disorder
                  b.   **Dissociative amnesia** occurs without any apparent organic cause
                        i.   Is anterograde, not retrograde
                        ii.   Is selective and includes memories most people would want to forget
                        iii. People much less disturbed over dissociative amnesia
                        iv.   People with dissociative amnesia remain well oriented to time and place; continue to learn new information
                        v.   Forgotten events are simply screened out and not lost altogether
            2.   Patterns of memory loss
                  a.   Localized amnesia--all events occurring during specific period of time are blocked
                  b.   Selective amnesia--only certain events forgotten during specific period of time
                  c.   Generalized amnesia--entire life forgotten
                  d.   Continuous amnesia--forgetting all events that occur after specific period up to present including events occurring after onset of amnesia
                  e.   Systematized amnesia--only certain categories of information forgotten
                  f.   Episodic memory is lost
                  g.   Semantic memory and procedural memory remain intact
                  h.   **Explicit memories** may be forgotten
                  i.   **Implicit memories** are still intact and continue to influence behavior

143

          j.   Onset of memory loss is typically gradual and remits gradually

    3.   Amnesia and Crime
         a.   Amnesia has created difficulties for legal system
         b.   Many people accused of crime cannot remember event; some are faking

C.   Dissociative Fugue
    1.   **Dissociative fugue** involves forgetting past and sudden travel away from home; traveling amnesia
    2.   Show purposeful activity; may create identity
    3.   Length and elaborateness of fugues vary considerably
    4.   Individual's memory remits suddenly and is amnesic for events while in fugue state

D.   Dissociative Identity Disorder
    1.   **Dissociative identity disorder** (formerly multiple personality disorder) characterized by personality breaking up into 2 or more distinct, well-integrated identities
    2.   One of more identities is amnesic
    3.   **Host** is original personality and **alters** are later developing personalities
    4.   Host and alters often have complex patterns of consciousness
    5.   Types of Personalities
         a.   Personalities often are polar opposites and include internal homicide
         b.   Personalities may divide up emotional life and other areas of functioning
         c.   Child personality is common
    6.   Childhood Abuse
         a.   Most common trauma is sexual abuse and incest
         b.   Disorder may be way that children use to distance themselves from abuse since most cases begin in childhood
         c.   Not clear if abused children are more likely to develop DID than nonabused children
         d.   Mechanism underlying DID is not known
    7.   Problems in Diagnosis
         a.   DID, once rare, reported more frequently and in North America
         b.   Some argue that DID is more a fad than legitimate syndrome
         c.   Rise in numbers could reflect better recognition of DID and increased awareness and reporting of childhood sexual abuse
         d.   Concern expressed over false cases; criteria is used to distinguish false cases

  e. Physiology of DID patients changes depending on which personality is in charge

E. Depersonalization Disorder

  1. **Depersonalization disorder** involves disruption of personal identity without amnesia

  2. Central feature is a sense of strangeness or unreality in oneself

  3. Often accompanied by **derealization**, feeling of strangeness about world

    a. May involve déjà vu

    b. May involve jamais vu

  4. Depersonalization can occur in course of normal life, as part of other psychological disorders, and near death experience

  5. Depersonalization is diagnosed when it interferes with person's life

F. Groups at Risk for Dissociative Disorders

  1. Prevalence as high as 3 percent in general population

  2. DID more common in females, and these tend to be already troubled

  3. Depersonalization is rare and more common in females, and is seen worldwide where it may be seen as a legitimate trance or spirit possession

III. Dissociative Disorders: Theory and Therapy

A. The Psychodynamic Perspective: Defense Against Anxiety

  1. Pierre Janet originated idea of mental dissociation

  2. Dissociation as Defense

    a. Freud argued dissociation disorders were neuroses that were extreme and maladaptive defenses

    b. Research supports anxiety-relief hypothesis

  3. Treating Dissociation

    a. Psychodynamic therapy most common treatment for dissociative disorders

    b. Treatment involves three stages

    c. In dissociative disorders, material is protected from exposure

      i. Repressed memory may be revealed through hypnosis

      ii. Hypnosis may bring on or exacerbate symptoms

      iii. Memory-retrieval may be retraumatized, especially when it takes form of abreaction

      iv. Memory is retrieved gradually, which may be long process, especially in DID

B. The Behavioral and Sociocultural Perspectives: Dissociation as a Social Role

1. Dissociative disorders seen as form of learned coping response with production of symptoms in order to obtain rewards or relief from stress
2. Results of person adopting a social role that is reinforced by its consequences
3. Sociocultural perspective views symptoms as product of social reinforcement
   a. Seen as strategy to evoke sympathy and escape responsibility for certain actions performed by nonresponsible part of self
   b. Patient, hypnosis and therapist's attention help to create disorder, and come to believe in its existence
   c. Research reveals that when situation demands it and appropriate cues are given, personalities can be manufactured
4. Nonreinforcement
   a. Way to treat dissociative symptoms is to stop reinforcing them
   b. Treatment involves expressing no interest in alters and expecting patient to take responsibility for actions committed by alters

C. The Cognitive Perspective: Memory Dysfunction
1. Dissociative disorders seen as disorders of memory, namely explicit memory for dissociated material
2. Retrieval Failure
   a. State-dependent memory established in extreme emotional state may be lost
   b. Control elements can activate or inhibit retrieval information
3. Improving Memory Retrieval
   a. Therapists use cognitive mechanism in treatment
   b. Therapists may improve implicit memory

D. The Biological Perspective: Brain Dysfunction
1. Some dissociative disorders may be neurological disorders
   a. May be by-products of undiagnosed epilepsy
   b. Hippocampus may be involved since it is involved in memory integration, which stress can affect
   c. Abnormality in serotonin functioning may be involved
2. None of neurological hypotheses rules out psychological causes
3. Drug Treatment
   a. Not many drug treatments developed
   b. Barbiturate sodium amytal and SSRI's have been used

IV. Somatoform Disorders
   A. **Somatoform disorders** involve psychological conflicts that take on a somatic form
   B. May involve complaints or actual loss or impairment of normal physiological function
   C. Body Dysmorphic Disorder
      1. **Body dysmorphic disorder** consists of extreme distress over physical appearance
      2. Most complain of facial flaws and thinning hair
      3. Individuals are not delusional, but do suffer great unhappiness
      4. Onset is usually gradual and may be begin with someone's negative comment; tends to be chronic
      5. Disorder is associated with social phobia, depression, and related to obsessive-compulsive disorder
   D. Hypochondriasis
      1. **Hypochondriasis** is gnawing fear of disease
      2. Fear is maintained by misinterpretation of physical signs and sensations as abnormal
      3. Symptoms are not faked; they truly feel the pains they report
      4. Fears do not have bizarre quality of delusions
      5. Different from obsessive-compulsion disorder where fears are groundless
      6. Developmental factors may predispose person to hypochondriasis
   E. Somatization disorder
      1. **Somatization disorder** characterized by numerous and recurrent physical complaints
      2. Resembles hypochondriasis, but focus differs
         a. Symptoms described as vague, dramatic, and exaggerated
         b. Complaints are many and varied
      3. Often accompanied by depression and anxiety
   F. Pain Disorder
      1. **Pain disorder** occurs when person has pain that is more severe or persistent than can be explained by medical causes
      2. Tend to have psychiatric symptoms
      3. Psychological factors may be result or cause of pain
      4. Indications of pain as being psychologically related
         a. Harder time localizing pain
         b. Pain is described in emotional terms
         c. Less likely to specify changes in pain
         d. See pain as the disorder rather than as symptom of a disorder
   G. Conversion Disorder
      1. In conversion disorder, there is actually disability, but no organic pathology

2. Symptoms vary considerably; most common are blindness, deafness, paralysis, and anesthesia
3. Symptoms are not supported by medical evidence; but also are not faked
4. Was formerly known as hysteria
5. Conversion disorder seen as result of some psychological conflict
   a. Blocks person's awareness of internal conflict; **primary gain**
   b. Excuses person from responsibilities and attracts sympathy and attention; **secondary gain**
6. Many patients show **la belle indifference** (beautiful indifference)
7. Evidence shows that person's body is capable of functioning properly, but are not consciously refusing to use body parts
8. Conversion, Malingering, or Organic Disorder?
   a. Differential diagnosis is difficult
   b. Malingering must be ruled out
   c. Actual organic disorders must be ruled out
      i. Glove anesthesia contradicts structure of nervous system
      ii. Symptoms are very similar to true organic disorders
   d. Criteria for differential diagnosis
      i. Rapid appearance of symptoms
      ii. La belle indifference
      iii. Selective symptoms
   e. Conversion disorder is rare; but diagnosis may be rare, symptoms may go unnoticed

H. Groups at Risk for Somatoform Disorders
1. Prevalence for body dysmorphic disorder is not clear
   a. Unmarried, average age of onset is 16
   b. Equally common in males and females
2. Somatization disorder more common in females and is common (2.8%); cultural differences with regard to complaints
3. Conversion disorder's prevalence questioned; 5 to 14% in general medical setting involved symptoms
   a. Twice as common in females
   b. SES status is factor
4. History of childhood trauma increases vulnerability

V. Somatoform Disorders: Theory and Therapy
A. The Psychodynamic Perspective: Defense Against Anxiety
1. Somatizing as Conflict Resolution
   a. Strong emotions not expressed would led to somatic symptoms
   b. Hostility and anxiety play role

   c. Disorders seen as defense against anxiety produced by unacceptable wishes

   d. Conflict-resolution theories have been proposed

  2. Uncovering Conflict

   a. Patient is induced to release repression of material

   b. Somatic symptoms will subside

   c. No evidence that psychodynamic treatment is any more effective than other therapies

   d. Supportive therapy, brief physical exams may be best approach

B. The Behavioral and Sociocultural Perspectives: The Sick Role

  1. Somatoform disorders are inappropriate adoptions of sick role

  2. Learning to Adopt the Sick Role

   a. Rewards of sick role more reinforcing than rewards of illness-free life

    i. Person must have experience with sick role directly or indirectly

    ii. Adoption of sick role must be reinforced

   b. Respondent conditioning of ANS may play role as anxiety riggers symptoms causing further anxiety

   c. Sociocultural theories focus on large cultural factors in adoption of sick role such as culture's attitudes toward unexplained somatic symptoms

  3. Treatment by Nonreinforcement

   a. Therapist withdrawals reinforcement for illness behavior

   b. Therapist tries to build up patient's coping skills involving social-skills training

   c. Therapist often tries to provide face-saving mechanism so that patient can give up illness

   d. Other techniques involve relaxation and contingency management

C. The Cognitive Perspective: Misinterpreting Bodily Sensations

  1. Overattention to the Body

   a. Cognitive style predisposes person to exaggerate normal bodily sensations and catastrophize minor symptoms

   b. Corresponding high rates of negative affect have been found in somatizers

  2. Treatment: Challenging Faulty Beliefs

   a. Cognitive therapy and behavior therapy may be effective for hypochondriasis and pain disorder

   b. Cognitive therapy focuses on patient testing explanations and confronting beliefs

D. The Biological Perspective: Brain Dysfunction

  1. Genetic Studies

        a.   Somatoform patients tend to have family histories of somatic complaints

        b.   Genetic family patterns have been reported; twins studies and adoption studies give preliminary support to genetic factor

2.   Brain Dysfunction and Somatoform Disorders

        a.   Possible problem lies in processing of sensory signals in cerebral cortex; appears suppressed

        b.   May be dysfunction in right cerebral hemisphere due to lateralization

        c.   Abnormality in serotonin functioning has been proposed

3.   Drug Treatment

        a.   Biological treatments are scarce

        b.   Antidepressant drugs seem to help some patients

Chapter Boxes

- Who Committed the Crime? Dissociative Identity Disorder and the Law
  - A. DID patient arrested for rape and was found not guilty by reason of insanity
  - B. DID arouses skepticism
  - C. Raises questions about responsibility of committing crime
  - D. If personality knew right from wrong at time of crime, DID patient is held responsible

- Recovered Memory of Childhood Abuse: A Modern Dilemma
  - A. Recovered memories are memories of childhood abuse that eventually return to consciousness
  - B. Recovered memories generates huge public interest
  - C. People can forget true episodes of abuse
  - D. Information stored in frontal cortex more susceptible to influence from media and therapists

Learning Objectives (LO)

By the time you have finished studying this chapter, you should be able to do the following:

1.   Compare and contrast dissociative and somatoform disorders, describing their similarities and differences (178).

2.   Define dissociative amnesia and describe five patterns of this disorder mentioned in the text (179-181).

3.   Define dissociative fugue and differentiate from dissociative amnesia (181-182).

4.   Define dissociative identity disorder and describe ways in which personalities can manifest themselves (182-184).

5.   Describe the problems with diagnosing dissociative identity disorder, and in determining the validity of cases of recovered childhood memories (184-187).

6.   Define depersonalization disorder and describe the symptoms that accompany it (185-188).

7.   Describe the characteristics of body dysmorphic disorder (194-195).

8   Describe the characteristics of hypochondriasis (195-196).

9.   Define somatization disorder and pain disorder and distinguish them from hypochondriasis (196-197).

10.   Define conversion disorder and list the characteristics that distinguish it from a biologically based disability (197-199).

11.   Describe how the psychodynamic perspective would explain and treat each of the disorders in this chapter (189-190, 200-201),

12.   Describe how the behavioral and sociocultural perspectives would account for and treat the disorders in this chapter (190-192, 201-202).

13.   Describe how the cognitive perspective would explain and treat each of the disorders in this chapter (192-193, 202-203).

14.   Describe biological research on, and treatment of, the disorders in this chapter (193-194, 203-204)

Lecture Leads (LL)

Debating dissociative identity disorders (LL 7-1)
Hochman and Harrison reviewed all articles appearing in several journals published in
the United States, Canada, Australia, New Zealand, and Europe between 1976 and 1995
on the subject of dissociation identity disorder. The focus of their analysis was to
determine how English-speaking clinicians around the word view the validity of DID.
The authors reported that psychiatrists in the United States have a much more positive
view on the validity of the disorder than their counterparts elsewhere.

Resources:
Hochman, J., & Harrison, G. Jr. (1997). Debating dissociative diagnoses. <u>American
Journal of Psychiatry</u>, <u>154</u>, 887-888.

Recovered memory of child abuse (LL 7-2)
Expand on the textbook's treatment of recovered memory of child abuse. As a starting
point, use the box on pages 184 and 185. For a review, see Martinez-Taboas (1996).

Resources:
Loftus, E. F. (1997). Creating false memories. <u>Scientific American,</u> 70-75.

Loftus, E. F., & Ketcham, K. (1994). <u>The myth of repressed memory</u>. New York: St.
Martin's Press.

Martinez-Taboas, A. (1996). Repressed memories: Some clinical data contributing
toward its elucidation. <u>American Journal of Psychotherapy</u>, <u>50</u>, 217-230.

More information on dissociative identity disorder (LL 7-3)
Because dissociative identity disorder has received so much attention in the popular
media, it may be surprising to learn that it is extremely rare. Fewer than 100 cases of
DID have been documented. Nevertheless, it fascinates students of psychology and the
general public alike. The average number of personalities is around five; the range
extends from two to twenty. As the textbook presents, often individuals with multiple
personalities have a history of having been sexually abused or tortured as children. The
famous multiple personality, Sybil--whose life was the subject of a popular movie--was
sexually abused by her schizophrenic mother (Schreiber, 1973). A multiple personality
named Debra was forced to engage in sexual relations with her father for a three-year
period beginning when she was about six years old (Bowman et al., 1985). Apparently,
multiple personality is one way for a person to cope with repeated abuse. One theory of
the etiology of multiple personality links its development to the capacity of young
children to actively fantasize and easily switch roles (Bowman et al., 1985). Although
originating as a childhood protective device, the role playing and fantasizing become part
of the adult personality and manifest themselves through the various secondary
personalities these individuals display. A fascinating recent focus of multiple personality
research is its use as a way of investigating the impact of psychological factors (mind) on

physiological ones (body). Goleman (1988) reports the rather amazing findings of different physiological patterns between the multiple personalities. One individual who had a low blood pressure of 90/60 when in one personality had higher blood pressure (150/110) in another. Other research has found differences in vision between personalities within the same person. Perhaps most bizarre is Goleman's (1988) description of a multiple personality named Timmy: "When Timmy drinks orange juice he has no problem. But Timmy is just one of close to a dozen personalities who alternate control over a patient with multiple personality disorder. And if those other personalities drink orange juice, the result is a case of hives. The hives will occur even if Timmy drinks orange juice and another personality appears while the juice is still being digested. What's more, if Timmy comes back while the allergic reaction is present, the itching of the hives will cease immediately, and the water-filled blisters will begin to subside." With the current interest among psychologists in the physiological impact of psychological variables such as personality and stressful life events, these results with multiple personalities suggest that psychological factors can indeed have a strong impact on physiological functioning.

Resources:

Boon, S., & Draijer, N. (1993). Multiple personality disorder in The Netherlands: A clinical investigation of 71 patients. American Journal of Psychiatry, 150, 489-494.

Bowman , E. S., Blix, S., & Cooper, P. M. (1985). Multiple personality in adolescents: Relationship to incestual experiences. Journal of Child Psychiatry, 24, 109-114.

Carpenter, A., MacLeod, J. C. (1995). Dissociative identity disorder an self-injury: A review of the literature and case history. Issues in Criminological & Legal Psychology, 22, 84-89.

Goleman, D. (June 28, 1988). Probing the enigma of multiple personality. The New York Times, C1, C13.

Schreiber, F. F. (1973). Sybil. Chicago: Regnery.

Case studies of dissociative and somatoform disorders (LL 7-4)
You may wish to augment those case descriptions of the dissociative and somatoform disorders presented in the textbook. This is an effective way to introduce the chapter. The literature is replete with varied, engaging, and fascinating cases. Rosik (1997) presents the case of a 68-year-old Hispanic female who was diagnosed with geriatric dissociative identity disorder. Apparently, her health care providers had misdiagnosed her dissociative symptoms for 3 decades. Rosik also discusses how ethnicity may affect the diagnosis of DID. The case of an individual with DID is described by Bryant. The patient, HS, was assessed regarding differences in autobiographical memories recalled by various alters. A 23-year-old male, described by Phillips, O'Sullivan, and Pope, presented with the chief complaint of a preoccupation with working out. The authors suggested

that this represented a form of body dysmorphic disorder characterized by compulsive weightlifting. The subject reported excessive concern that his body was too small and he lacked adequate muscularity. The subject's excessive concern forced him to miss social events, lose most of his friends, and dropped out of college. After using clomipramine, his obsessions regarding his appearance moderately decreased. In a case of conversion disorder, a 21 year-old female married against her family's wishes. After several years of marriage, the young wife experienced intermittent blindness, muteness, deafness, and "aimless wandering." A 12-year-old female complained of globus hystericus, which is a form of conversion disorder where the individual perceives a lump in their throat. She would refuse to sallow solid foods for fear that she would choke. She was successfully treated using behavior therapy focusing on weight gain.

Resources:

Bryant, R. A. (1995). Autobiographical memory across personalities in dissociative identity disorder: A case report. Journal of Abnormal Psychology, 104, 625-631.

Donohue, B., Thevenin, D. M., Runyon, M. K. (1997). Behavioral treatment of conversion disorder in adolescence: A case of globus hystericus. Behavior Modication, 21, 231-251.

Mazumdar, P. K., Najib, M. A., Varma, S. L. (1996). Hysteria revisited. European Psychiatry, 11, 106.

Phillips, K. A., O'Sullivan, R. L., & Pope, H. G., Jr. (1997). Muscle dysmorphia. Journal of Clinical Psychiatry, 58, 361.

Rosik, C. H. (1997). Geriatric dissociative identity disorder. Clinical Gerontologist, 17, 63-66

Simeon, D., Gross, S., & Guralnik, O., & Stein, D. (1997). Feeling unreal: 30 cases of DSM-III-R depersonalization. American Journal of Psychiatry, 154, 1107-1113.

Gender differences in body dysmorphic disorder (LL 7-5)
Do men and women have different complaints in body dysmorphic disorder? In analysis of 93 women and men with the disorder Phillips and Diaz found several differences. For instance, women were more likely to be excessively concerned with their hips and their weight and be comorbid with anorexia nervosa. Women tended to hide unpleasant facial features with makeup and pick their skin. Body build, genitals, and hair thinning were common complaints among men, who also tend to wear hats to hide their thinning hair. The authors point out that although there are several gender differences, men and women do not differ significantly on clinical features. Perugi et al. found women to be preoccupied with breasts and legs, while men were excessively concerned with height and excessive body hair, with a lifetime comorbidity with bipolar disorder.

Resource:

Perugi, G. et al. (1997). Gender-related differences in body dysmorphic disorder. Journal of Nervous and Mental Disorders, 185, 578-528.

Phillips, K. A., & Diaz, S. (1997). Gender differences in body dysmorphic disorder. Journal of Nervous and Mental Disorders, 185, 570-577.

Understanding origin of pain (LL 7-6)

While the layperson may consider somatoform disorders are as "just being in a person's head," there are important implications for medical and psychological treatment. To the person with a somatoform disorder, the concern or the pain is real, and the sufferer seeks to treat it. In a two-year longitudinal study, Dionne, Koepsell, and Von Korff found psychosocial factors to be the best predictors of chronic back pain. Based on their interviews with 1,213 adult members of an HMO, they found somatization and depression to be two of the four predictors of chronic impairment. Similarly, the American Psychological Association (1997) stated that an NIH-funded study by Robert Gatchel found the following four psychosocial factors to be predictors of pain: reports of high intensity of pain; high scores on Scale 3 of the MMPI; receipt of workers' compensation or involvement in a personal injury suit; and being female. The reinforcement value of receiving monetary compensation is clearly a motivator for not returning to work, although remaining inactive obviously increases pain since there is more time to think about it, fewer distractions from it, and less activity to alleviate it. It is important to determine the underlying reasons for the chronic pain. Persons identified as "adaptive copers" tend to experience less pain and function at a higher level than persons who report high pain, limited activity, and a sense that they lack control over their lives, or persons who feel a lack of social support (APA, 1997). While adaptive copers are likely to improve with biomechanical and educational interventions, the other two groups also need psychological intervention to prevent relapse. A technique developed by Smith, Rost, and Kashner had excellent results in lowering annual medical expenses (including psychiatrists' fees) by 33 percent. This involved providing psychiatric treatment for somatization disorder, a letter from the psychiatrist to the doctor making the following recommendations: Schedule brief appointments and physical examinations every four to six weeks, but only at set times and not on demand; avoid laboratory tests, surgery, and hospitalization unless absolutely necessary; avoid suggesting to the patient that the problem is all in her or his mind. The importance of understanding and assessing somatoform disorders is important not only with respect to the improving patient's psychological wellbeing, but also to ensure the basic medical credo, "First do no harm.' If the problem is psychogenic, treating it as a physical illness, even to the extent of performing unnecessary and possibly dangerous surgery (as surgery is always), does nothing to help the patient but inevitably creates potential for greater harm.

Resources:

American Psychological Association. (1997). Mind & body. Psychosocial factors
    provide clues to pain. Available: WWW URL
    http://helping.apa.org/psychosocial.html.

Dionne, C. E., Koepsell, T. D., & Von Korff, M. (1997). Predicting long-term functional
    limitations among back pain patients in primary care settings. Journal of Clinical
    Epidemiology, 50, 31-43.

Smith, G. R., Rost, K., &, Kashner, T. M. (1995). First aid for somatizers. The Harvard
    Mental Health Letter, 1, 6-7.

Pseudoseizure as conversion disorder (LL 7-7)
Conversion disorder represents a difficult diagnostic challenge for clinicians. Of
particular concern is ruling real organic causes. Burack, Back, and Pearlman describe a
fascinating case of the use of deception to diagnosis a case of pseudoseizure.
Pseudoseizure, or nonepileptic serizure, is regarded as a conversion disorder. RB had
seizures several times a day, but did not have many of the classic signs of an epileptic
seizure. Thorough medical and neurological evaluation revealed nothing abnormal.
While in the hospital, one of his seizures was observed; his physicians believed that his
seizures were nonepileptic in nature. To test this hypothesis, saline was administered
intravenously, but was described to RB as a drug that may trigger a seizure. RB had a
seizure that lasted 2 minutes, but the EEG revealed no abnormality. The authors discuss
the ethics involved in using a placebo diagnostic tool.

Resources:

Burack, J. H., Back, A. L., Pearlman, R. A. (1997). Provoking nonepileptic serizures:
    The ethics of deceptive diagnostic testing. The Hastings Center Report, 27, 24-
    33.

Harden, C. L. (1997). Pseudoseizures and dissociative disorders: A common
    mechanism involving traumatic experiences. Seizure, 6, 151-155.

Talking Points (TP)

Dissociative versus associative (TP 7-1)
As you introduce dissociative disorders, start by asking students to define associative or to associate. Then move to the dissociative. Those psychological functions that are affected in the dissociative disorders go to the very essence of being an individual, such as consciousness, memory, and identity.

Dissociative disorders on soap operas (TP 7-2)
Lead a discussion about why soap opera characters are so prone to dissociative disorders. Ask the students for specific examples of the stars' unfortunate afflictions. Have the students give detailed descriptions of the behaviors, including the inevitable recovery. Discuss if these depictions are accurate. If they are not, what could be changed to make them fit the criteria for dissociative disorders?

Amnesia and fugue (TP 7-3)
The media have reported the return of a person who has been missing for months or even years. Many times these individuals state that they had completely forgotten their former lives until their memories were suddenly triggered. Discuss the possibility of this occurrence in terms of dissociative amnesia and dissociative fugue.

Dissociative identity disorder (TP 7-4)
A fascinating topic to the students is Dissociative Identity Disorder (DID) (formerly Multiple Personality Disorder). The media and the film industry have highlighted this disorder. There are several good clips of this disorder available in the films and video section at the end of this chapter. As an introduction to your lecture show one or more of these brief clips or rent *Sybil* or *The Three Faces of Eve*. One effective way to convey the essence of DID is to point to a student describing that this student has one body. Next point to several students saying, "These individuals with their personalities, memories, skills, mannerism, and attitudes are in this one body" as you point back to the one student.

Sybil (TP 7-5)
Many students will be familiar with the movie *Sybil*. They may not be aware that Sybil was in treatment for over eleven years and still suffered some symptoms long after her treatment ended. The psychodynamic approach has been the most widely used therapy for this disorder. Discuss the implications of having this perspective as the method of understanding this disorder. Have the students discuss other possible explanations of these symptoms in terms of the other major perspectives.

Role of childhood abuse in DID (TP 7-6)
Have the students debate whether they believe an event like childhood abuse can be so traumatic that the child must create another "person" to protect her/him or take the punishment for her/him. Drawing on evidence in the text and from other sources, select

158

students to debate both sides. Then have the class discuss what seems most believable for them. How would they determine whether someone really does have many different alters? How would a therapist "plant" alters in a client's mind? How would this not be likely? What purpose do the alters serve? What purpose would it serve someone to claim that she/he does/does not have dissociative identity disorder?

Prevalence of DID (TP 7-7)
Students often overestimate the actual prevalence of Dissociative Identity Disorder (DID). Discuss what appears to be the increasing prevalence of this diagnosis in terms of secondary gain for both the patient and the treatment provider. Also discuss the possibility of malingering or comorbidity with other personality disorders.

Integrate alters? (TP 7-8)
While many therapists in the past have believed it is best to integrate all of the alters into one primary personality, this is not necessarily the case today. Some therapists (and their clients) choose instead to maintain separate identities for the personalities but have them communicating with each other. Truddi Chase (see her autobiography, *When Rabbit Howls,* or interviews with Oprah Winfrey), for example, has stated that the original Truddi died when her stepfather threw her into a well and then dropped snakes on top of her; a therapist has described a client who chose to retain her three personalities of student/bookkeeper/ homemaker because each came out as appropriate and maximized time and enjoyment for the client. What would the students choose to do if they were the client and/or the therapist?

Somatoform disorders (TP 7-9)
Just a reminder to use the case histories presented in the textbook as you are introducing the disorders. They can be very effective in illustrating the symptoms and the disruptive nature of psychological disorders.

A bad hair day (TP 7-10)
Does having a bad hair day constitute body dysmorphic disorder? What would it "take" for some to be diagnosed with the disorder focused on hair?

Hypochondriasis (TP 7-11)
Many students confuse hypochondriasis with malingering. Outline the differences between the two on an overhead and ask for student input. Ask students for specific examples from different cultures that might help emphasize cultural differences in both hypochondriasis and malingering. Emphasize the real fear the hypochondriac has of illness and the diligence he or she exhibits in seeking treatment.

amnesia in the case of **Jane Doe**...	p. 178
brief **spells** of memory loss or identity confusion...	p. 179
may be caused by a **blow to the head**	p. 179
all events...are **blocked out.**	p. 179
the man might recall the **fire engines** coming...	p. 180
may wander about **aimlessly**...	p. 181
Three Faces of Eve...Sybil...	p. 182
"nice" personality and..."**naughty**" personality.	p. 183
trauma syndromes in general--that grew out of the **Vietnam War.**	p. 185
These findings, however, do not **rule out** iatrogenesis.	p. 185
the are functioning like **robots** or living in a dream.	p. 185
depersonalization often occurs after "**near-death experiences**"...	p. 188
a young girl who has an **imaginary companion**...	p. 189
Many of these patients [have] rich **fantasy lives.**	p. 192
Sirhan Sirhan, the man convicted of killing **Robert F. Kennedy.**	p. 192
to say which of a list of cities "**rings a bell**"...	p. 193
they may **drop out of school**, quit their jobs, avoid dating, and become **house-bound.**	p. 195
somatization patients tend to engage in "**doctor shopping**"...	p. 196
he or she hopes to received attention, "**babying**":...	p. 200
People who are ill are justified in adopting the "**sick role.**"	p. 201
teach people how to manage social **give-and-take** without such **blackmail**.	p. 202

160

Activities and Demonstrations (ACT/DEMO)

What's the matter with me? (ACT/DEMO 7-1)
Objective: To engage students in asking relevant questions about dissociative disorders
Materials: A 3 x 5 index card for each student; masking tape
Procedure: Hand out one card per student. Ask them to write on the card one of the dissociative disorders. Collect the cards and then randomly distribute the cards, again one to each student. Ask the students keep the cards face down. Next, students should help each other by taping the index card on their foreheads with the disorder label face up. Students are now to walk around the classroom asking questions of others attempting to determine what disorder is taped to their head. Obviously, students cannot directly ask what disorder they have.
Discussion: Based on the answers they receive from their questions, they should be able to identify which disorder has been assigned to them.

Guest speakers (ACT/DEMO 7-2)
Objective: To illustrate the differences between the perspectives
Materials: None
Procedure: Invite speakers who specializing in any of the disorders to your class to discuss how diagnosis and treatment play out in professional practice. Specifically, invite a psychiatrist and a psychoanalyst with experience to class. Of particular interest to students will be DID. Make sure they have done their homework on recovered memories. Make sure you schedule this presentation early, since many mental health professionals are very busy.
Discussion: Beforehand, instruct students to review this chapter and be prepared to ask questions of their guest speakers. Afterwards, ask students to compare and contrast the speakers' presentations and textbook material.

Role playing somatoform disorders (ACT/DEMO 7-3)
Objective: To demonstrate the types of behaviors associated with somatoform disorders
Materials: None
Procedure: Have the students individually or in small groups select one of the disorders from the packets. Give students or group the packet and have them develop a role play for the specific disorder. Tell the students that they have at least overnight to prepare for their disorder and that they will be expected to role play the disorder in front of the class. If using groups, one person plays the role of the subject, and other group members can play family members, employers, friends, and clinician.
Discussion: Give feedback on the accuracy of the role play. Ask the students how they developed their role and who they used as a model. Was there any influence from the media? If so, what specific individuals did they use as models? You could show a video at this point that will reinforce the correct behaviors and change the incorrect ones.

Somatoform and Dissociative disorders and the popular press (ACT/DEMO 7-4)
Objective: To demonstrate the use and misuse of the criteria for diagnosing of somatoform and dissociative disorders
Materials: Magazines and tabloid newspapers from your local checkout line (e.g. National Inquirer; Sun).
Procedure: The day before you do this activity, ask students to bring to class tabloid newspapers and articles dealing with dissociative disorders. Place students in groups; each group should have three to four articles. Have them evaluate these articles in terms of the criteria used in developing the stories on somatoform and dissociative disorders. Ask the students how the authors have interpreted or misinterpreted the data from the DSM series. the students should decide on what the correct symptoms should be for each article. A spokesperson from each group should discuss their findings.
Discussion: Project a copy of the article on the overhead and ask the spokesperson from the group to describe the article. Summarize the findings on the article and correct any incorrect notions. Why is this research so easily misinterpreted? What effect does these misinterpretations have on the general public?

Films and Videos

48 Hours. CBS. The CBS news magazine aired a segment on MPD that looked at the disorder and various forms of treatment, including some that are somewhat controversial.

Body Dysmorphic Disorder. Films for the Humanities & Sciences looks at this disorder that leads people to become obsessed with drastically changing their appearance. The film includes interviews with two women who have battled the disorder, as well as with an expert who attempts to explain what causes the disorder.

Case Study of Multiple Personality. PSU, Audio-Visual Services. Consists of original footage of the interviews with the original "Eve" (Chris Sizemore) and her psychiatrists, Drs. Cleckley and Thigpen. It is fascinating for students to watch the real person. Although her personalities were ultimately integrated, subsequent to this first story, Ms. Sizemore split several more times beyond the initial three personalities of Eve White, Eve Black, and Jane.

Hypochondriasis and Health Care: A Tug of War. PSU. Simulated interviews with hypochondriacs and lectures on ways of dealing with them.

Multiple Personality. PSU. A patient interviewed has exhibited 53 personalities, several of which suggest different brain patterns during their respective appearances.

The Brain Teaching Modules, Module No. 23, Multiple Personality Disorder. PBS. Provides some physiological evidence to support the reality of this disorder, despite current controversy that it may be iatrogenically induced.

Using Movies and Mental Illness as a Teaching Tool

There are dramatic and compelling scenes in *Agnes of God* that can be used to start a classroom discussion of the way the mind influences the body, and it may be useful to have some students conduct out-of-class research to document that stigmata are a bona fide and well documented phenomenon.

Additional selected scenes from *Mask, The Elephant Man* or *My Left Foot* will help you focus a class discussion of body image and its relationship to body dysmorphia disorder. Your students will also enjoy compiling a list of film vignettes supporting a diagnosis of hypochondriasis for Woody Allen's film persona.

There are several scenes in *Primal Fear* that illustrate rapid changes in personality and behavior associated with dissociative disorders. Of course, by the end of the film we realize that the lead character does *not* have a dissociative disorder but is only malingering. The film can be used as a springboard for class discussion about the prevalence of dissociative disorders and the likelihood that a patient faking a dissociative disorder could actually delude a therapist or an attorney.

It may be helpful to go over the mental status examination for Norman Bates (*Psycho*) in class, raising the question of whether or not the character would actually present in the manner Wedding and Boyd suggest. (A general discussion of the accuracy of the fictitious interview can be used as a pedagogical tool with almost every chapter in *Movies and Mental Illness*.)

Movie	Link to Chapter	Page Reference to Wedding and Boyd
• The Great Dictator • Overboard • Mirage • Spellbound	dissociative amnesia (p.179)	p. 25 p. 26 p. 28 p. 35
• Identity Unknown • Paris, Texas	dissociative fugue (p. 181)	p. 29 p. 35
• Psycho • Voices Within: The Lives of Truddi Chase • Three Faces of Eve • Sybil • Dr. Jekyll and Mr. Hyde	dissociative identity disorder (p. 182)	p. 21 p. 28 p. 30 p. 31 p. 32
• Altered States	depersonalization (p.185)	p. 35
• Cyrano de Bergerac • Roxanne	body dysmorphic disorder (p.194)	p. 41 p. 41
• Hannah and Her Sisters	hypochondriasis (p. 195)	p.36
• Freud • Sorry, Wrong Number • Persona	conversion disorder (p. 197)	p. 38 p. 40 p. 40

Classroom Assessment Techniques (CAT)

One-Sentence Summary (CAT 7-1)
Ask student to summarize a specific piece of information in this chapter by responding to the question, "Who does/did what to whom, when, where, how and why?" Ask students to write a one-sentence summary for the various treatment approaches.

Focused Listing (CAT 7-2)
Select an important point from this chapter and ask students to write five words or phrases that describe the point.

Definition Matrix (CAT 7-3)
Using the handout, students should identify each perspective definition of abnormality presented in the textbook. For each perspective, students should provide a definition, an example, and advantages and disadvantages of the criterion. Students should attempt to write only a few words or phrases.

Suggestions for Essay Questions

- What concerns have been raised regarding the diagnosis of Dissociative Identity Disorder?
- Contrast and compare hypochondriasis, somatization disorder, and body dysmorphic disorder.
- Create a fictitious case study of a person with conversion disorder. Include demographic information in your case. What symptoms characterize conversion disorder?

Definition Matrix
Classroom Assessment Technique

Perspective	Definition	Example	Treatment Options
Psychodynamic			
Behavioral/ Sociocultural			
Cognitive			
Biological			

Chapter 8

Psychological Stress and Physical Disorders

Chapter Map

Section	Instructor Manual Components
Mind and Body Psychological States • Defining Stress • What Determines Responses to Stress	*Careers in health psychology (LL 8-1)* *Therapy for Type A's (LL 8-2)* *Good stress, bad stress (TP 8-1)* *Rethinking stress (TP 8-2)* *Type A's (TP 8-3)* *Community resources (ACT/DEMO 8-1)*
How Stress Influences Illness • Changes in Physiological Functioning • Changes in High-Risk Behavior	*Immune functioning in young adults (LL 8-3)* *Final exams and colds (TP 8-4)* *Uplifts and hassles (ACT/DEMO 8-2)* *Stress and minor illness (ACT/DEMO 8-3)*
Psychological Factors and Physical Disorders • Coronary Heart Disease • Hypertension • Cancer • AIDS • Headache • Obesity • Sleep Disorders	*Types of migraine headaches (LL 8-4)* *Increasing the risk of CHD in women (LL 8-5)* *Attitude and long-term survival with AIDS (LL 8-6)* *Effects of menstrual cycle in migraine headaches (LL 8-7)*

Groups at Risk	Individual responses specificity (TP 8-5)
• Gender • Race • Socioeconomic Status	
Stress and Illness: Theory and Treatment • The Behavioral Perspective • The Cognitive Perspective • The Psychodynamic Perspective • The Family Systems Perspective • The Sociocultural Perspective • The Biological Perspective	Stress reduction (TP 8-6) Coping with stress and faith (TP 8-7) Cognitive appraisal and exams (TP 8-8) Changing thoughts (TP 8-9) Demonstrating biofeedback (ACT/DEMO 8-4) Guest speakers (ACT/DEMO 8-5)

Chapter Outline

I. Introduction
    A.   **Psychophysiological disorders** are illnesses influenced by emotional factors
        1.   Widely diverse medical conditions are affects, if not caused by psychological factors
        2.   DSM-IV has comprehensive category that may be applied to any illness
        3.   Researchers recognize that physically-caused illness can cause stress, which affects course of illness
    B.   **Health psychology** reflects holistic concept of body and mind

II. Mind and Body
    A.   **Mind-body problem** refers to question of relationship between mind and body
    B.   Historically, mind and body were seen as separate, as in dualism
        1.   Plato originated idea
        2.   Laid foundation of modern science rationalism; nature explained through empirical evidence
        3.   Organic causation was the rule in explaining illness
        4.   Once thought involuntary physiological functions could be influenced voluntarily
        5.   Mind and body are one; psychological and physical refer to different ways of talking about same phenomenon
    C.   Psychological Stress
        1.   Defining Stress
            a.   **Stress** can be defined as a stimulus: stress consists of environmental demands that lead to physical responses
           b.   Stress can be defined as response; general adaptation syndrome with three stages
           c.   Stress can be defined as interaction between stimulus and person's appraisal of it
        2.   What Determines Responses to Stress?
           a.   Stimulus Specificity
               i.   **Stimulus specificity** refers to different kinds of stress that produce different kinds of physiological responses
              ii.   Subtle distinctions can be made; reactions differ if we are expecting a stressful event or are undergoing the event
              iii.   Reactions are very complex since different stressors produce different patterns of responses

        b.   Individual Response Specificity
            i.   People have characteristic patterns of physiological response called **individual response specificity**
            ii.   Some people respond to stress more intensely
        c.   Stimulus Versus Individual
            i.   Person and stressor operate simultaneously
            ii.   Degree of increase and decrease subject to individual response specificity

D.   How Stress Influences Illness
    1.   Connection exists between stress and illness
    2.   Changes in Physiological Functioning
        a.   Stress and the Autonomic Nervous System
            i.   ANS controls smooth muscles, glands, and internal organs
            ii.   Sympathetic division mobilizes body; parasympathetic division returns body to resting state
            iii.   ANS contributes to fight-or-flight response
        b.   Changes in the Immune System
            i.   **Immune system** is body's system of defense against infectious disease and cancer
            ii.   **Psychneuroimmunology** is the study of the immune system's link between stress and illness
            iii.   Studying subjects following naturalistic major events, minor events, and laboratory stressors suggests decreases in cellular immunity and reduced immune functioning
        c.   Feedback Loops
            i.   Body systems provide **feedback** or information about relating the system
            ii.   **Negative feedback** is important in theories of stress and illness
            iii.   Disregulation model argues that stress-related illness occurs when there is disruption in negative feedback
            iv.   Oscillations are rhythmic back and forth cycle of body systems
            v.   Stress may disrupt rhythms affecting other systems
    3.   Changes in High-Risk Behavior
        a.   Stress may cause people to adopt behavior that puts them at risk of illness
        b.   Stress can interfere with preventive measure against disease
        c.   Stress may encourage its victims to report illness

III. Psychological Factors and Physical Disorders
    A. Coronary Heart Disease
        1. **Coronary heart disease** caused by atherosclerosis and is manifested as heart attack or sudden cardiac death
        2. A number of risk factors have been identified
        3. Link exists between social environment/status and atherosclerosis
        4. Relationship between social and occupational stress and development and progression of coronary heart disease
        5. Cardiovascular reactivity thought to contribute to development and expression of coronary heart disease
        6. Research suggests relationship between some qualities (e.g., hostility, anger) seen in **Type A** people and heart disease
    B. Hypertension
        1. Chronically high blood pressure is known as **hypertension**
        2. Hypertension increases risk for other cardiovascular disorders
        3. The regulatory mechanism involving feedback breaks down and blood vessels remain chronically constricted
        4. **Essential hypertension** occurs where there is no known organic cause
            a. Hypertensives may live in environments where stimuli that increase blood pressure are common
            b. Individual response specificity may play role in essential hypertension
        5. Many people with hypertension are unaware of the condition
    C. Cancer
        1. Cancer is associated with psychological stress
        2. Social support and group therapy help patients with breast cancer and malignant melanoma
        3. Active coping may be an benefit of group therapy
    D. AIDS
        1. Acquired immune deficiency syndrome (AIDS) is caused by the **human immunodeficiency virus (HIV)**
        2. Virus, found in several bodily fluids, attacks the immune system, leaving the person open to various infections (e.g., Kaposi's sarcoma)
        3. The relationship between stress and the course of AIDS is unclear
        4. Avoidance behavior has been seen as a benefit of psychological treatment
    E. Headache
        1. **Migraine headaches** and **muscle-contraction headaches** are related to stress, but differ from each other in several ways
        2. Theories of migraine have shifted away from psychological to organic causes
            a. Involves dysfunction in operation of serotonin

b.   Precise nature of serotonin dysfunction is not known

c.   Genetic, hormonal factors may play role

d.   Stress can trigger migraine headache

F.   Obesity

    1.   Eating behavior can be affected by disruption in the normal regulatory cycle

    2.   Anorexia nervosa is extreme malnourishment

    3.   **Obesity**, as a socially defined condition, refers to an excessive amount of fat on the body

    4.   Physical and social consequences of obesity

    5.   Genetic differences and behavioral differences contribute to obesity

    6.   Obesity also due to interaction of physiological and psychological factors such as more responsiveness to taste of food and problem of feedback from stomach to brain

    7.   Weight loss programs shifting emphasis from dieting to exercise

    8.   Most effective program focus on several components

    9.   Some have argued for a more broad definition of physical attractiveness

G.   Sleep Disorders

    1.   Insomnia

        a.   **Insomnia** is the chronic inability to sleep

        b.   There are three broad patterns of insomnia--problems with falling asleep, awakening repeatedly during night, waking up too early

        c.   Concern for sleep disturbance leads to anticipatory anxiety

        d.   Many factors are related to insomnia such as drugs, alcohol, and stress

        e.   The definition of sleep affects whether insomniacs are actually sleeping

        f.   Hypnotics are used, which cause several problems

            i.   Altering architecture of sleep leading to REM rebound

            ii.   Withdrawal from drug leads to insomnia

        g.   An illegal market for benzodiazepines has emerged

        h.   A new hypnotic may be promising, but with fewer side effects

        i.   Most hypnotics are not effective over the long-term

    2.   Circadian Rhythm Disorders

        a.   **Circadian rhythm disorders** occur when people try to sleep at times that are inconsistent with their circadian rhythms

        b.   Common among shift workers, but not limited to them

c.   Target bedtime and light therapy appear to be effective treatments

IV.   Groups at Risk
    A.   Gender
        1.   Risk for coronary heart disease is higher among men
            a.   May be due to reproductive hormones
            b.   May be due to men more likely to engage in potentially heath-damaging behaviors
        2.   Others suggest gender differences in experience of stressors
    B.   Race
        1.   African-Americans have higher rates for hypertension, and morbidity and mortality rates for several disorders
        2.   Data on racial differences in cardiovascular disorders is unclear
        3.   Socioeconomic status and race are related
    C.   Socioeconomic Status
        1.   Socioeconomic status is a factor in determining health
        2.   Association may be function of greater emotional impact of stressful life events
        3.   Socioeconomic status affects development and progression of coronary heart disease
        4.   Work environment where there is low control over decisions and low skills requirements may be important
        5.   A relationship may exist between survival and recovery and socioeconomic status

V.   Stress and Illness: Theory and Therapy
    A.   The Behavioral Perspective
        1.   Respondent Versus Operant
            a.   Respondent conditioning can have powerful effect on physiological responses
            b.   Physiological responses (e.g., blood pressure, urine formation) can be modified by operant conditioning
                i.   Learning could operate in development of physical disorders
                ii.   Learning can be used to relieve the disorder
        2.   Biofeedback, Relaxation, and Exercise
            a.   Biofeedback training can give patients ability to control physiological functions
            b.   Patients given immediate feedback in **biofeedback training**
            c.   **Relaxation training** used extensively in stress-relief programs; uses progressive relaxation
            d.   Exercise may be effective in reducing stress

B.   The Cognitive Perspective
    1.   Predictability and Control
        a.   Predictable stimuli are less stressful than unpredictable stimuli
        b.   Control helps to reduce stress
        c.   Coping can solve problems that create stress; it can also affect our physiological response to stress
        d.   Coping is connected to cognitive processes and is determined by cognitive styles
        e.   Lazarus' model sees stress as dynamic reciprocal, interactive relationship involving six basic factors
            i.   Environmental event
            ii.   Primary appraisal of event
            iii.   Secondary appraisal
            iv.   Coping
            v.   Outcomes of coping
            vi.   Health outcomes
    2.   Stress Management Intervention
        a.   Goal of stress management programs is to pinpoint the sources of stress and to build up skills to cope with stressors
        b.   People taught muscle relaxation
        c.   Programs developed for Type As, cardiac rehabilitation programs
        d.   Cognitive-behavioral stress management programs developed and includes relaxation training, cognitive restructuring, assertiveness training, and health education
C.   The Psychodynamic Perspective
    1.   Psychological Inhibition
        a.   Refers to stress-related physical disorders as organ neuroses
        b.   Disorders caused by repression, anxiety, and defense
        c.   Family interactions central to stress-related physical disorders
        d.   Inhibition of expression of emotion, behavioral, and social impulses contributes to development of "psychosomatic" disorders
    2.   The Value of Catharsis
        a.   Research confirms value of emotional catharsis to physical health
        b.   Journaling may have effect on immune system by allowing expression of negative emotion
D.   The Family Systems Perspective

1. Major source of physical illness is the stress imposed by modern industrial society
2. No regular social support prevents protection against illness
3. Strong evidence to show that people without social support are more prone to disease
4. Marital status is a risk factor for physical illness

E. The Sociocultural Perspective
   1. Changes in society affect susceptibility of certain groups to particular illnesses
   2. Gender and race are important risk factors

F. The Biological Perspective
   1. Genetic Predisposition
      a. Stress-related physical disorders tend to run in families
      b. Early identification of those at risk is important
   2. PNI and Interactive Theories
      a. Different perspectives represent differences of focus
      b. Stress and illness are interactive

Chapter Boxes

- Minor Stress and Illnesses
    - A.   Daily hassles of life may be more stressful than major unpleasant events
    - B.   Stress affects body's defenses against herpes viruses
    - C.   Stress affects one's of being infected with herpes in the first place

Learning Objectives (LO)

By the time you have finished studying this chapter, you should be able to do the following:

1. Define the relationship between psychology and health and summarize your text's position on the mind-body problem (208-210).

2. Define stress, and explain how stimulus specificity and individual response specificity interact to determine a person's reaction to stress (210-211).

3. Summarize the impact of stress on body regulatory processes, behavior, the functioning of the immune system, and the susceptibility to illness (211-216).

4. Describe the relationship between coronary heart disease and stress, making reference to the impact of social status, gender, and personality characteristics (216-218).

5. Describe essential hypertension, and discuss its possible stress-related causes (219-220).

6. Summarize research on psychological factors affecting patients' susceptibility to and survival of diseases like cancer and AIDS (220-222).

7. Define migraine headache and discuss current thinking on the biogenic versus psychogenic nature of this disorder (222-223).

8. Define obesity and discuss the biological and psychological factors assumed to be responsible for the problem (223-224).

9. Describe the physiological and psychological factors associated with sleep disorders such as insomnia and circadian rhythm disorder (224-227).

10. Describe how gender, race, and socioeconomic status relate to the risk for stress-related disorders (227-228).

11. Discuss how behavioral psychologists explain and treat stress-related disorders through the mechanisms of learning (228-230).

12. Summarize the cognitive perspective's view of stress-related disorders (230-231).

13.   Describe the psychodynamic perspective's concept of "organ neurosis" as an explanation for stress-related disorders, and discuss the usefulness of catharsis in treatment (231-232).

14.   Describe the family-systems and sociocultural understandings of stress-related disorders (232).

15.   Summarize biological theories on the stress-related disorders (232-233).

Lecture Leads (LL)

Careers in health psychology (LL 8-1)

Gatchel, Baum, and Krantz point out, "With the growing realization that psychological variables are important in health and illness...a new association between psychology and medicine has develped, as psychologists have begun to participate more actively in the diagnosis, treatment, and prevention of medical problems." Students may be trained in health psychology at the undergraduate and postgraduate levels. Undergraduates may go into medicine, becoming physicians and nurses. The training in health psychology before entering the medical field often gives a person an ability to understand and manage social as well as psychological aspects of problems they treat (Taylor, 1995). For example, a person with a background in health psychology may well realize that self-care plans set up for a chronically ill person will not be successful unless immediate family members are included in the education of the regimen as well. Some students at the undergraduate level move into allied health professional fields: social work, occupational therapy, dietetics, physical therapy, and public health. Many undergraduates interested in health psychology decide to attend graduate school in psychology. There they learn theory, research, teaching, and intervention skills necessary to practice health psychology (Sheridan et al., 1989). In fact, Sayete and Mayne (1990) found that in a survey of clinical psychology programs, behavioral medicine/health psychology was the most common clinical subspecialty for research and training. Upon completion of their graduate degree, some health psychologists become teachers and train people in a variety of health related fields. Other health psychologists decide they want to work with medial patients in a hospital setting and become clinicians (Enright et al., 1990). These individuals set up health programs one-on-one with patients, for use when the patient returns home. More and more health psychologists are working with corporations (some as consultants), advising employers on issues such as which health care system to select, stress reduction for employees, and employee weight-reduction programs.

Resources:

Enright, M. F., Resnick, R., DeLeon, P. H., Sciara, A. D., & Tanney, F. (1990). The practice of psychology in hospital settings. American Psychologist, 45, 1057-1058.

Gatchel, R. J., Baum, A., & Krantz, D. S. (1989). An introduction to health psychology (2d ed.). New York: Random House.

Matarazzo, J. D. (1980). Behavioral health and behavioral medicine: Frontiers for a new health psychology. American Psychologist, 35, 807-817.

Sayete, M. A., & Mayne, T. J. (1990). Survey of current clinical and research trends in clinical psychology. American Psychologist, 15, 1263-1266.

179

Sheridan, E. P., Perry, N. W., Johnson, S. B., Clayman, D., Ulmer, R., Prohaska, T., Peterson, R. A., Gentry, D. W., & Beckman, L. (1989). Research and practice in health psychology. Health Psychology, 8, 777-779.

Taylor, S. E. (1995). Health psychology (3rd ed.). New York: McGraw-Hill.

Therapy for Type A's (LL 8-2)
Executives and professionals no longer have to drive to the psychologist's office. They can be picked up by a "therapy mobile" and driven to work, home, or their next appointment. This new form of therapy was recently reported by Berger (1995) as way to fit therapy sessions into the busiest of schedules. For $175 a uniformed driver will pick you up in a van, outfitted with a burgundy couch, two-bucket seats, a small table, and a therapist. The driver, who is sealed off from the conversations that take place during the sessions, will drive you to your next appointment. Dr. Lennox and Dr. Strauss, who started the business (named Mobile Psychological Services), state that more serious cases are handled in a conventional office. However, cases of substance abuse and phobias can certainly be handled in the van, although they admit that they have yet to treat a case of claustrophobia in the van. The therapists noted that for clients who are Type A personalities, the van therapy may actually feed into their neuroses, gratifying their need to squeeze even more things into their pressured lifestyle. The problem is, as one client pointed out, that their schedule is so packed that it is either this or nothing. Dr. Lennox and Dr. Strauss do hope that van clients see the value of therapy and begin to schedule visits in their conventional office. Will this actually become a part of our future? These psychologists reported that as of January 1995 (in just 10 months) they were up to 50 clients, 6 therapists, 3 drivers, and 4 vans. They are even considering franchising.

Resource:
Berger, J (January 13, 1995). Psychologists come up with idea of chauffeured sessions for patients. The New York Times, B1.

Immune functioning in young adults (LL 8-3)
It has been fairly well established that psychological factors can influence virtually any physical condition. Theorists have hypothesized that repeated exposure to stress in particular decreases immune system functioning, which increases susceptibility to nearly any illness, but research results have been inconsistent. A recent study by Schleifer, Keller, Bartlett, Eckholdt and Delaney examined immunological changes in a group of young adults, all of whom were diagnosed as having unipolar depression (and were unmedicated) as determined by the Structured Clinical Interview for the DSM-III-R. In comparison to a group of matched control subjects with no evidence of depression, the subjects in the depressed group demonstrated changes in immune system functioning; specifically a decrease in what is referred to as "natural killer" cell activity. The researchers point out that these changes are similar to, but not identical to the immune system changes already observed in elderly depressed patients. These finding do indicate that depression can have an effect on immune system function in the young as well.

Resource:
Schleifer, S. J., Keller, S. E., Barlett, J. A., Eckholdt, II. M., & Delaney, B. R. (I 996).
    Immunity in young adults with major depressive disorder. American Journal of
    Psychiatry, 153, 477-482.

Types of migraine headaches (LL 8-4)
Although the basic dynamics of vascular changes are the same, migraine headaches can
be classified into five groups: classic migraine, common migraine, cluster migraine,
hemiplegia or opthalmaplagic migraine, and lower-half migraine (AHCCH, 1962).
Classic migraine, experienced by about 10% of all those who suffer from migraines, is
characterized by an aura or prodromal stage (i.e., preheadache) that is usually indicated
by visual disturbances (e.g., scotomata, fortification spectra) (Adams et al., 1980;
Williamson, 1981). Though the prodromal stage generally lasts about 10 to 30 minutes,
the headache phases may last for 6-8 hours or up to several days. In the headache stage, a
unilateral, throbbing pain, located contralateral to the visual aberrations, is experienced
(Raskin, 1978; Adams et al., 1980). The temporal, orbitial, supraorbital, and occipital
regions of the head are the most frequent sites of pain (Williamson, 1981). Autonomic-
like symptoms (e.g., vomiting, sweating, chills) are common accessories of a classic
migraine (Dalessio, 1980). Occuring in about 85% of all migraine subjects, common
migraines are different from the classic migraine in their lack of a clearly delineated
prodromal stage (Adams et al., 1980). Moreover, the pain is usually more bilateral
(Williamson, 1981) and of longer duration (AHCCH, 1962). Anorexia, nausea, and
vomiting usually supplement the head pain (Dalessio, 1980; Blanchard & Andrasik,
1982). Lacking in a prodromal stage, the cluster migraine head pain tends to be unilateral
and may last 8-12 weeks in regular intervals (Adams et al., 1980). Associated symptoms
include sweating, running nose, and increased tear production (AHCCH, 1962).
Hemiphegia or opthalmaplegia migraine involves a disturbance of the oculomotor cranial
nerve which produces UPJ lateral pain and palsy of the face (Adams et al., 1980).
Lower-half migraine associated pain stems from the lower face (AHCCH, 1962).

Resources:
Ad Hoc Committee on Classification of Headache. (1962). Classification of headache.
    Journal of the American Medical Association, 179, 717-718.

Adams, H. E., Feuerstein, M., & Fowker, J. L. (1980). Migraine headache: Review of
    parameters, etiology, and intervention. Psychological Bulletin, 87, 217-237.

Dalessio, D. J. (ed.). (1980). Wolff's headache and other head pain. New York: Oxford
    University Press.

Increasing the risk of CHD in women (LL 8-5)

Brezinka and Kittel reviewed the literature on psychosocial factors associated with CHD in women. They identified several risk factors. For example, women who come from lower socioeconomic classes, do not engage in exercise, smoke, and experience increased stress are at high risk for CHD. Moreover, Brezinka and Kittel found that women are more likely to experience psychosocial impairment and depression than men following a heart attack.

Resource:

> Brezinka, V., & Kittel, F. (1996). Psychosocial factors of coronary heart disease in women: A review. <u>Social Science and Medicine, 42</u>, 1351-1365.

Attitude and long-term survival with AIDS (LL 8-6)

A group of patients who had AIDS for at least three years was studied to determine the variables of long-term survival. Barroso found that five dimensions described their survivability. Most relevant to this chapter was the attitude termed " focusing on living." Barroso reported that a focus on living referred to having a positive attitude, forward looking planning, and using one's energy for constructive purposes. As the article suggests, "focusing on living" has important implications for treating and supporting AIDS patients.

Resource:

Barroso, J. (1996). Focusing on living: Attitudinal approaches of long-term survivors of AIDS. <u>Issues in Mental Health Nursing, 17</u>, 395-408.

Holm, Bury, and Suda studied 12 women with migraine. The study examined subjects' stress levels and coping strategies at premenses, menses, and ovulation. They found that the menstrual cycle affected the women's use of coping strategies, in addition to a relationship between stress and migraine. The authors suggest that the relationship between stress and migraine is exacerbated with the menstrual cycle.

Resource:

Holm, J. E., Bury, L., & Suda, K. T. (1996). The relationship between stress, headache and the menstrual cycle. <u>Headache, 36</u>, 531-537.

Talking Points (TP)

Good stress, bad stress (TP 8-1)
Unfortunately, most of us assume that stress is always bad. But stress can also be quite adaptive. Ask students for examples of when stress prepared them. This chapter focuses on the distress or the "bad stress." Stress is like cholesterol. There is good and bad cholesterol, just like stress.

Rethinking stress (TP 8-2)
Ask your students to evaluate the following statements: Stress is rational and irrational, stress is normal and abnormal, and stress is universal (adapted from Auerbach and Gramling, 1998).

Type A's (TP 8-3)
Ask the students for examples involving friends or, more likely, their parents and relatives with type A personality. Other examples of Type A personality can be gleaned from television, movies, and politics.

Final exams and colds (TP 8-4)
An example of PIN that should hit home with many students is the occurrence of colds during final exam week. Ask your students how many of them experience stress during finals and how many typically get colds or other psychophysiological symptoms (e.g., headache, stomachache) during finals. This illustrates psychoneuroimmunology in the lives of students. By the way, on some campuses, cults are especially active during finals week. Ask your students to explain why.

Individual responses specificity (TP 8-5)
Many people have specific stress responses and will respond with very specific symptoms when under stress, such as a headache or an upset stomach. List several examples from student volunteers on an overhead transparency. Have students discuss the possible etiology of such stress responses. How can we either manage or eliminate these unwanted responses? What are the methodologies that we could employ to minimize the responses?

Stress reduction (TP 8-6)
Outline both positive and negative stress reduction techniques. Because of the increasing prevalence of alcohol abuse on many college campuses, describe its negative effects in both physiological and psychological terms. Have the students give examples of both physiological and psychological problems that they have witnessed in their fellow students. Be sure to keep this discussion anonymous.

Coping with stress and faith (TP 8-7)
No doubt there are students of faith in your classroom. Ask for volunteers to describe how faith can help to manage stress.

Cognitive appraisal and exams (TP 8-8)
How do students perceive exams? Do they appraise them as a challenge, as a way to demonstrate their knowledge. Or do they appraise exams as threats? Ask for a show of hands. Do you see any relationships between appraisal type and performance of exams?

Changing thoughts (TP 8-9)
Each student should select two or three stressful events that they experience on a relatively frequent basis, or on a less frequent basis if it is something that really distresses them. They should think about how each event is stressful and exactly what their thoughts are about each of these events. Then they should take each event and put it into a more positive light, deciding exactly how they can use it to enhance their lives or how they can see each event in a more positive, growth-enhancing manner.

subjects were given **nose drops** containing **cold** viruses	p. 208
most reports of psychological influence on physical health as **"anecdotal".**:	p. 208
In this view, nature was a vast, **self-powered machine.**	p. 209
the list of "psychophysiological disorders" were **drawn up.**	p. 209
can be stressful enough to **tax one's health**...	p. 210
the usefulness of minor positive events such as **gossiping** with friends...	p. 210
colds strike when we are **"run-down"**...	p. 211
each adapted for different virus, bacterium, or other **invader.**	p. 212
Most of use have heard of people dying of a **"broken heart"**...	p. 213
the daily **hassles** of life...	p. 214
This irregularity **takes its toll**...	p. 215
found to be more than twice as likely as others to experience a **cardiac event**...	p. 218
Eventually, they developed **strong bonds.**	p. 220
in the **womb.**	p. 221
often involving strange visual sensations such as...**blind spots.**	p. 222
unleashed a **great flurry** of research...	p. 222
the thinness of today's **fashion models**...	p. 223
Hence, insomnia is a classic example of the **vicious cycle.**	p. 225
Sometimes the disorder is due to work shifts.	p. 226
This principle was borne out during the **London blitz** of World War II.	p. 230
the **working out** of better defenses.	p. 231
these disorders tend to **run in families.**	p. 231
In addition to the **breakup of the family**...	p. 232

185

Activities and Demonstrations (ACT/DEMO)

Community resources (ACT/DEMO 8-1)
Objective: To identity community resources
Materials: None
Procedure: Have students research community resources that are available for persons who suffer from or are at-risk for psychophysiological disorders. Create a resource manual categorized according to the particular disorder, including name of each group, contact person(s), phone numbers, the types of services they offer, and whether any fee is involved. Students may also wish to explore the Internet for information or resources that are available.
Discussion: Students will learn that there are many resources available. A resource manual would be a valuable asset to the community.

Uplifts and hassles (ACT/DEMO 8-2)
Objective: To identity daily hassles and uplifts
Materials: None
Procedure: For this activity students are to form small groups and identify daily hassles and uplifts. Tell the students to keep in mind that these hassles and uplifts are mostly thoughts that they have. After approximately 15 to 20 minutes, have a representative from each group read off the daily hassles and uplifts for that group. Finally, discuss which the students feel impact our mental and psychological well-being more, uplifts or hassles.
Discussion: Kenner et al. also suggest that daily uplifts (positive aspects of our life) can act as a buffer against hassles. The most often cited hassles include concerns about weight, health of family members, rising prices of commonly purchased items, home maintenance, too many things to do, losing things, crime, and physical appearance. The most frequently cited uplifts include relating well with significant others, completing a task, feeling healthy, getting enough sleep, eating out, meeting responsibilities, visiting someone, phoning (writing) someone, and spending time with family.

Resource:

Kanner, A. D., Coyne, J. C., Schaefer, C., & Lazarus, R. S. (1981). Comparison of two modes of stress management: Daily hassles and uplifts versus major life events. Journal of Behavioral Medicine, 4, 1-39.

Stress and minor illness (ACT/DEMO 8-3)
Objective: To demonstrate the relationship between minor stress and illness
Materials: Hassles and Uplifts Scale
Procedure: Bring the mild stress inventory to class. Have students fill out the inventory. Ask them to list the number of illnesses they have had in the past month on the form.

Either collect the forms and do a correlation for the next class period or perform an eyeball correlation and display on an overhead transparency.

Discussion: Discuss the relationship between the mild hassles and uplifts and the stated illnesses that students have experienced. Is there a temporal relationship between mild stress and illness? Do students become sicker at the end or the beginning of the semester. When they are freshmen or seniors? Repeat this demonstration the last week of class and compare the results if possible.

Demonstrating biofeedback (ACT/DEMO 8-4)
Objective: To demonstrate biofeedback principles
Materials: Biofeedback machines
Procedure: Many psychology departments will have biofeedback machines from the 1970s when the research was at a high mark. If you can find some working machines, check to see that the operation of the machines is still satisfactory. An alternative is that simple biofeedback machines can be inexpensively obtained at some electronics stores such as RadioShack; these will be much more crude than the departmental research machines but will still be useful. Bring such a machine to class and ask for a volunteer to demonstrate the effects of decreased anxiety levels. Take base line readings with the equipment and then have the students close their eyes and relax as much as possible.
Discussion: What were the effects of the relaxation? Did the subjects change the parameters of the data being collected? Early data from biofeedback studies were very promising but faded upon further investigation.

Guest speakers (ACT/DEMO 8-5)
Objective: To illustrate the type of treatments used in clinical practice
Materials: None
Procedure: Invite speakers to your class to discuss the various physical disorders presented in the chapter. If there are different obesity/weight loss programs in your community, consider inviting a representative. Check with the local hospitals for sleep disorders clinics and cardiac rehabilitation units. Make sure you schedule this presentation early, since many mental health professionals are very busy.
Discussion: Beforehand, instruct students to review this chapter and be prepared to ask questions of their guest speakers. Afterwards, ask students to discuss speakers' presentations.

Films and Videos

AIDS. Changing the Rules. PBS. A compelling educational documentary aimed at protecting adult heterosexuals against AIDS.

AIDS: Face to Face. FHS. Donahue converses with AIDS patients about courage, fear, remorse, and resignation.

187

AIDS. No Sad Songs. FML. Focuses on the emotional and psychological effects of AIDS on victims, friends, and family.

AIDS. The Women Speak. FHS. Deals with mothers who lose a child to AIDS, social workers who work with AIDS patients, foster mothers of HIV-positive babies, and women infected with AIDS.

Controlling Pain. FHS. Examines risk for stress-related diseases, the effects of prolonged stress, and ways to handle it.

Getting a Handle on Stress. FHS. Program host Jim Hartz undergoes a stress evaluation test that uses a battery of physical and psychological tests to determine whether the subject is a "hot reactor"--someone whose body overreacts to stress. The program explains the effects of stress, how stress can be managed, and visits a stress management course that teaches stress reduction techniques.

Headaches. MTI. Distinguishes among the many kinds of headaches and examines a variety of treatments.

Headaches: When the Pain Won't Stop. FHS. Distinguishes among tension, cluster, and migraine headaches; how to diagnose serious problems and how to treat headaches.

Hypertension: Your Blood Pressure Is Showing and Stress: Is Your Lifestyle Killing You? PBS. Explores the causes and effects of high blood pressure and deals with ways to control stress that affects one's health.

Insomnia. FHS. Explains the characteristics of different types of levels of sleep/sleeplessness; explains circadian rhythm and the consequences of its disturbance, sleep apnea and treatments for it. REM behavior disorder, narcolepsy, and the effects of sleeping pills.

Managing Stress. FHS. This program distinguishes between positive stress, which can strengthen the immune system, and negative stress, which can increase the likelihood of heart disease, high blood pressure, and cancer. It shows the effects of different types of stress and how an individual can reduce stress.

Managing Stress. PSU. Basic research on stress is covered. Techniques to successfully manage stress are highlighted.

Maximizing Performance. FHS. Using relaxation to reach the full potential of our minds is explored with exercises called affirmations and visualizations; a psychotherapist discusses biofeedback; and a student describes how relaxation response has dramatically changed his life.

Mind over Body. TLF. 1972. Shows the influence of a person's psychological state on routine illness and body injuries.

Mind/Body Wellness. RMI. Examines the relationships between our emotional and personal well-being and our health.

New Stress. FHS. Since it was first coined by Canadian scientist Hans Selye, the word *stress* has been part of our everyday vocabulary. But what exactly is stress? This program explains that it is a biological response of an organism to its environment, and indispensable to survival. However, when stress becomes chronic, as is often the case in contemporary life, stress can lead to sickness, or even death. In addition, stress is not limited to living organisms: the concept of stress is used by engineers to define the tension forces in structures such as bridges, as well as the mechanical strains in biological tissues such as bone and muscle. Using this stress concept, biochemical technicians can increase strength and resilience in prostheses designed for the handicapped.

Stress and Immune Function. FHS. This program examines the relationship between stress and illness and the studies that link stress to immune system malfunctions: higher cancer mortality, respiratory infections, herpes, and autoimmune disorders

Stress and Immune Functions. FHS. Examines the relationship between stress and illness and the studies that link malfunctions of the immune system to stress.

Stress. FHS. This program demonstrates proven methods of coping with stress.

Stress: A Disease of Our Time. TLF. Experiments with rats, soldiers, and children in classrooms illustrate the concept of stress.

Techniques for Mind/Body Wellness. RMI. Teaches methods to achieve emotional and physical well-being.

The Mind, No. 5-Pain and Healing. PBS. Explores the mind's role in healing the body and controlling pain.

The Relaxation Response. FHS. The relaxation response is explained and students are guided through exercises designed to trigger the response; a student who has been cured of insomnia with relaxation is profiled; and flotation tanks are discussed.

Western Medicine Meets East. FHS. Examines the use of acupuncture and other traditional Eastern medical techniques as anesthetics during surgery and as treatment for such ailments as arthritis and backache.

189

Using Movies and Mental Illness as a Teaching Tool

Your students will appreciate a classroom opportunity to watch the classic scene in which Captain Queeg (Humphrey Bogart) deteriorates while on the witness stand in *The Caine Mutiny*. More contemporary examples of stress reactions are available from selected scenes in *Falling Down* or *Glengarry Glen Ross*.

Darlene Cates is superb playing the role of "Momma" in *What's Eating Gilbert Grape*. Showing excerpts from the film will force your students to examine their reactions to film characters – and presumably people they encounter in real life – who are obese (e.g., the scene in which food is brought to Momma because she is too fat to walk to the table) or mentally retarded (e.g., the scene in which Leonardo DiCaprio, playing the younger brother, climbs the town's water tower and can't get down).

In a similar way, selected scenes from *Passion Fish* and *The Waterdance* can be used to get your students thinking about what life must be like for someone who suddenly must cope with life in a wheelchair. The later film is especially effective in examining the issue of the changes in sexual functioning associated with paralysis. Some of the anxiety associated with spinal cord injuries and sexuality can also be illustrated with scenes from *Born on the Fourth of July* and *Coming Home*.

Movie	Link to Chapter	Page Reference to Wedding and Boyd
• Duet for One • The Caine Mutiny • Falling Down • The Waterdance • Jerry Maguire • The Men • The Accidental Tourist	stress (p. 210)	p. 43 p. 47 p. 47 p. 47 p. 47 p. 47 p. 47

Classroom Assessment Techniques (CAT)

Focused Listing (CAT 8-1)
Select an important point from this chapter (e.g., mind-body problem, individual response specificity, psychoneuroimmunology) and ask students to write five words or phrases that describe the point.

Learning Review (CAT 8-2)
Students are to write in order five of the most important ideas they learned in this chapter.

Muddiest Point (CAT 8-3)
Instruct students to write about an issue, concept, or definition presented in Chapter 8 that they find most confusing or difficult to understand.

Minute Paper (CAT 8-4)
Ask your students to write about important questions they have that remain unanswered.

Suggestions for Essay Questions

❑ How does the research on psychophysiological disorders support the idea that mind and body are one?
❑ Explain how two people who experience the same stressors can have different psychological reactions to it.
❑ Describe how psychological variables influence cancer and hypertension.
❑ If you are a psychologist who subscribes to the cognitive perspective, what is your explanation of psychophysiological disorders?

Hassles and Uplifts Scale

Place an "X" next to each event that has happened to you in the last month.

Hassles

1. Misplacing or losing items
2. Troublesome neighbors
3. Social obligation
4. Inconsiderate smokers
5. Thoughts about death
6. Health of a family member
7. Not enough money
8. Concerns about owing money

Uplifts

1. Practicing your hobby
2. Being lucky
3. Saving money
4. Liking fellow workers or students
5. Successful financial dealings
6. Being rested
7. Feeling healthy
8.   Finding something lost

List the number of minor health problems you have had in the same period.

(Adapted from Kanner et al. 1981)

Chapter 9

Mood Disorders

Chapter Map

Section	Instructor Manual Components
Depressive and Manic Episodes • Major Depressive Episode • Manic Episode	*Experiencing mood disorders (LL 9-1)* *Famous people with mood disorders (TP 9-1)* *Continuum (TP 9-2)* *Normal depression vs abnormal depression (TP 9-3)* *Mania (TP 9-4)* *Role playing mood disorders (ACT/DEMO 9-1)*
Mood Disorder Syndromes • Major Depressive Disorder • Bipolar Disorder • Dysthymic Disorder and Cyclothymic Disorder • Dimensions of Mood Disorder • Comorbidity: Mixed Anxiety-Depression	*Loneliness (LL 9-2)* *How depression affects us (TP 9-6)* *Free association (TP 9-7)*
Suicide • The Prevalence of Suicide • Groups at Risk for Suicide • Myths About Suicide • Suicide Prediction • Suicide Prevention	*The right to commit suicide (TP 9-8)* *Suicide myths (TP 9-9)* *Community resources (ACT/DEMO 9-2)* *Developing a suicide awareness and prevention program (ACT/DEMO 9-3)*

Mood Disorders: Theory and Treatment	Rational emotive therapy (LL 9-3)
• The Psychodynamic Perspective • The Behavioral Perspective • The Cognitive Perspective • The Sociocultural Perspective • The Biological Perspective	Beck: Working with depressed individuals (LL 9-4) More on depressive realism (LL 9-5) Cultural factors in SAD (LL 9-6) Carbohydrate craving, serotonin, and tryptophan in SAD (LL 9-7) Setting circadian rhythms (LL 9-8) Electroconvulsive therapy (TP 9-10) Light therapy (TP 9-11) Replacing maladaptive statements (ACT/DEMO 9-4) Script writing (ACT/DEMO 9-5)

Chapter Outline

I.   Introduction
    A.   **Depression** and **mania** in mild and temporary forms are part of ordinary existence
    B.   **Mood disorders** are conditions of mood where mood swings are prolonged and extreme that life is seriously disrupted
    C.   Mood disorders have been of interest since beginning of history of medicine

II.   Depressive and Manic Episodes
    A.   Mood disorders have an episodic quality
    B.   Nature of the episode and duration determine diagnosis and often treatment
    C.   Major Depressive Episode
        1.   **Major depressive episode** develops gradually over weeks or months, last several months, and ends gradually
        2.   Most areas of person are affected by depression
        3.   Major depressive episode has several characteristics
            a.   Depressed mood; deeply depressed people see no way that it can be help called **helplessness-hopelessness syndrome**
            b.   Loss of pleasure or interest in usual activities; loss of pleasure is known as **anhedonia** and is far-reaching
            c.   Disturbance of appetite
            d.   Sleep disturbance
            e.   Psychomotor retardation or agitation; in **retarded depression**, person seems overcome by fatigue; **agitated depression** involves incessant activity and restlessness
            f.   Loss of energy
            g.   Feelings of worthlessness and guilt
            h.   Difficulties in thinking
            i.   Recurrent thoughts of death or suicide
    D.   Manic Episode
        1.   Manic episode typically begins suddenly over a few days and is usually shorter than a depressive episode
        2.   Manic episode may last days to several months and ends abruptly
        3.   Manic episode has several characteristics
            a.   Elevated, expansive, or irritable mood
            b.   Inflated self-esteem
            c.   Sleeplessness
            d.   Talkativeness
            e.   Flight of ideas
            f.   Distractibility
            g.   Hyperactivity

        h.   Reckless behavior
4.   For diagnosis, manic episode must have lasted at least a week and seriously interfered with person's functioning
5.   A briefer, less severe manic condition is called a hypomanic episode
6.   Individuals who meet diagnostic criteria for both manic episode and major depressive episode simultaneously are diagnosed with mixed episode

III.   Mood Disorder Syndromes
    A.   Major Depressive Disorder
        1.   People who experience one or more major depressive episodes with no mania are diagnosed with **major depressive order**
        2.   One of the greatest mental health problems in United States
            a.   Prevalence is 4% of men and 6% of women
            b.   Lifetime risk is 17%
            c.   Second only to schizophrenia for admissions to mental hospitals
            d.   Often are more debilitating than many other chronic medical conditions
            e.   Major depression is fourth leading cause of disability and premature death worldwide
        3.   Course
            a.   In 80% of cases, first episode is not the last
            b.   Median number of episodes is 4 with median duration of 4.5 months
            c.   Course varies considerable; some come in clusters
            d.   Some return to their premorbid adjustment
             e.   Depressive episodes generate stressful life events which can maintain depression
        4.   Groups at Risk for Depression
            a.   Race and marital status are risk factors
            b.   Risk for women is one to three times higher than for men
                 i.   Men and women respond to depressed moods differently
                 ii.   Women wonder why depression is occurring; men distract themselves
            c.   The young are at greater risk than the old for depression
            d.   Symptoms differ depending on age group
    B.   Bipolar Disorder
        1.   **Bipolar disorder** involves both manic and depressive phases
        2.   Common pattern is that initial manic episode followed by normal phase, then a depressed episode, then normal period

3.   In rapid-cycling type, there are swings between depressive and manic or mixed episodes over long period with little or no normal functioning between

4.   Other differences exist between bipolar and major depression
     a.   Bipolar disorder much less common
     b.   Two disorders show different demographic profiles
     c.   Married or those in intimate relationships less likely to develop major depression; does not matter in bipolar disorder
     d.   People with major depression tend to have histories of low self-esteem, dependency, and obsessional thinking; those with bipolar tend to have history of hyperactivity
     e.   Depressive episodes in bipolar more likely to show s pervasive slowing down
     f.   Two disorders differ in their course
     g.   Two disorders differ in their prognosis
     h.   Bipolar disorder more likely to run in families

5.   DSM-IV divides bipolar disorder into two groups
     a.   Bipolar I disorder--person has had at least one manic or mixed episode and usually, not necessarily, at least one major depressive episode
     b.   Bipolar II disorder--person has had at least one major depressive episode and at least one hypomanic episode, but does not meet criteria of manic or mixed episode

6.   Dysthymic Disorder and Cyclothymic Disorder
     a.   **Dysthymic disorder** involves a mild, persistent depression
     b.   Cyclothymic disorder is a chronic pattern of hypomanic and depressive behavior
     c.   Both disorders have slow gradual onset often in adolescence
     d.   Individuals with these disorders tend to have relatives with mood disorders
     e.   Prevalence and gender difference tend to mirror their graver counterparts

7.   Dimensions of Mood Disorder
     a.   Psychotic Versus Neurotic
          i.   Depressive and manic episodes can have psychotic features where the individual loses touch with reality
          ii.   Many cases remain at the neurotic level
          iii. Some argue that neurotic and psychotic level mood disorders are different entities altogether
          iv.   The **continuity hypothesis** says that distinction is more quantitative than qualitative
     b.   Endogenous Versus Reactive

       i.   Some regard that neurotic forms of mood disorders are psychogenic and psychotic forms as biogenic

       ii.   Depression linked to external event was called **reactive**

       iii.   Depression not linked to external event was called **endogenous**

       iv.   Reactive and endogenous actually refer to different patterns of symptoms and reflect other differences

  c.   Early Versus Late Onset

       i.   The earlier the onset of disorder, the more likely person's relative share, or had had mood disorders

       ii.   Early onset affects person with early onset

       iii.   Findings suggest that early onset have higher "genetic loading" for mood disorders

       iv.   Could also mean that environmental factors account for onset

  d.   Cormorbidity: Mixed Anxiety-Depression

       i.   **Comorbidity** is the co-occurrence of disorders

       ii.   Symptomatology of anxiety and depression show overlap

       iii.   Findings raise questions about disorders being two distinct entities or different manifestations of same underlying disorder

       iv.   It has been proposed to include new category in DSM reflecting mixed anxiety-depression

IV.   Suicide

  A.   A common reason for suicide is depression

  B.   Lifetime risk of suicide in people with mood disorders is 19%; 55% were depressed before fatal attempt

  C.   The Prevalence of Suicide

     1.   Many people who commit suicide make their deaths look accidental

     2.   Eight people attempt suicide for every one who commits suicide

     3.   Suicide is 8th most common cause of death in United States

  D.   Groups at Risk for Suicide

     1.   Certain demographic variables are strongly correlated with suicide

     2.   The modal suicide attempter is native-born Caucasian woman, a homemaker in her 20s or 30s who attempts suicide by swallowing barbiturates and gives the reason as martial difficulties or depression

     3.   The modal suicide committer is native-born Caucasian man in his 40s or older for reasons of ill health, depression, or martial difficulties commits suicide by shooting or hanging himself or by carbon monoxide poisoning

4. Recent shifts have been observed in suicide-related variables, particularly with age and race
5. Teenage Suicide
    a. Suicide rate has risen 200% since 1960
    b. Teenagers exposed to situations as stressful as those facing adults, but lack resources such as emotional self-control
    c. Trouble within family another major risk factor
    d. Problems of suicidal teenagers rooted in families' problems and feel there is no solution to their problems
6. Myths About Suicide
    a. More than half of all suicide victims had clearly committed their suicidal intent within 3 months of fatal act
    b. About 40% of all suicides made previous attempts or threat
    c. Most clinicians agree that encouraging patients to talk about suicidal wishes helps them overcome their wishes
7. Suicide Prediction
    a. Suicide is often directly related to stress; preceded by "exit" events
    b. Cognitive variables, such as hopelessness, may be useful predictors
    c. A suicidal scenario is made up of several elements
        i.   Pain, related to thwarted psychological needs
        ii.   Self-denigration
        iii. Constriction of the mind
        iv.   Sense of isolation
        v.   Hopelessness
        vi.   Decision that egression is only solution to problem
    d. Suicide notes express suffering and neutral statements
    e. Most suicide attempters do not really wish to die, but are communicating intensity of their feelings
8. Suicide Prevention
    a. Telephone hot lines established in later 1950s
    b. School-based workshops are given that present warning signs
    c. Efforts have not been very successful, with only slight drops or not reaching those at risk for suicide

V. Mood Disorders: Theory and Therapy
    A. The Psychodynamic Perspective
        1. Reactived Loss
            a. Depression was due to massive defense mounted by the ego against intrapsychic conflict
            b. Abraham suggests that depression arises when one loses a love object toward whom one had ambivalent feelings
                i. The positive feelings give rise to guilt

           ii.   The negative feelings give rise to intense anger

           iii.   Anger is turned inward, producing self-hatred and despair

   c.   Modern theorists have revised theory

           i.   Depression is rooted in a very early defect

           ii.   The primal wound is reactivated by recent setback or blow and person experiences infantile trauma

           iii.   Regression leads to hopelessness and helplessness

           iv.   Ambivalence toward love object is fundamental to emotion

           v.   Loss of self-esteem is primary feature of depression

           vi.   Depression has functional role

   d.   Some research support for dependency on others and role of parental loss and poor parenting

2.   Repairing the Loss

   a.   Therapist tries to uncover childhood roots of depression and to explore ambivalent feelings about lost object

   b.   Interpersonal Psychotherapy has been used and consists of identifying core problem and discussion of solutions

B.   The Behavioral Perspective

   1.   Extinction

       a.   Many behaviorists regard depression as result of extinction

       b.   Amount of positive reinforcement person receives is dependent on several factors

           i.   Number and range of stimuli that are reinforcing to person

           ii.   Availability of such reinforcers in the environment

           iii.   Person's skill in obtaining reinforcement

       c.   Some studies have produced supporting results

   2.   Aversive Social Behavior

       a.   Depressives are more likely to elicit negative reactions from others

       b.   This has formed basis for interpersonal theories of depression

           i.   Depressives try to force caring behavior from others

           ii.   Reactions tend to be ineffective, which aggravates their depression

           iii.   Some studies have found that rejecting responses do maintain or exacerbate depression

           iv.   Poor social skills help to maintain depression

   3.   Increasing Reinforcement and Social Skills

       a.   Treatments involve at increasing patient's rate of reinforcement

       b.   Another approach is social-skills training

      c.   Most behavioral treatments are multifaceted that include monitoring self-statements and training in variety of areas

      d.   None of behavioral therapies are more effective than drugs

      e.   With rise of cognitive therapy, behavioral therapies without cognitive components were abandoned

C.   The Cognitive Perspective

    1.   The way the person thinks about themselves, the world, and the future gives rise to other factors in depression

    2.   Helplessness and Hopelessness

      a.   Depression may be link to **learned helplessness,** where the critical factor is the expectation of lack of control over reinforcement

      b.   Hopelessness theory says that depression depends on a helplessness expectancy and a negative outcome expectancy

      c.   Source of expectations of helplessness and negative outcomes are the attributions and inferences people make about stressful life events

          i.   Causes are permanent rather than temporary

          ii.   Generalized rather than specific to one area of their functioning

          iii.   Internal rather than external

    3.   Negative Self-Schema

      a.   Negative bias--seeing oneself as a "loser" is fundamental cause of depression

      b.   Stress can activate the negative schema

      c.   Research finds that depressives have very negative self-schemas

      d.   Studies indicate that depressives selectively attend to and remember more negative than positive information about themselves

      e.   Sometimes, depressives may be more pessimistic, but more realistic than our optimism

    4.   Cognitive Retraining

      a.   Multifaceted therapy developed to modify dysfunctional thinking and to change schemas

      b.   In Beck's therapy, alteration of the schema inoculate the person against future depression

      c.   Another treatment, reattribution training, is attempt to correct negative attributions

      d.   Cognitive therapies have been found to be at least as effective as drug therapy and perhaps superior at 1-year follow-up

          i.   Combining cognitive therapy and drug therapy may be superior

                    ii.   Cognitive therapy has relapse-prevention effect, unlike drug therapy

D.   The Sociocultural Perspective
    1.   Society and Depression
        a.   Durkheim saw suicide as an act that occurs within society and under control of society
        b.   Socioeconomic conditions affect suicide rate
        c.   Prevalence of depression in United States has increased and age of onset has dropped
             i.   Social change may account for the prevalence
             ii.   Family structures, moving away, moving down socioeconomic ladder may be related
    2.   Suicide prevention programs have not been especially effective
    3.   Perhaps better approach is to attack social problems associated with suicide such delinquency, teenage pregnancy, and family distress

E.   The Biological Perspective
    1.   Genetic Research
        a.   Family studies suggest genetic component in mood disorders; first-degree relatives of those with mood disorder are more likely to develop disorders
        b.   Concordance rates for bipolar disorder was 72% among MZ twins and 14% for DZ; for unipolar disorder, 40% for MZ twins and 11% for DZ
        c.   Genetic factors are more important in bipolar disorder than in depression
        d.   Environmental factors such as individual-specific environments are important; less important are shared environmental factors
        e.   Adoption studies provide most impressive evidence for the heritability of mood disorders
        f.   Linkage analysis provides mixed results
    2.   Neurophysiological Research
        a.   Mood disorders may be related to biological rhythms such as sleep disturbances like shortened REM latency
        b.   One theory suggests that when important social zeitgeber is removed from person's life, its removal is a loss, but also disrupts body's circadian rhythms leading to consequences
        c.   **Seasonal affective disorder** is closely related to biological rhythms
             i.   For diagnosis of SAD, person must meet criteria for major depressive episode, remission and onset tied to seasons, and pattern must have lasted for at least 2 years
             ii.   Winter version of SAD tied to shorter photoperiod

   iii. Women are at greater risk with average age at onset of 23
   iv. Theory suggests that lag in circadian rhythms causes SAD
   v. Most SAD patients report improvement with light therapy

3. Neuroimaging Research

  a. CT and MRI studies suggest mood disorders involve abnormalities in brain structure (e.g., ventricles, frontal lobe, cerebellum, basal ganglia)

  b. Suggests that these brain areas are involved in mood regulation

4. Biochemical Research

  a. Hormone Imbalance

   i. Depression is due to malfunction in hypothalamus

   ii. Dysfunction may be related to control of hormone production

   iii. Depression can sometimes be treated by altering hormone levels

   iv. Hormone imbalances are characteristic of endogenous and psychotic depression

   v. **Dexamethasone suppression test** used to differentiate between endogenous and reactive cases

   vi. Hormone imbalances occur both in major depression and in depressive episodes of bipolar disorder, but does not seem to be a primary cause

  b. Neurotransmitter Imbalance

   i. Catecholamine hypothesis argues that increased levels of norepinephrine produce mania, while decreased levels produce depression

   ii. Tricyclic drugs block reuptake of norepinephrine and serotonin

   iii. Serotonin involved in mood disorders and suicide by indirect evidence

   iv. Another theory suggests that atrophy of certain neurons in the hippocampus triggers depression; antidepressant drugs may influence brain-derived neurotrophic factor

  c. A summary of biochemical findings

5. Antidepressant Medication

  a. The major classes of antidepressant medication are **MAO inhibitors, the tricyclics, and selective serotonin reuptake inhibitors (SSRIs)**

  b. Drugs work by increasing levels of neurotransmitters by interfering with an enzyme or reuptake

    c.   Balancing symptoms relief with side effect an important consideration

    d.   Tricyclics effective 50 to 70 percent of patients with depression

    e.   Selective serotonin reuptake inhibitors block neurotransmitter reuptake

         i.   Prozac gaining popularity, but can have side effects

         ii.   Often patients will increase dose which can led to overdosing

    f.   Main antimanic drug is **lithium**

         i.   Effective in ending about 70% of manic episodes

         ii.   Lithium's effectiveness is primarily preventive

         iii.   Regular blood tests important to monitor level of drug

6.   Electroconvulsive Therapy

    a.   Electric shock in **electroconvulsive therapy** can relieve severe depression

    b.   Treatment involves 9 or 10 sessions over period of several weeks

    c.   Most common side effect is memory dysfunction

    d.   Many patients are very frightened of ECT

Chapter Boxes

- Why Do Gender Differences in Depression Emerge In Adolescence?
  - A. Women are twice as likely to develop serious depression.
  - B. Women tend to have number of characteristics that put them at risk for depression
  - C. In adolescence, new risk factors emerge
  - D. Girls who adopted narrowed role prescribed for women at higher risk for depression

- Streams of Fire: Bipolar Disorder and Creativity
  - A. Artists show unusually high rate of mood disorder
  - B. Jamison has studied artists and describes creative benefits of mania

- Drug Therapy Versus Psychotherapy
  - A. Some concern expressed for attempting to "biologize" psychological disorders
  - B. Root cause of some depressions may be related to biology
  - C. Most effective treatment is combination of drug therapy and psychotherapy
  - D. Relapse is more likely to follow sole use of drug therapy
  - E. Psychological disorder is never just biochemical

Learning Objectives (LO)

By the time you have finished studying this chapter, you should be able to do the following:

1. List and describe nine characteristics of a major depressive episode (238-239).

2. List and describe eight characteristics of a manic episode (240).

3. Describe the patterns of mood episodes that are characteristic of major depressive disorder and bipolar disorder (242-244).

4. Summarize the population data that differentiate major depression from bipolar disorder (241-243).

5. Define dysthymia and cyclothymia, and distinguish them from major depressive disorder and bipolar disorder (244-246).

6. Distinguish between neurotic versus psychotic disorders, endogenous versus reactive disorders, the effects of early versus late onset, and describe the phenomenon of comorbidity (246-248).

7. Summarize the population data concerning suicide (248-250).

8. List some common myths about suicide and the major behavioral, environmental, and cognitive predictors of suicide, and evaluate the effectiveness of suicide prevention (251-252).

9. Explain the "reactivated loss" and "anger in" hypotheses held by the psychodynamic perspective, and describe psychodynamic attempts to treat mood disorder (252-254).

10. Explain how behavioral psychologists account for mood disorders and suicide in terms of learning processes and extinction, and describe behavioral treatments for mood disorder (254-256).

11. Explain how cognitive theorists account for mood disorders and suicide in terms of destructive thinking, learned helplessness, and poor self-schemas, and describe cognitive treatments for mood disorder (256-259).

12. Summarize sociocultural factors that may impact on mood disorders and suicide, and describe what the sociocultural perspective would recommend to solve these problems (259-260).

13. Summarize recent biological research on mood disorder, making reference to genetic studies, neurophysiological studies, neuroimaging work, and biochemical research (260-265).

14. Discuss biological treatments for mood disorder, including drug treatments and electroconvulsive shock treatments (265-268).

Lecture Leads (LL)

Experiencing mood disorders (LL 9-1)
Although the textbook does present some first person accounts of depression, you may wish to provide more detail. Joel Smith, a university president, describes his ordeal with depression. He laments about the isolation depression causes and how "hope is gone." He describes a dangerous consequence of profound depression by saying that "it suddenly seems perfectly clear that I should die. This is not tragic. It's the opposite. This is a good feeling, not euphoric but authentic and pernicious. My ultimate guardian-- namely, myself--has not just gone off duty but, so much more dangerously, has become the advocate, the agent of destruction." Locate biographies or autobiographies of people who have suffered from mood disorders. First person descriptions seem to convey the essence of psychological disorders, especially mood disorders, so much more personally and tragically than clinical transcripts.

Resources:

Endler, N. (1990). Holiday of darkness: A psychologist's journey out of his depression. Toronto: Wall & Thompson.

Smith, J. P. (1997). Depression: Darker than darkness. The American Scholar, 66, 495-499.

Loneliness (LL 9-2)
Most people see the relationship between loneliness and depression as obvious, yet do not recognize the magnitude of the problem. In a national study, as many as 26 percent of Americans reported being very lonely or being removed from others. The reasons given for being lonely generally fall into one of five categories: 1) unattached, no spouse or sexual partner, 2) alienated, feeling misunderstood or different, 3) being alone, the "empty house" feeling, 4) forced isolation, hospitalization, or housebound due to a lack of transportation, and 5) dislocation, being in a new situation without or outside of social support systems. Many students are surprised, often pleasantly, since they don't feel so weird, to find that it is the young and not the elderly who are more often lonely. Not surprisingly, married persons report less loneliness, and separated, divorced, or widowed persons are most lonely. Interestingly, choiceful singleness, including those who "just never married," do not report being more lonely than the general population. Brehm reports that gender does affect loneliness, but interactively rather than directly. For example, married females report a higher level of loneliness than do married males, whereas males report greater loneliness among those who never married, those whose spouse has died, and those who are separated or divorced. Specifically, Brehm believes that men and women differ in their vulnerability to two different types of loneliness. Since marriage is more likely to reduce a woman's social network than a male's, women report a lack of a network of friends and acquaintances (social isolation) as being more loneliness-inducing, whereas men seem more responsive to the loss of a single intense relationship (emotional isolation). Coping strategies tend to fall into one of four

208

categories: 1) sad passivity (e.g., sleeping, overeating, watching TV), 2) social contact, 3) active solitude (e.g., studying, reading, exercise), or 4) distractions (e.g., shopping).

Resources:
Brehm, S. (I 985). Intimate relationships. New York: Random House.

de Jong-Gierveld, J. (1987). Developing and testing a model of loneliness. Journal of Personality and Social Psychology, 53, 67-82.

Meers, J. (1985, July). Loneliness. Psychology Today, pp. 28-33.

Rational emotive therapy (LL 9-3)
One of the cognitive restructuring therapies that is probably the most well known is Ellis' rational emotive therapy (RET). Ellis proposed his system of therapy at about the same time that some behaviorists were questioning the S-R model of behavior. Attention was being attracted by the basic premise of RET, which states that psychological disorders are due to maladaptive thoughts that manifest themselves within the individual as patterns of explicit or implicit self-verbalizations. Ellis proposes that irrational thoughts include any type of self-verbalizations that have self-defeating of self-destructive consequences. As an example, consider what types of maladaptive behaviors would be spawned by the irrational thoughts of believing that it is necessary for an adult to be loved by everyone for every action that is taken. Ellis would argue that most of the problems that we experience are products of our innate tendency towards irrational thought patterns, such as demanding that we should and must behave in a prescribed way and that people should and must behave in a specific way. RET's concept is described in the A-B-C-D-E paradigm. "A" is thought of as an activating event (e.g., loss of a loved one), "B" is the chain of self-verbalizations that the individual experiences (e.g., "this is horrible, I can't go on living"), and the consequences of the event are symbolized by "C" (e.g., emotional distress). One observation that is imperative to note in Ellis' system is that "B", the chain of self-verbalizations, produces "C", emotional distress; in other words, the actual event per se does not directly elicit emotions, but the interpretations nested in self-verbalizations. Ellis termed the A-B-C component as emotional reactivity. The actual workings of the therapy are reflected in the D-E portion of the paradigm mentioned above. A brief description of the process in RET would involve the therapist pointing out the illogic inherent in the individual's irrational thoughts by the "logico-empirical method of scientific questioning, challenging and debating."

Resources:
Ellis, A. (1962). Reason and emotion in psychotherapy. New York: Lyle Stuart

Ellis, A. (1979). The practice of rational-emotion therapy. In A. Ellis & J. Whiteley (Eds.). Theoretical and empirical foundations of rational-emotion therapy. Monterey, CA: Brooks/Cole.

Ellis, R. (1993). Reflections on rational-emotive therapy. <u>Journal of Consulting and Clinical Psychology</u>, <u>61</u>, 199-201.

Beck: Working with depressed individuals (LL 9-4)

The cognitions of depressed people are believed to be typified by pervasive misconceptions and false beliefs. Misconceptions and false beliefs, according to Beck, are characterized by 1) arbitrary inference-jumping to unsupported conclusions, 2) magnification-exaggerating the meaning of an event, 3) personalization-attributing an external event to one's self, 4) polarized thinking--either/or interpretations, 5) overgeneralization--drawing a conclusion on a single occurrence, and 6) selective abstraction--disregarding an important event's context while focusing on details. Beck considers these processes as being in excess of a particular quality, or in other words, as being "too extreme" or "too absolute." He also proposes that specific disorders are characterized by specific interactions of maladaptive cognitions. For example, obsession is construed as thoughts that focus on doubts of past performances, anxiety is viewed as thoughts of preeminent danger, and depression are thoughts centering on a negative self-worth, negative interpretation of the present, and a negative expectancy of the future. Maladaptive behaviors, such as crying or suicidal threats in depression, are related to self-verbalizations that are promoted by the existence of the distorting processes mentioned above. The therapeutic process of treating depression commences by what Beck terms as "successive approximations" to combat the client's perception of oneself as "a loser." Graduated activities (successfully boiling an egg one day to successfully preparing a meal the next day to successfully keeping within the constraints of a budget) provide the client opportunities to successfully engage in behaviors that facilitate the reevaluation of one's self-worth in a more positive light. Progressively, the focus of therapy is redirected to the cognitions of the client. Maladaptive cognitions are exposed to the client by way of "introspection." The therapist's emphasis, at this stage, is one of directing the client to incorrect misconceptions and their maladaptive outcome. At some point in therapy, the individual is trained to note maladaptive behavior-generating self-verbalizations and in effect, to put "distance" between one's self and those self-verbalizations to achieve objectivity. It is hoped by allowing the client to objectively focus on his/her thoughts, an understanding of the relationship between thought and behavior is established. Finally, with the assistance of the therapist, more appropriate and adaptive self-verbalizations are presented.

Resources:

Beck, A. T. (1985). Cognitive therapy of depression: New perspectives. In P. Clayton (Ed.), <u>Depression</u>. New York: Raven.

Beck, A. T. (1991). Cognitive therapy. <u>American Psychologist</u>, <u>46</u>, 368-375.

Beck, A. T., Rush, A. J., Shaw, B. F., Emery, G. (1979). <u>Cognitive therapy of depression</u>. New York: Guilford.

More on depressive realism (LL 9-5)
As the textbook describes, people who are happy or optimistic are less accurate in their ratings of certain events than are those who are depressed. Alloy and Abramson first identified this in 1979, initially labeling it the sadder-but-wiser effect. Alloy and Abramson originally wanted to test the learned helplessness theory of depression. They recruited groups of depressed and nondepressed persons. The subjects were then, one at a time, placed behind a series of lights and buttons. At specified intervals, they were given a choice of whether or not to push one of the buttons. A light came on every other button-pressing choice, whether they pressed or not. The participants were asked at the end of the study to estimate their control over the light. From the helplessness theory, it was predicted that the depressed would do worse at the tasks. Surprisingly, the depressed persons were very accurate, whereas the nondepressed grossly overestimated their degree of control over the light. Other studies have shown that nondepressed people consistently overestimate their control over positive events and underestimate their control over negative events.

Resources:
Alloy, L. B., & Abramson, L. Y. (1979). Judgment of contingency in depressed and nondepressed students: Sadder but wiser? Journal of Experimental Psychology: General, 108, 441-485.

Hapgood, F. (1985, August). The sadder-but-wiser effect. Science, 85, 86-88.

Cultural factors in SAD (LL 9-6)
Although biology clearly does play a role in seasonal affective disorder, there is some epidemiology evidence that suggests cultural factors operate as well. The incidence of SAD in Florida and New York is 1.4 and 7.3, respectively. Iceland, which is obviously more north than Florida and New York, has a SAD incidence of 3.9%. The amount of sunlight has been identified as playing a significant role in SAD. This is the curious thing about SAD. Residents of Iceland receive far less sunlight in the winter than either New York or Florida, yet has a lower rate of SAD. Magnusson and Stefansson suggest that Icelanders live in a harsh environment that encourages the development of emotional resiliency thereby modulating the stress of winter. Also important is the obvious difference in population density between New York and Iceland.

Resources:
Magnusson, A., & Stefansson, J. G. (1993). Prevalence of seasonal affective disorder in Iceland. Archives of General Psychiatry, 50, 941-946.

Rosenthal, N. E. (1993). Diagnosis and treatment of seasonal affective disorder. Journal of the American Medical Association, 270, 2717-2720.

Carbohydrate craving, serotonin, and tryptophan in SAD (LL 9-7)
Beside depression, a common symptom of seasonal affective disorder (SAD) is
carbohydrate craving. Increased consumption of carbohydrates will result in excessive
weight gain during the winter. It has been hypothesized that the reduction in the duration
of daylight in winter could be an important factor in SAD. Although it is not yet clear
how a reduction in daylight could translates into depression, a possible biochemical
mechanism has recently been proposed. The theory involves the regulation of brain
levels of the neurotransmitter serotonin. Briefly, it is thought that serotonin regulation in
the brain is disturbed during the winter months in individuals suffering from SAD. The
source of serotonin in the brain is the amino acid tryptophan, which is found in the blood.
Tryptophan from the blood enters the brain where it is converted into serotonin in certain
neurons. Interestingly, the rate at which tryptophan enters the brain is influenced by the
level of carbohydrate intake. To simplify, high carbohydrate intake increases the amount
of tryptophan that enters the brain, thus increasing the amount of serotonin that gets
synthesized. It may be that the increased serotonin produced by the carbohydrate
ingestion may provide mild relief of the symptoms of SAD. Supportive of this view is
the fact that delta-fenfluramine, a drug that *enhances* serotonin transmission can relieve
the depression and carbohydrate craving that occurs in SAD. Students should also be
interested to learn that the disorder of premenstrual syndrome (PMS) has also been linked
to a disturbance in serotonin regulation similar to that found with SAD. However,
whereas sufferers of SAD cycle into and out of depression over the course of several
months, PMS sufferers have monthly bouts of depression and carbohydrate craving,
usually a couple of days before menstruation. Once again, delta-fenfluramine has been
found to be of some benefit for PMS sufferers.

Resources:
Nelson, M. J., Bandura, L. L., & Goldman, B. R. (I 990). Mechanisms of seasonal cycles
of behavior. Annual Review of Psychology, 41, 81-108.

Wurtman,R.J.,&Wurtman, J. J. (1989). Carbohydrates and depression. Scientific
American, 262, 68-75.

Setting circadian rhythms (LL 9-8)
A recent study by Campbell and Murphy suggests that light exposure to the back of the
knee can affect circadian rhythms. Subjects' body temperature and melatonin levels were
monitored. A relationship was found between the indices of biological rhythms and the
light exposure to the back of the knee. The authors discuss the implications that this
discovery has for treating sleep and circadian rhythm disorders.

Resource:
Campbell, S. S., & Murphy, P. J. (1998, January 16). Extraocular circadian
phototransduction in humans. Science, 279, 396-399.

Talking Points (TP)

Famous people with mood disorders (TP 9-1)
To mention famous people with mood disorders is to tell students that even the rich and famous are not immune from psychological disorders. That is especially true of mood disorders, given Seligman's description of depression as the "common cold" of abnormal behavior. Those who suffered from mood disorders include Abraham Lincoln, Ernest Hemingway, Joan Rivers, Curt Cobain, Dan Rather, Moses, Marilyn Monroe, Mike Wallace, Patty Duke, Dick Cavett, Drew Carey, Rod Steiger, Winston Churchill, Ezra Pound, Vincent van Gogh, and Jim Abbott. By the way, ask students what they think the characterization of depression means.

Continuum (TP 9-2)
When developing a lecture on depression, emphasize that depression and mania exist on a continuum. On one extreme is that common emotion of the "blahs" or "feeling down." Of course, on the other extreme is major depression. The same holds true of mania.

Normal depression vs abnormal depression (TP 9-3)
Students may not readily distinguish between clinical depression and normal depression, the kind we all feel at some point in our lives. Using the *DSM-IV* as a guide, discuss some of the relevant distinctions. Stress that learning to cope with normal depressions may actually strengthen the students' ability to deal with future stressful events

Mania (TP 9-4)
Elevated mood, feeling wonderful, seeing the world as an excellent place. All these are characteristics of mania. Many students might react to them with , "That sounds great. Who wouldn't want to feel that good?" It is very important that students understand that mania is not healthy, that it is not a good thing. You may, however, point out that Kay Jamison thinks that mania has given many artists the energy to inspire and create.
.
How depression affects us (TP 9-6)
Using the characteristics in the chapter as a guide, ask students how depression they've experienced (i.e., nonclinical; blues) affects their lives. The economic cost of depression is somewhere around $45 billion per year (Johnson & Indvik, 1997).

Free association (TP 9-7)
As you introduce depression and mania, ask students to free associate, that is, to name what comes to mind when they think of the two disorders. Next, ask for relevant examples or applications of the symptoms.

The right to commit suicide (TP 9-8)
Although the right to die has become a relatively "hot" topic in the past few years, particularly with respect to terminal illness, this is not a new phenomenon. There has consistently been much cultural diversity with respect to suicide and attitudes about

suicide. In some cultures, such as traditional Japanese, it has been an honorable way to save face for oneself or one's family in many situations. In the United States today there is ongoing debate about whether a terminally ill person should be forced to continue to suffer when there is no hope of a cure and when the person's illness is creating extraordinary financial hardship for that person's family. Debate whether there are instances when suicide is acceptable; students who believe it is never acceptable should present ways to overcome the hardships that are endured by the person who wishes to end his/her life and the families involved with respect to costly terminal illnesses. You can easily lead into a discussion of physician-assisted suicide.

Suicide myths (TP 9-9)
Before you introduce the topic of suicide, ask students to write down three to five things they "know" about suicide. Have students generate a list of myths associated with suicide. Discuss the etiology of these myths. Also mention your local treatment centers and crisis centers that the students can use for emergency treatment of mood disorders. Stress the importance of getting professional help for individuals with mood disorders.

Electroconvulsive therapy (TP 9-10)
Before students read the material on ECT, ask how many would consider receiving ECT themselves, given their understanding of it. Would they encourage a family member or friend to receive ECT? After discussing ECT, ask the same questions? Do students think differently about ECT?

Light therapy (TP 9-11)
Students should understand that light from an ordinary lamp is not sufficient to treat SAD. You may wish to contact a company that supplies lights for phototherapy. An example of a company that supplies a 10,000 LUX desklamp is Northern Light Technologies, (3070 Brabant-Marnieau, Montreal, Canada H4S IK7; phone number is 800-263-0066.

where life seems **grey** and nothing seems worth doing.	p. 238
a person who has been functioning normally is **plunged into despair** or is **scaling the heights** of mania.	p. 238
Depression can usually be **"read"** immediately in the person's motor behavior...	p. 239
Their frequent complaints about loss...**material goods**...	p. 239
Manics often seen other people as slow, **doltish spoilsports**...	p. 240
buying sprees, reckless driving, careless **business investments**...	p. 240
difficult for people coming out of a depressive episode to resume their **former lives.**	p. 241
is **haunted by fears** of death...	p. 242
Dysthymics are typically **morose**...	p. 244
with their **mental powers** newly sharpened...	p. 245
normal **"blues"** are simply different points on a single continuum.	p. 246
then having no diagnostic label gives us a **false picture** of the field.	p. 248
How can people who **"have their whole lives ahead of them"** want ...	p. 249
One **"psychological autopsy"** compared...	p. 250
have given it the status of **"unmentionable"** in the minds of many...	p. 251
the first telephone **"hot lines"** for potential suicides were established...	p. 252
no longer regarding anger as the **hub** of depression...	p. 253
it seems to work just as well, at least **in the short run**....	p. 254
shallow reassurance of the **"now, now"** variety...	p. 255
the nuts and bolts of socializing.	p. 255
tendency to see oneself as a **"loser"**...	p. 257
away from their birthplaces, and up and down the **socioeconomic ladder.**	p. 260
light therapy...can actually prevent a **full-blown relapse**...	p. 262

215

Activities and Demonstrations (ACT/DEMO)

Role playing mood disorders (ACT/DEMO 9-1)
Objective: To show the types of behaviors associated with mood disorders
Materials: None
Procedure: Have the students individually or in small groups select one of the mood disorders. Their task is to develop a role play to illustrate the disorder as well as other information (e.g., effect on family, demographics, suspected etiology, treatment perspectives). Tell the students that they have at least overnight to prepare for their disorder and that they will be expected to role play the disorder in front of the class. If using groups, one person plays the role of the subject, and other group members can play family members, employers, friends, and clinician.
Discussion: Give feedback on the accuracy of the role play. Ask the students how they developed their role and who they used as a model. Was there any influence from the media? If so, what specific individuals did they use as models? You could show a video at this point that will reinforce the correct behaviors and change the incorrect ones.

Community resources (ACT/DEMO 9-2)
Objective: To identity community resources
Materials: None
Procedure: Have students research community resources that are available for persons who suffer from or are at-risk for mood disorders and/or suicide. Create a resource manual categorized according to the particular disorder, including name of each group, contact person(s), phone numbers, the types of services they offer, and whether any fee is involved. More specifically, the resource manual could include what steps a suicidal person should take to get help.
Discussion: Students will learn that there are many resources available. A resource manual would be a valuable asset to the community.

Developing a suicide awareness and prevention program (ACT/DEMO 9-3)
Objective: To encourage students to think about suicide prevention
Materials: None
Procedure: This activity can be conducted with students working individually or in small groups. Students are to take the role of policy makers. Their charge is to develop national, state, or local programs aimed at suicide awareness and prevention.   The programs ought to incorporate what is known about suicide, suicide prevention, and mood disorders. Each program should include an objective and goals that describe how the objective will be reached. The goals should be explicitly linked to the literature summarized in the textbook.
Discussion: Select several programs to be presented and discussed. The critical question is the degree to which the programs take into account the research on suicide and mood disorders. One avenue of discussion might be to compare and contrast what students developed to what is typically included in suicide prevention programs.

Replacing maladaptive statements (ACT/DEMO 9-4)
Objective: To demonstrate an important component of cognitive therapy
Materials: Maladaptive Statements Handout
Procedure: Each student should translate the maladaptive, irrational beliefs that are believed to be involved in depression into more healthy, adaptive statements. After all students have completed the worksheet, they are to pair up with someone and compare their adaptive statements.
Discussion: Select a few adaptive statements to discuss in class. Give feedback on the appropriateness of the statements. You may wish to solicit personal examples of the maladaptive and adaptive statements from students. Ask students how the use of maladaptive statements may be related to depression.

Script writing (ACT/DEMO 9-5)
Objective: To explain treatment approaches suggested by the various theoretical perspectives
Materials: None
Procedure: Students should be placed in groups of no more than three. Each group should be assigned a particular theoretical perspective and a mood disorder. Their goal is to write a script summarizing how their assigned perspective would understand the mood disorder and treatment approach. For instance, the script might be between two psychologists describing their views on etiology, or it could be between client and therapist as they discuss the treatment.
Discussion: You should select several scripts for presentation or for analysis. Ask other students for their feedback on the accuracy of the script, given the material presented in the textbook.

Films and Videos

Beating the Depression Blues. MTI. Discusses the incidence of depression, its causes, and its treatment.

Childhood Depression. FHS. This program profiles a three-year-old and his parents, of whom all have depressive disorders. Mother and son visit Dr. Donald McKew, noted author, who explains how genetic disorders and chemical imbalance can cause mood disorders.

Childhood's End: A Look at Adolescent Suicide. FML. Explores the emotional and complex issues surrounding adolescent suicide.

Dead Serious. MTI. Examines the major factors that contribute to teenage suicide.

Depression. FHS. Explains the differences between occasional mood changes and depression.

Depression. PBS. Examines depression and bipolar disorders, suicide, and explanations of depression based on research.

Depression: A Study in Abnormal Behavior. MGH. The case of a depressed schoolteacher is discussed, using several models of depression. Diagnostic and treatment issues are reviewed.

Depression and Suicide. PBS. Focuses on two high schools at which a student has recently committed suicide.

Depression: Back from the Bottom. FHS. This program explains the symptoms of depression and the range of treatment options, from antidepressant medication to electroconvulsive therapy (ECT). It also explains the differences between the old and new ECT procedures, showing how ECT is thought to stimulate the brain's neurotransmitters, restoring the brain's chemical balance. Two patients, both suffering from severe depression, explain what it feels like to be severely depressed and how they manage to go on.

Depression: Beyond the Darkness. IM. Examines misconceptions about the nature of depression and explores various theories about its causation.

Depression: Biology of the Blues. FHS. The biological causes of depression, the difference between sadness and depression, the functions of drug therapies and electroconvulsive therapy, and the neurotransmitter imbalances that are involved.

Depression: Biology of the Blues. FHS. This program focuses on the biological rather than the psychosocial causes of depression--a crippling mental illness that can cause death through suicide, starvation, and secondary illness brought on by lack of care. Researchers in the field of mood disorders explain the difference between sadness and depression, the function of drug therapies, and the findings that point to neurotransmitter imbalances as a cause of depression; the use of electroconvulsive therapy on seriously depressed patients; and the ongoing research into genetic components of depression.

Depression: The Shadowed Valley. NET. An overview of the etiology and manifestation of depressive symptoms.

Dying to Be Heard...Is Anybody Listening? FHS. This program offers specific advice on how to recognize teens in danger of committing suicide and successfully intervene. It talks to teens who have attempted suicide, about their reasons for trying and about their lives after treatment, and it profiles a Texas community that banded together to stop a rash of teen suicides, showing how it turned tragedy into triumph.

Elderly Suicide. FHS. Suicide is an increasingly common choice as the perceived alternative to chronic disease and pain, waning mental and physical powers, economic

218

stress, and fear of helplessness and total dependence. In its wake, it often leaves family members with unassuageable guilt.

Gifted Adolescents and Suicide. FHS. Explains the suicide risks of over-achieving teens.

Grief. FHS. An in-depth look at paintings depicting grief by Giotto, Grunewald, El Greco, David, and Bacon.

Interview with a Depressive. PSU. This video is part of a continuing series. It depicts a man suffering from some of the classic symptoms of depression.

Men, Depression, and Desperation. FHS. Men can be overwhelmed by crisis--death, divorce, job loss--and often seek escape through isolation, drugs, or even suicide.
Mysteries of the Mind. FHS. Explores the neurochemical and genetic components of manic-depressive and mood disorders.

Suicide and The Police Officer. FHS. Suicide among police officers is an example of what can happen when those who protect others fail to protect and care for themselves. This program, produced by the New York City Police Foundation, focuses on the underlying problems, such as alcohol or drug abuse and severe relationship problems, that can lead to suicide. Discussion guide included.

Suicide: The Teenager's Perspective. FHS. This program deals with peer groups and one promising solution to the increasing number of teen suicides. Teenagers are accustomed to going to their friends with their problems; in this case, the friends have been trained to recognize the signs of impending suicide. In this program, Jim Wells, a nationally recognized expert on suicide, says that even as teens are taking their own lives, they do not really want to die. The purpose of this program is to provide some help before an attempt is made.

Suicide: The Parents' Perspective. FHS. When grief is compounded by guilt, all of the problems of bereavement are multiplied. This program seeks to help parents listen to their teenagers with greater awareness, not to place blame on parents for not hearing, but to help them identify the symptoms of serious trouble, and to recognize that all parents can do is their best, which is sometimes not enough to prevent suicide.

Teenage Suicide. FHS. This documentary explores some of the reasons teens commit suicide and the recent increase in suicides and describes some of the behavior patterns to which family and friends should be alerted. A young man who attempted suicide describes his calls for help and how he hoped they would be heeded.

Unmasking Depression. FHS. This program follows the lives of four adults in their prime years. We hear about their fears and emotional pain and their thoughts of suicide. The best part of the program comes when they explain how they overcame depression in ways that others can learn from.

Using Movies and Mental Illness as a Teaching Tool

The chapter on mood disorders in *Movies and Mental Illness* is replete with examples of depression, bipolar disorder, and suicide; many of the films discussed in the text have vivid and dramatic scenes that will serve to trigger class discussion.

The scene in which *Mr. Jones* is climbing on the center beam of a house provides a good illustration of the euphoria and disregard for personal safety sometimes seen in people with bipolar disorder.

Any of the films on the life of van Gogh (e.g., *Lust for Life, Vincent, Vincent & Theo*) will serve to get students thinking and talking about the life and untimely death of this fascinating artist, and it is a rewarding pedagogical exercise to have students debate his probably diagnosis. Numerous medical and psychiatric diagnoses have been proposed to explain the tragedy of van Gogh's life, but each diagnosis is based on speculation and conjecture. Van Gogh was treated at a mental hospital in Saint-Remy and committed suicide near the hospital at the age of 37. If a film is *not* shown in class, you may want to consider using Don Mclean's song *Vincent* as a prelude to the class discussion of this man's unhappy life.

It will be useful to have your students discuss the ways in which bystanders handled suicidal characters in films like *Scent of a Woman* and *The Hospital*. These films will also support a discussion of risk and lethality. For example, Colonel Slade (Al Pacino) is at dramatically increased risk for suicide because of his apparent alcoholism, his love of guns and his military history; Dr. Herbert Bock (George C. Scott) is at high risk because of his alcoholism, his profession, and his special knowledge of pharmacology and easy access to lethal medications.

The biographical film *Mishima* ends with a ritualistic stabbing that may serve as a springboard for discussion of cross-cultural attitudes about suicide. The extraordinary Italian film *Umberto D.* presents a poignant examination of suicide as a realistic alternative to a life of poverty and loneliness. Both films contain multiple scenes that will be appropriate to use as triggers to generate class discussion.

Any professor dealing with suicide scenes from films needs to be prepared to deal with the strong emotions the films can produce in the student who has lost a loved one to suicide.

Movie	Link to Chapter	Page Reference to Wedding and Boyd
• Scent of a Woman • The Hospital • The Bell Jar	major depression (p. 240)	p. 53 p. 54 p. 58
• Mr. Jones • Call Me Anna • Lust for Life • A Woman Under the Influence • Mommie Dearest	bipolar disorder (p. 242)	p. 49 p. 52 p. 58 p. 62 p. 62
• The Hospital • One Flew Over the Cuckoo's Nest • Dead Poets Society • Night, Mother • Scent of a Woman • Ordinary People • The Tenant • Network • The End	suicide (p. 248)	p. 54 p. 55 p. 59 p. 60 p. 53 p. 61 p. 63 p. 63 p. 63
• An Angel at My Table • One Flew Over the Cuckoo's Nest	electroconvulsive therapy (p. 268)	p. 55 p. 55

Classroom Assessment Techniques (CAT)

Memory Matrix (CAT 9-1)
Students should use the handout provided to review the purposes, functions, and importance of key terms.

Focused Listing (CAT 9-2)
Select an important point from this chapter (e.g., depression, premorbid adjustment, catecholamine hypothesis) and ask students to write five words or phrases that describe the point.

Learning Review (CAT 9-3)
Students are to write in order five of the most important ideas they learned in this chapter.

Muddiest Point (CAT 9-4)
Instruct students to write about an issue, concept, or definition presented in Chapter 9 that they find most confusing or difficult to understand.

Suggestions for Essay Questions

- How is clinical depression different from the "blues" that most people experience?
- Describe the differences and similarities between major depression and bipolar disorder.
- One of your friends is clinical depressed. She asks you about the effectiveness of drug therapy versus psychotherapy. What is your reasoned response to you?
- Describe the genetic research examining mood disorders.

Memory Matrix
Classroom Assessment Technique

Key Terms	Function/Purpose/Importance
depression	

Maladaptive Statements
Handout

Maladaptive Statement	Adaptive Statement
In order to be happy, I have to be successful in whatever I undertake.	
If I make a mistake, it means that I am inept.	
If somebody disagrees with me, it means he doesn't like me.	
Everyone I interact with must like me, otherwise it means I'm not a good person.	
I need to get an "A" in all my classes.	
When bad things happen, I must dwell on them.	
Things outside of my control cause unhappiness.	
I have no control over how I feel.	
If I failed in something in the past, chances are I will fail at it again.	

Chapter 10

Personality Disorders

Chapter Map

Section	Instructor Manual Components
Eccentric Personality Disorders • Paranoid Personality Disorder • Schizotypal Personality Disorder • Schizoid Personality Disorder	*A new classification system for personality disorders (LL 10-1)* *Experiencing components of personality disorders (TP 10-1)* *Causing problems (TP 10-2)* *Helpful traits (TP 10-3)* *Insight into problem (TP 10-4)* *Fringe beliefs (TP 10-5)* *Differential diagnosis for personality disorders (TP 10-6)* *Create your own personality disorder (ACT/DEMO 10-1)*
Dramatic/Emotional Personality Disorder • Borderline Personality Disorder • Histrionic Personality Disorder • Narcissistic Personality Disorder	*Transitional objects and borderline personality disorders* *(LL 10-2)* *Gender bias in personality disorders (TP 10-7)* *Mnemonic for borderline personality disorder (TP 10-8)* *Differential diagnosis and overlap (ACT/DEMO 10-2)*
Anxious/Fearful Personality Disorder • Avoidant Personality Disorder • Dependent Personality Disorder • Obsessive-Compulsive Personality Disorder	*Examples of personality disorders (TP 10-9)* *Role playing personality disorders (ACT/DEMO 10-3)*

Groups at Risk • Comorbidity • The Dispute over Gender Bias • Cultural Bias	*Comorbidity in personality disorders (LL 10-3)* *Suicide risk and personality disorders (LL 10-4)*
Personality Disorders: Theory and Treatment • The Psychodynamic Perspective • The Behavioral Perspective • The Cognitive Perspective • The Sociocultural Perspective • The Biological Perspective	*Object relations in personality disorders (LL 10-5)* *Personality disorders and therapist-client sex (LL 10-6)* *Nature and nurture in personality disorders (LL 10-7* *Getting inside the heads of the personality disorders (ACT/DEMO 10-4)*

Chapter Outline

I.   Introduction
    A.   **Personality disorders** are conditions that involve stable traits of entire personality
        1.   Personality traits are enduring patterns of perceiving, relating to, and thinking about environment and oneself exhibited in wide range of contexts
        2.   Personality traits when inflexible and maladaptive and cause significant functional impairment or subjective distress, constitute personality disorder
    B.   Debate over diagnostic value of personality disorders
        1.   Not particularly reliable
        2.   Diagnostic criteria more specific to address diagnostic overlap
        3.   Assumes stable personality traits

II.   Odd/Eccentric Personality Disorders
    A.   Paranoid Personality Disorder
        1.   Defining characteristic of **paranoid personality disorder** is suspiciousness
            a.   Suspiciousness causes constant scanning environment for evidence to support suspicions
            b.   Suspiciousness affects emotional adjustment and social relationships
            c.   Individual sees problems originating from others, not themselves
        2.   Paranoid personality disorder differs from paranoid schizophrenia or delusional disorder; paranoid personality disorder is less disabling
    B.   Schizotypal Personality Disorder
        1.   **Schizotypal personality disorder** characterized by odd speech, behavior, thinking, and/or perception, but not odd enough for schizophrenia
        2.   Often have histories of being teased and participation in fringe groups
        3.   Disorder added to improve diagnosis of schizophrenia
    C.   Schizoid Personality Disorder
        1.   Defining characteristic of **schizoid personality disorder** is severely restricted range of emotions associated with social detachment
        2.   Appear to have little/no interest in relationships; do not seem to experience ordinary emotions such as pleasure, warmth
        3.   Appear to take pleasure in solitary activities; may appear to be self-absorbed

4. Do not show typical patterns of thoughts, behaviors, speech of schizophrenia
5. There may be biological relationship to schizophrenia

III. Dramatic/Emotional Personality Disorders
    A. Borderline Personality Disorder
        1. **Borderline personality disorder** proposed by psychodynamic
        2. Syndrome has four core elements
            a. Difficulties in establishing secure self-identity
            b. Distrust
            c. Impulsive and self-destructive behavior
            d. Difficulty in controlling anger and other emotions
        3. May be due to abnormalities in limbic system
        4. Some have argued borderline personality disorder related to depression
        5. Is one of most frequently diagnosed personality disorders
    B. Histrionic Personality Disorder
        1. Self-dramatization is essential feature of **histrionic personality disorder**
        2. Emotional displays often manipulative to gain attention and sympathy
        3. Interpersonal relationships are fragile
            a. In relationships, can become demanding
            b. Typically flirtatious and sexually provocative
        4. Most of those diagnosed with histrionic personality disorder are women
    C. Narcissistic Personality Disorder
        1. In **narcissistic personality disorder** individual has grandiose sense of self-importance, sometimes with feelings of inferiority
        2. Bragging of talent and achievements often accompanied by fragile self-esteem
        3. Individuals are poorly equipped for friendship or love
            a. Demand great deal from others such as affection, favors
            b. Typically have long histories of erratic interpersonal relationships
        4. Resembles histrionic personality disorder
            a. What narcissistic type wants is admiration
            b. What histrionic type wants is concern
        5. Psychoanalytic theory suggests cause is compensation for inadequate affection and approval from parents in early childhood
        6. Social learning theory suggests parents' inflated views of their children's talents leading to unrealistic expectation is cause

IV. Anxious/Fearful Personality Disorders
    A. Avoidant Personality Disorder

1. **Avoidant personality disorder** marked by social withdrawal
2. Social withdrawal based on fear of rejection
    a. Has hypersensitivity to possibility of rejection, humiliation, or shame
    b. Tends to avoid relationships unless sure of other's uncritical affection
3. Avoidant personalities have low self-esteem
4. Difficult to differentiate from social phobia
    a. Social phobia restricted to specific situations
    b. Avoidant personality disorder affects almost every day of person's life
B. Dependent Personality Disorder
    1. Dependence on others characterizes **dependent personality disorder**
    2. Fear of abandonment underlies dependency
    3. May grow tolerate of unacceptable behaviors of others leading to a vicious cycle leading to more helpless feelings
    4. Overlap with borderline personalities, borderline personality is more disabling
C. Obsessive-Compulsive Personality Disorder
    1. Excessive preoccupation with orderliness, perfectionism, and control describe **obsessive-compulsive personality disorder**
    2. Overly concerned with mechanics of efficiency
    3. Obsessive-compulsive personality disorder differs from obsessive-compulsive disorder
        a. Personality disorder is milder and more pervasive
        b. Personality disorder is more common
    4. While seen as "workaholics," typically perfection prevents them from making decisions and meeting deadlines
    5. Treatment is sought only after personal tragedies like divorces, loneliness, and stress

V. Groups at Risk
    A. Comorbidity
        1. Personality disorders rare in general population, but may be common in clinical populations
        2. People at risk for personality disorders are those who are in psychological treatment for other disorders
            a. Most do not seek treatment for personality disorders
            b. Treatment is sought for more specific problems; in treatment personality disorder is identified
    B. The Dispute over Gender Bias
        1. Men are at higher risk for some personality disorders (i.e., paranoid, schizotypal, schizoid, narcissistic, obsessive-compulsive, antisocial)

2. Women are at higher risk for some personality disorders (i.e., borderline, dependent)
3. Diagnosticians view men and women differently
    a. Disorders that involve emotionalism more frequently diagnosed in women
    b. Disorders that involve self-importance or callousness more frequently diagnosed in men
    c. Differences may be due to idiom of distress
4. DSM-IV changes reflect recognition of gender bias and to create sex-blind criteria

C. Cultural Bias
1. Diagnosis assumes behavior is significantly different from expectations of one's culture
2. Diagnosticians must know individual's culture, but may bend over backwards to respect culture

VI. Personality Disorders: Theory and Therapy
A. The Psychodynamic Perspective
1. Character Disorders
    a. Personality disorders due to disturbances in parent-child relationship
    b. Severe personality disorders originate in separation, individual process
    c. Results in weakened ego and poor adaptive functioning
    d. Fall between neurotics and psychotics in terms of ego strength
        i. Normal coping behavior has broken down
        ii. Replaced by erratic, distorted or deviant behavior
        iii. Breakdown affects broad range of ego functions
    e. Introjection believed to play role in personality disorders
2. Psychotherapy for Personality Disorders
    a. Individuals generally resistant to treatment
    b. Psychodynamic therapy takes more directive, more parental approach with personality disorders than with other disorders
    c. Insight still believed to be mechanism of change

B. The Behavioral Perspective
1. Skills, Acquisition, Modeling, and Reinforcement
    a. Families often expect children to be cheerful; parents do not coddle; child never able to get sympathy for minor upsets
    b. As children, individuals never learn emotional skills that would allow them to take problems to parents
    c. Reinforcement and modeling may play role in personality disorders

2.   New Learning
      a.   Patients need social skills training and assertiveness training
      b.   **Dialectical behavior therapy** used with borderline patients combining social skills training and how to regulate emotions and tolerate distress

C.   The Cognitive Perspective
    1.   Faulty Schemas
      a.   Personality disorders seen as product of distortions or exaggerations in underlying schemas
      b.   Schemas are not perceived to be faculty; person will generate and perceptions and situations that confirm schemas
      c.   Beliefs are acquired by learning and modeling in response to developmental conditions
      d.   In personality disorders, schemas which are seen as being on continuum, involved schemas pushed to end of range
    2.   Altering Schemas
      a.   Goal of therapy is to alter the schema
      b.   Therapists attempt to convince patient to modify, reinterpret, or camouflage schema
          i.   Reinterpretation refers to putting it to more functional use
          ii.   Schematic camouflage refers to helping patient to act in more socially acceptable ways

D.   The Sociocultural Perspective
    1.   Personality disorders due to large-scale social processes
    2.   Therapy should focus on changing society

E.   The Biological Perspective
    1.   Genes and Personality
      a.   Genes play influential role in development of normal personality
      b.   Studies reveal relationship of personality disorders to Axis I disorders that have genetic component
    2.   Drug Treatment
      a.   Personality disorders can be alleviated by drugs used for their Axis I counterparts
      b.   Some personality disorders have no drug treatments as yet
      c.   Drugs and Diagnosis
          i.   Evidence raises diagnostic questions about reclassified patients with Axis I disorders
          ii.   Drugs treat a symptom common to both personality disorders and Axis I disorders

Chapter Boxes

- Impulse-Control Disorders
    - A. **Impulse-control disorders** involve the failure to resist impulses to act in a way harmful to oneself or others
    - B. Most common are trichotillomania and pathological gambling
    - C. Pathological gambling occurs in stages resulting in a compulsion to gamble and desperation
    - D. Trichotillomania involves pulling out body hair

- Politics and Personality Disorders
    - A. Gender imbalance in personality disorder may result in politics
    - B. Histrionic personality disorders resembles age-old stereotype of women
    - C. When women act in stereotypic ways, society labels them as disturbed
    - D. DSM-IV reflects gender politics; for example self-defeating personality disorder and sadistic personality disorder
    - E. Evidence suggests that some abused women may behave in ways that might constitute personality disorders
    - F. Person whose behavior is considered abnormal is excused from moral and criminal responsibility
    - G. Diagnoses influenced by politics
    - H. Question of diagnosis must be, does it describe a condition that actually exists

Learning Objectives (LO)

By the time you have finished studying this chapter, you should be able to do the following:

1. Define a personality disorder according to *DSM-IV* criteria, and discuss the reliability of this diagnostic category (274).

2. List and describe the essential characteristics of the three odd/eccentric personality disorders [paranoid, schizotypal, and schizoid] (275-277).

3. List and describe the essential characteristics of the three dramatic/emotional personality disorders [borderline, histrionic, and narcissistic] discussed in the chapter (277-280).

4. List and describe the essential characteristics of the three anxious/fearful personality disorders [avoidant, dependent, and obsessive-compulsive] (280-282).

5. Distinguish between paranoid personality disorder, delusional disorder, and paranoid schizophrenia, and distinguish between obsessive-compulsive personality disorder and obsessive-compulsive disorder (276, 282).

6. Summarize the population statistics regarding personality disorders, and give four examples of impulse-control disorders (282-284).

7. Discuss the psychodynamic perspective on the development of personality disorders, and summarize the psychodynamic approach to the treatment of these problems (286-287).

8. Discuss personality disorders and their treatment from the behavioral and cognitive perspectives (287-289).

9. Explain the sociocultural perspective's view of personality disorder, including reference to political issues that complicate attempts to define and diagnose these disorders (284-286, 289-290).

10. Summarize genetic and biochemical research into the causes and treatment of personality disorders (290-291).

Lecture Leads (LL)

A new classification system for personality disorders (LL 10-1)
Even thought the current classification system for personality disorders has face validity, the overlap between disorders makes its practical use difficult. Peter Tyrer suggests a new classification based on severity, with the disorders divided into three clusters (i.e., flamboyant, withdrawn/eccentric, anxious/fearful). There would be four severity levels: no personality disorder, personality difficulty, personality disorder in one cluster, and personality disorder in one or two or more clusters. The author argues that the reliability of assessment would be greatly improved.

Resource:
Tyrer, P. (1996). New ways of classifying personality disorders. <u>Psychiatriki</u>, <u>7</u>, 43-48.

Transitional objects and borderline personality disorders (LL 10-2)
Laporta confirmed others' observations that many individuals who are admitted and later diagnosed with borderline personality disorder carry-in either blankets or stuffed animals. This provides support for the role that objects may play in personality disorder.

Resource:
Laporta, L. D. (1997). Borderline personality disorder and transitional objects. <u>American Journal of Psychiatry</u>, <u>154</u>, 1484-1485.

Comorbidity in personality disorders (LL 10-3)
As the textbook describes, there is significant overlap between personality disorders and Axis I disorders. A study by Tyrer, Gunderson, Lyons, and Tohen investigated the degree of relationships found in the overlap. They reported that the strongest association was among substance abuse with cluster B (dramatic/erratic), the anxiety disorders with cluster C (fearful/anxious), and somatization and clusters B and C personality disorders. The importance of further study lies in the possibility that comorbidity between Axis I and personality disorders may affect the outcome of treatment in unknown ways. Tyrer et al. suggested that there are certain personality traits that predispose the individual to particular mental disorders that are indicated on Axis I.

Resource:
Tyrer, P., Gunderson, J., Lyons, M., & Tohen, M. (1997). Extent of comorbidity between mental state and personality disorders. <u>Journal of Personality Disorders</u>, <u>11</u>, 242-259.

Suicide risk and personality disorders (LL 10-4)
Suicide is a clinical concern in some instances when a client is diagnosed as having a personality disorder. In an attempt to better understand the relationship between personality disorders and suicide risk, Isometsa et al. (1996) took a random sample of 229 subjects who committed suicide during a 12-month period in Finland. The researchers

conducted psychological autopsies on each of the victims and identified 67 that met the DSM-III-R criteria for personality disorders. An interesting initial finding was that of the 67, 43 of the victims would have been diagnosed with a cluster B personality disorder (i.e., dramatic/erratic), 23 would have been diagnosed with a cluster C disorder (i.e., anxious/fearful), and one would have been diagnosed with a cluster A disorder (i.e., eccentric/odd). In comparison to a matched set of suicide victims who did not meet the criteria for personality disorders, the researchers found that suicide victims with personality disorders were more likely than the matched controls to have depressive symptoms, psychoactive substance use disorders, or both. Further, it was found that those victims with cluster B disorders were more likely than comparison subjects to have psychoactive substance abuse disorders and a history of previous nonfatal suicide attempts. Although this research is retrospective in nature, the results highlight which combination of factors may be more likely to predict suicide in clients diagnosed with personality disorders.

Resource:
Isometsa, E. T., Henrikson, M. M., Heikkinen, M. E., Aro, Fl. M., Marttunen, M. J., Kuoppasalmi, K. I., & Lonnqvist, J. K. (I 996). Suicide among subjects with personality disorders. <u>American Journal of Psychiatry</u>, <u>153</u>, 667-673.

Object relations in personality disorders (LL 10-5)
Since personality disorders are often manifested in terms of relationships with others, it makes sense that some of the maladaptive traits seen in individuals with personality disorders could potentially have their origins in early relationships with parents and other adults. Recent research by Nigg et al. indicates that the internal "object world" of individuals with borderline personality disorder (BDP) is littered with malevolent object representations. The authors assessed the object representations of clients with BDP using the Early Memories Test (EMF). For comparison, the authors also assessed the object representations of a group of individuals with major depressive disorders and a group of individuals without any psychiatric diagnoses. The results indicate that the object representations of clients with BDP were more likely to contain themes of malevolence in relation to their "objects". Consider the following Early Memory narrative: {My earliest memory?} First day of kindergarten, I imagine-running out of the classroom and being stopped by the superintendent. I remember him pushing me down on the bench and hitting my head on the wall, and crying, and my brother came from another classroom to help, and the superintendent made him go back into his classroom and I had to stay outside. (Nigg et al., 1992, p. 60). This kind of behavioral inconsistency from individuals children regard as models may be the source of BDP. The authors contend that these kinds of object representations need to be considered in any explanation of the causes of BDP.

Resource:
Nigg, J. T., Lotir, N. E., Westen, D., Gold, L. J., & Silk, K. R. (1992). Malevolent object representations in borderline personality disorder and major depression. <u>Journal of Abnormal Psychology</u>, <u>101</u>, 61-67.

Personality disorders and therapist-client sex (LL 10-6)

Research on the effects of therapist-client sex is fraught with methodological limitations to the extent that conclusions regarding the level of harm caused are not clear. It has been suggested that Therapist-Patient Sex Syndrome may result from such a relationship, and includes guilt, feelings of isolation, lability, identity and boundary disturbances, and an inability to trust. Williams outlines three reasons why it is difficult to accurately assess the level of harm following sexual relationships among therapist and client. One of the reasons centers on the nature of borderline and histrionic personality disorders. It is argued that these two personality disorders often resemble the Therapist-Patient Sex Syndrome. The implication here is the question of whether actual sex between therapist and patient caused Therapist-Patient Sex Syndrome. As Williams pointed out, "if such patients are in fact at greater risk for therapist-patient sex, this would create sampling bias by assuming that many or most patients who had sex with their therapists would manifest harm that may have predated the sexual abuse."

Resource:

Williams, M. H. (1995). How useful are clinical reports concerning the consequences of therapist-patient sex? American Journal of Psychotherapy, 49, 237-243.

Nature and nurture in personality disorders (LL 10-7)

It is important to recognize nature and nurture as interacting rather than polar forces in contributing to the development of personality (Rutter, 1997). Perhaps one of the more common of the personality disorders is borderline personality disorder which involves extreme emotional lability. Paris suggests a combination of biological factors, such as innate temperamental traits of high impulsivity and emotional instability, as well as lower levels of serotonin. Psychological histories for these individuals are inconsistent, while some clients describe extreme neglect, or physical and/or sexual abuse, others claim to have had normal childhoods. Social factors may be involved in terms of not providing emotional security or consistency. Paris suggested that it is the interaction of all three of these elements that lead to the disorder. Different treatment modalities are necessary, depending on the specific disorder, which includes its genetic and environmental antecedents. Without understanding the interactive causes of these disorders, we are not only taking a shot in the dark at whether we are effectively treating a disorder, it but may, as Rice noted, take a chance that the a cure will backfire. As the "nature versus nurture" debate continues, perhaps, as Rutter suggested, it is time to stop seeing each of these factors as being mutually exclusive of the other, but rather, to look to their interaction with each other.

Resources:

Paris, J. (1997). Borderline personality disorder: What is it, what causes it? How can we treat it? The Journal, 8, 1-3. Available: URL WWW http://www.mhsource.com/hy/j8l.html.

Rutter, M. L. (1997). Nature-nurture integration. American Psychologist, 52, 390-398.

Talking Points (TP)

Experiencing components of personality disorders (TP 10-1)
One of the things that makes diagnosis of personality disorders difficult is that we all have shown characteristics of the personality disorders. Truth be known, each of us has some quirks and mannerisms that come close to schizotypal personality disorder. Probably, most of us have had suspicions about others that were not valid. Now and then, we are dramatically and emotionally labile. Ask students for more specific examples of how normal behavior may reflect personality disorders.

Causing problems (TP 10-2)
It is often said that people with personality disorders cause more problems for their significant others and friends than they do for themselves. Lead a discussion to explore why this statement is probably true.

Helpful traits (TP 10-3)
Ask your students to think of situations, occupations, or contexts where having certain personality traits is quite helpful. An actor, for example, would be well served if he or she possessed some histrionic traits. An author who is schizotypal might be more successful when writing horror stories. A forest wilderness lookout could have avoidant traits. Would paranoid personality disorder be adaptive for a CIA undercover operative? How about obsessive-compulsive personality disorder in an accountant or a quality assurance specialist? Are there other examples?

Insight into problem (TP 10-4)
When asked if they have any psychological problems, many individuals with personality disorders will say that they do not have any problems. Discuss the reason for this feeling. Possible areas for discussion could center on the definition of personality disorder as long standing maladaptive behaviors. Ask the students how they would convince the individual that he or she has a problem.

Fringe beliefs (TP 10-5)
Many New Age religions incorporate magical thinking, beliefs in the power of crystals, talking to past (dead) ascended masters, and belief in reincarnation. Discuss whether these people are simply schizotypal or have some other types of disorders. You may want to discuss faking of this power for other gains also.

Differential diagnosis for personality disorders (TP 10-6)
One case underscores how it may be difficult to accurately diagnose personality disorders. A sixty-five-year-old man was showing behavior consistent with paranoid personality disorder. These changes in his personality and behavior were not due to any personality disorder, but to frontal lobe dementia. Once again, ask students to consider the importance of accurate assessment and diagnosis.

Gender bias in personality disorders (TP 10-7)

Before you introduce the topic of gender bias, use an overhead transparency to list the stereotypic behaviors and traits of males and females. On the same transparency write the behaviors and traits of personality disorders and the prevalence rates for each gender. Ask students to draw any conclusions based on the information on the transparency. Discuss the importance of gender role and patient expectations in the etiology of these disorders, as well as therapist expectation in their diagnosis. Many of the personality disorders seem to reflect what in our culture has been defined as either more masculine or feminine traits

Mnemonic for borderline personality disorder (TP 10-8)
Senger (1997) has developed a mnemonic for borderline personality disorder: "IMPULSIVE"-- Impulsiveness, Moodiness, Paranoia, Unstable self-image, Labile intense relationships, Suicidal gestures, Inappropriate anger, Vulnerability to abandonment, and Emptiness.

Examples of personality disorders (TP 10-9)
Ask students for illustrations of personality disorder portrayed on TV, soap operas, movies, fiction, and nonfiction. Here are some possible examples: Sam Malone (*Cheers*) narcissistic personality disorder, J. R. Ewing (*Dallas*) antisocial personality disorder; Kramer (*Seinfeld*); schizotypal personality disorder; George (*Seinfeld*) paranoid personality disorder; the Anal Retentive Chef (*Saturday Night Live*) obsessive-compulsive personality disorder; Marsha Brady (*The Brady Bunch*) borderline personality disorder; Jim Ignatowski (*Taxi)* schizotypal personality disorder, Whitley Gilbert (*A Different World*) histrionic personality disorder. You could develop this into a classroom activity.

Cross-Cultural Teaching

decisive break in reality contact that characterizes those very **grave** conditions.	p. 275
the neighbors are **blaring music** at night...	p. 276
others join **fringe political groups.**	p. 276
often become embroiled in hostile disputes, which may **escalate to lawsuits.**	p. 276
self-proclaimed **alien abduction survivors**...	p. 276
joy, happiness, **gaiety,** and pleasure is completely lacking	p. 277
may appear absentminded--"**out of it**"...	p. 277
dominate the entire dinner party with the tale of their **faith healing**..	p. 278
a **meteoric rise** thought the **company ranks**	p. 279
they are generally **stiff** and formal in their dealings with others...	p. 282
continues to win as **beginner's luck**...	p. 283
whether it is possible to create "**sex-blind**" criteria...	p. 286
may seem "**macho**"...	p. 286
Such parents do not **coddle.**	p. 287
other "**goody-goody**" behaviors...	p. 288

239

Activities and Demonstrations (ACT/DEMO)

Create your own personality disorder (ACT/DEMO 10-1)
Objective: To illustrate the difficulty of classifying personality disorders and how culture and background influences classification
Materials: None
Procedure: In this activity, students are to create their own personality disorder. They are to describe a syndrome, name it, and put it into one of the three DSM-IV clusters. Next, students ought to get into small groups and share their creation. The groups should analyze how their culture, experiences, and background have influenced their personality disorder. Specifically, does the "disorder" reflect religion bias, gender bias, regional bias (e.g., rural vs urban), student bias (e.g., fraternity, major), political correctness, and political bias?
Discussion: Each group should select one person to present their disorder to the rest of the class. In this large group, you should keep track of how students have created and described their own disorders.

Differential diagnosis and overlap (ACT/DEMO 10-2)
Objective: To demonstrate the difficulty of diagnosis.
Materials: Ambiguous description of an individual with a mental disorder.
Procedure: Develop a description based on your own expertise and preferences for a personality disorder. Start with a discussion of and short lecture on the different personality disorders. Have the students form small groups of four or five students each. A problem with the DSM-IV is the overlap in symptoms between personality disorders. For example, impulsivity is a symptom in many of the disorders. Have each group try to decide on a diagnosis based on the DSM-IV criteria.
Discussion: Have a group spokesperson present the group diagnosis. On an overhead transparency summarize each group's decision. Many of the groups will have different diagnoses depending on how well you have chosen the description. Lead a discussion on the difficulties in differential diagnosis. Have students generate more exclusive criteria that might be useful in these diagnoses. Ask for relevant cultural examples, where the diagnoses could be affected.

Role playing personality disorders (ACT/DEMO 10-3)
Objective: To identify the types of behaviors and thoughts associated with personality disorders
Materials: None
Procedure: Have the students individually or in small groups select one of the personality disorders. Their task is to develop a role play to illustrate the disorder as well as other information (e.g., effect on family, demographics, suspected etiology, treatment perspectives). An example might be a psychologist interviewing a client; the interview could illustrate comorbidity issues. Another example of a role play could be an interaction of a histrionic personality with others at a party. Tell the students that they have at least overnight to prepare for their disorder and that they will be expected to role play the disorder in front of the class. If using groups, one person plays the role of the

240

subject, and other group members can play family members, employers, friends, and clinician.

Discussion: Give feedback on the accuracy of the role play. Ask students to comment on the accuracy of the role play and to guess what disorder was being portrayed.

Getting inside the heads of the personality disorders (ACT/DEMO 10-4)
Objective: To identify the types of personality disorders
Materials: Handout
Procedure: Each student is to develop a thought that would be characteristic of each of the personality disorders presented in the chapter. For example, what would an individual with paranoid personality disorder think that would be descriptive of the disorder? When all are done, have the students get into groups to review and critique their responses.
Discussion: Select a sample of responses. Write the "thoughts" on an overhead transparency linking them to the diagnostic criteria.

Films and Videos

Personality. CRM. Explores the complexity of personality development.

Personality Disorders. ANN/CPB. A section of the *World of Abnormal Psychology* series.

The Psychopath/Antisocial Personality. Nature or Nurture. PBS. One of the Mind Video Modules. Looks at the characteristics of a psychopathic criminal and how he came to be that way.

Closet Narcissistic Disorder. The Masterson Approach. CRM. Series of videos that demonstrates various forms of treatment for a wide range of disorders. This video does a reenactment of therapy sessions with a patient presenting with chronic chest pains, although there is no physiological basis for the pain. Axis I diagnosis is undifferentiated somatoform disorder, Axis II diagnosis is personality disorder not otherwise specified.

Diagnosis According to the DSM-IV. FHS. Presents a diagnostic interview demonstrating antisocial personality disorder (Program 3). After the interview, there is a round-table discussion by the clinicians participating in the entire series to highlight their reactions and the specific behaviors that led to the diagnosis.

Using Movies and Mental Illness as a Teaching Tool

Students love watching and discussing *Fatal Attraction*, and the film is a provocative and useful introduction to the complexities of the diagnosis of borderline personality. Students can debate the accuracy of Wedding and Boyd's Patient Evaluation, they can complain about the contrived ending to the movie, and they can use the film as a starting place of a debate over whether or not personality disorders are bona fide examples of mental illness. Class time will be well spent if the class instructor goes through the "Questions to Consider" at the beginning of the chapter on Personality Disorders in *Movies and Mental Illness.*

Students will enjoy reviewing the list of films selected by Wedding and Boyd to illustrate personality disorders (Appendix B). The main character in many of these films will be found to have an antisocial personality. A film like *Silence of the Lambs* can be used as a wonderful starting place for a discussion of *evil* and whether or not the concept has any utility for psychologists and psychiatrists. (It is also fun to speculate with your students about whether or not Hannibal Lecter could *really* have completed a medical education and a psychiatric residency.)

There are some wonderful scenes of a histrionic Katharine Hepburn in *Long Day's Journey Into Night*. The film also allows the class to discuss whether or not there is a relationship between personality disorders and substance abuse.

242

Movie	Link to Chapter	Page Reference to Wedding and Boyd
• The Caine Mutiny	Paranoid Personality Disorder (p.275)	p. 76
• sex, lies, and videotape • Jeremiah Johnson • The Accidental Tourist	Schizoid Personality Disorder (p. 276)	p. 70 p. 77 p. 77
• Harold and Maude • Taxi Driver	Schizotypal Personality Disorder (p. 277)	p. 71 p. 77
• Fatal Attraction	Borderline Personality Disorder (p. 277)	p. 65
• Long Day's Journey Into Night • La Cage aux Folles	Histrionic Personality Disorder (p. 278)	p. 73 p. 74
• Bugsy • The Doctor	Narcissistic Personality Disorder (p. 279)	p. 74 p. 74
• What About Bob?	Dependent Personality Disorder (p. 281)	p. 75
• The Odd Couple	Obsessive Compulsive Personality Disorder (p. 281)	p. 76

Classroom Assessment Techniques (CAT)

Learning Review (CAT 10-1)
Students are to write in order five of the most important ideas they learned in this chapter.

Muddiest Point (CAT 10-2)
Instruct students to write about an issue, concept, or definition presented in Chapter 10 that they find most confusing or difficult to understand.

Minute Paper (CAT 10-3)
Ask your students to write about an important question they have that remains unanswered.

Suggestions for Essay Questions

- ❑ Why are personality disorders difficult to diagnose?
- ❑ If Freud could describe his understanding of the personality disorders, what would he say?
- ❑ Write a case study of an individual with borderline personality disorder. Make sure you integrate appropriate background and assessment information into your case study.

Getting inside the heads of the personality disorders
Handout

Personality Disorder   **Characteristic Thought**

Paranoid personality disorder

Schizotypal personality disorder

Schizoid personality disorder

Borderline personality disorder

Histrionic personality disorder

Narcissistic personality disorder

Avoidant personality disorder

Dependent personality disorder

Obsessive-compulsive personality disorder

Chapter 11

Substance Use Disorders

Chapter Map

Section	Instructor Manual Components
The Nature of Substance Dependence and Abuse	*Real people (TP 11-1)* *Drug use vs. drug abuse (TP 11-2)* *Keeping track (TP 11-3)*
Alcohol Dependence • The Social Cost of Alcohol Dependence • The Personal Cost of Alcohol Dependence • The Development of Alcohol Dependence • Groups at Risk for Alcohol Abuse and Dependence • Treatment of Alcohol Dependence	*Development of a drinking problem (LL 11-1)* *Gender differences in drinking patterns (LL 11-2)* *Alcohol's cost (TP 11-4)* *Messages in alcohol and cigarette print ads* *(ACT/DEMO 11-1)*
Nicotine Dependence • The Antismoking Movement • Legal Remedies • Nicotine Dependence: Theory and Therapy	*Natural history of smoking (LL 11-3)* *Hearing loss and smoking (LL 11-4)* *Nicotine: The "skeleton key" (TP 11-5)* *Preventing smoking (TP 11-6)* *Smoking cessation (TP 11-7)*

Other Psychoactive Drugs • Depressants • Stimulants • Hallucinogens • Marijuana and Hashish • Groups at Risk for Abuse of Illegal Drugs	*Caffeinism (LL 11-5)* *Comorbidity: PTSD and cocaine dependence (LL 11-6)* *Drug factory in your head (TP 11-8)* *Coca-Cola was literally coke (TP 11-9)* *Resolved: Marijuana should be decriminalized* *(ACT/DEMO 11-2)*
Substance Dependence: Theory and Treatment • The Psychodynamic Perspective • The Behavioral Perspective • The Family Systems Perspective • The Cognitive Perspective • The Sociocultural Perspective • The Biological Perspective	*Relapse prevention and the AVE (LL 11-7)* *Culture and drug abuse (LL 11-8)* *High-risk situations (TP 11-10)* *The abstinence violation effect (TP 11-11)* *Drug testing (TP 11-12)* *Alcohol's heritability and its implication (TP 11-13)* *The 12 Steps of AA (TP 11-14)* *Pregnancy and drug use (TP 11-15)* *Support groups and self-help (LL 11-3)* *Debate on drug testing (LL 11-4)* *Community resources (ACT/DEMO 11-5)* *Developing a drug prevention program (ACT/DEMO 11-6)* *Guest speakers (ACT/DEMO 11-7)*

Chapter Outline

I.   Introduction
      A.   Most Americans use some form of **psychoactive drugs,** which are
           substances that alter psychological state
           1.   Legal drugs can be as harmful as illegal drugs
           2.   Psychoactive drugs can be very helpful
           3.   Some drugs are part of social and religious rituals
      B.   Drugs have become major focus of social concern
      C.   In many cases drugs are not used individually

II.   The Nature of Substance Dependence and Abuse
      A.   Clear and consistent terminology does not exist that affects discussion of
           drug abuse
           1.   Physiological and psychological need was differentiated
                a.   **Addiction** refereed to state when body requires drug in
                     order to feel normal
                b.   Psychological dependence refereed to user's tendency to
                     center life on the drug
                c.   All psychoactive drugs have both physiological and
                     psychological effects that cannot be separate
           2.   Substance dependence and abuse focuses on way person uses drug
                in that use causes problems
      B.   **Substance dependence** must meet three of several criteria
           1.   Preoccupation with drug
           2.   Unintentional overuse
           3.   **Tolerance--**the usual dose no longer produces desired effect
           4.   **Withdrawal--**when drug level is reduced, psychological and
                physical disruptions occur
           5.   Persistent desire or efforts to control drug use
           6.   Abandonment of important social, occupational, or recreational
                activities
           7.   Continued drug use despite serious drug-related problems
      C.   **Substance abuse** refers to drug use pattern that has not progressed to
           dependence and meets one of several criteria
           1.   Recurrent, drug-related failure to fulfill major role obligations
           2.   Recurrent drug use in physically dangerous situations
           3.   Drug-related legal problems
           4.   Continued drug use despite social or interpersonal problems

III. Alcohol Dependence
      A.   Alcohol is most widely used of all psychoactive drugs
      B.   Can be purchased legally in most parts of United States
      C.   The Social Cost of Alcohol Problems

1. Impossible to calculate social cost of alcohol problems
2. Easier to calculate monetary cost of alcohol problems
   a. Alcohol-related automobile accidents cost $13.8 billion in 1994
   b. Decreased work productivity cost $70 billion
   c. Treatment and support services for alcoholics cost $20 billion
   d. Alcohol-related motor vehicle accidents cost $12 billion
      i. Effects of alcohol dependent on **blood alcohol level**
      ii. Blood alcohol level expressed in terms of amount of alcohol in relation to specific volume of blood
      iii. Gender differences seen in blood alcohol level
      iv. Blood alcohol level of 0.10% considered to be intoxication; as level rises, impairments increase
      v. Most men killed in accidents were drunk at the time
      vi. Relationship exists between bad driving record and alcohol abuse; alcohol increases likelihood of injuries on job

D. The Personal Cost of Alcohol Dependence
   1. The Immediate Effects of Alcohol
      a. Alcohol is depressant
      b. Initial effect of alcohol may be to stimulate rather than to depress
         i. Changes in mood and social behavior
         ii. Changes in judgment
      c. Actual changes are related to expectancies regarding effects of alcohol and broader context
   2. The Long-Term Effects of Alcohol Abuse
      a. Alcohol often used to cope with stress
      b. Abuse can cause problems that leads to more stress and more drinking
      c. Physical problems can occur ,such as cirrhosis of the liver, malnutrition, Korsakoff's psychosis
      d. Delirium tremens are rare and is part of withdrawal
   3. The Development of Alcohol Dependence
      a. There is variability in development of dependence
      b. Most develop it slowly, through social drinking, blackouts, sneaking drinks, and morning drinking
      c. Most experience trouble stopping themselves once they start drinking and go on spree drinking and benders
   4. Groups at Risk for Alcohol Abuse and Dependence
      a. Different groups have different patterns of alcohol consumption
      b. Gender
         i. Men are more involved with alcohol than women

249

        ii.   There are gender differences in the patterns of use and abuse

        iii.   It is unclear if these differences reflect social role or biological differences

    d.   Race, Ethnicity, and Religion

        i.   There are racial differences, but they are often confounded by age and gender

        ii.   There are ethnic patterns of alcohol use and abuse; gender and age also influence patterns

        iii.   Native Americans are especially at risk and risk may be related to cultural norms, protest, and poverty

        iv.   Religion also related to alcohol abuse with conservative Protestants very resistant to alcohol problems

        v.   Catholics have high percentage of alcohol use and abuse

    e.   Age

        i.   Adults are drinking less, young people drinking more

        ii.   Almost half of all college students binge drink

        iii.   Advertisement and mixed messages may play role

5.   Treatment of Alcohol Dependence

    a.   Treatment of alcohol dependence begins with **detoxification** which is getting alcohol our of person's system and getting through withdrawal

    b.   Detoxification can take place at home, under outpatient care, or in the hospital

    c.   Multimodal Treatments

        i.   Effective multimodal treatments include occupational therapy, relaxation training, group and individual therapy, family and marital therapy, and job counseling

        ii.   May include Antabuse which interferes with metabolic processing of alcohol causing unpleasant reactions; patient may stop taking drug

    d.   Support Groups: Alcoholic Anonymous

        i.   Social support provides reminder that help is available

        ii.   Most widely known is Alcoholics Anonymous

        iii.   AA: once an alcoholic, always an alcoholic

        iv.   AA: an alcoholic can never go back to normal drinking

        v.   Regular meetings, sponsor system, and Twelve Steps are important to recover

           vi.   AA has extremely high dropout rate; those who stay with it do get better

           vii.   Those who are highly motivated, most confident, and most active in coping likely to continue and benefit

   e.   Outpatient and Brief Treatments

           i.   Residential, outpatient, and day-hospitals expanding

           ii.   Appears to be no difference in relapse between inpatient and outpatient programs

           iii.   Brief treatments such as **motivational interviewing** increases motivation of person to change; follows several principles; FRAMES describes treatment process

   f.   Relapse Prevention

           i.   **Relapse prevention** important since most alcoholics who stop drinking eventually relapse again

           ii.   Relapse prevention approach has created treatment programs for addictions often used in conjunction of other models of treatment

           iii.   Relapse begins with high-risk situations that generate internal reactions

           iv.   Effective coping skills protect person from relapse

           v.   Abstinence violation effect causes slips to turn into relapse

   g.   Matching

           i.   Treatment may be more effective by **matching** where patients are directed to programs that best fit their characteristics

           ii.   Motivation level, demographics, intelligence, severity of abuse are used in matching patients to programs

           iii.   Project MATCH's results question matching

IV.   Nicotine Dependence

   A.   Nicotine dependence refers to those who want to stop smoking but cannot

   B.   Nicotine has paradoxical effects on the nervous system

       1.   Nicotine can stimulate nervous system

       2.   Nicotine can have a calming effect

   C.   The Antismoking Movement

       1.   Surgeon General's Report in 1964 started public concern over smoking's health hazard

       2.   Secondhand smoke is a health hazard as well

3.   Cigarette advertisements have been banned on radio and television; warning labels have been placed on packaging; smoking banned in many public places

4.   Tobacco companies have vigorously opposed antismoking legislation

5.   Proportion of Americans who smoked has decreased from 45% in 1954 to 25% in 1997

      a.   Fewer people are starting to smoke

      b.   Some are using smokeless tobacco, which is linked to cancer

D.   Legal Remedies

1.   Tobacco companies pressured by federal and state governments

2.   Agreement between federal government and tobacco companies requires payment and more federal control with disallowing lawsuits

3.   Many argue that agreement was not enough

E.   Nicotine Dependence: Theory and Therapy

1.   Learning or Addiction?

      a.   Behaviorist sees tobacco addiction as learned habit maintained by reinforcers

      b.   Research found that smokers smoke to avoid withdrawal, suggesting there is physiological addiction

      c.   Smokers self-regulate nicotine levels to prevent withdrawal from occurring

2.   Treatment

      a.   High relapse rates seen in treatment programs, and is higher among those who try to quit on their own

      b.   A number of new treatments have been developed such as cognitive behavioral therapy and chewing gum

      c.   A number of motivational, cognitive, social factors predict who will remain abstinent

          i.   Self-efficacy predicts continued abstinence

          ii.   Use of coping mechanisms predicts abstinence

          iii.   Antidepressants are being tried as a smoking-cessation aid

          iv.   Bad moods weaken resistance

          v.   Environmental effects such as advertisements and smoker's immediate environment affect likelihood of relapse

V.   Other Psychoactive Drugs

A.   Drugs have been available for many years legally and illegally

1.   Use of illegal drugs has been variable

2.   Use of legal drugs has remained fairly constant

B.   Depressants

1. **Depressant** is a drug that reduces pain, tension, anxiety, and slows intellectual and motor reactivity
   a. Opiates, sedatives, and tranquilizers
   b. Tolerance develops; withdrawal symptoms occur; high dosages depress vital systems
2. Opiates
   a. Opiates are drugs that induce relaxation and reverie and provide relief from anxiety and pain
   b. **Opium** is a chemically-active substance derived from opium poppy
   c. **Morphine** used as an analgesic and is dangerously addictive
   d. **Heroin** is much stronger than morphine
   e. **Methadone** is a synthetic chemical and differs from other opiates
      i. Effective when taken orally
      ii. It is longer-lasting and takes effect slowly
      iv. Satisfies craving without an equivalent euphoria
   f. Heroin is most widely abused opiate in United States
      i. Normally taken by injection
      ii. There is a rush and euphoria
      iii. Addiction and tolerance develop
      iv. Withdrawal can be very unpleasant
   g. Drug use represents means of adapting to stress
3. Barbiturates
   a. **Barbiturates** have a sedative effect, relieving tension and bringing relaxation and sleep
   b. Used by suicide attempters and can have **synergistic effect** when taken with alcohol
   c. Use by the young generally recreational and sporadic
   d. Use by older people as way of relieving insomnia
   e. Effects are very similar to alcohol
4. Tranquilizers and Nonbarbiturate Sedatives
   a. Tranquilizers used in treatment of anxiety disorders and stress-related physical disorders
   b. Nonbarbiturate sedatives replaced barbiturates as prescription sleeping medication
   c. Have same problems as the barbiturates
   d. Dependence on nonbarbiturates sedatives often begins with sleeping problem
      i. Initial use may bring relief
      ii. Tolerance develops after about two weeks
      iii. May cause drug-induced insomnia and suppression of REM leading to REM rebound
      iv. Addiction develops

253

C. Stimulants
    1. **Stimulants** provide energy, alertness, and feelings of confidence
    2. Amphetamines
        a. **Amphetamines** are group of synthetic stimulants
        b. Most common are Benzedrine, Dexedrine, and Methedine
        c. Irregular use and low doses appear not to pose any behavioral or psychological problems
            i. Problems arise from regular use and high doses
            ii. Tolerance develops and higher doses become necessary
        d. Effects of amphetamine abuse and paranoid schizophrenia are similar
    3. Cocaine
        a. Cocaine is a natural stimulant and is active ingredient in coca plant
        b. Became fashionable in 1970s and peaked in mid-1980s
        c. Can be injected, smoked, but usually snorted
        d. Crack cocaine is within buying power of more people
        e. Cocaine intoxication includes excitement, euphoria
        f. Tolerance develops with regular use of cocaine and heavy withdrawal symptoms
            i. First phase is the crash
            ii. Withdrawal is second phase
            iii. Extinction is final phase
D. Hallucinogens
    1. **Hallucinogens** act on CNS to cause distortions in sensory perception
    2. Achieve effect without substantial changes in arousal
    3. LSD
        a. **LSD (lysergic acid diethylamide)** was synthesized in 1938
        b. Interferes with processing of information
        c. Effects include perceptions of colors and images, changes in body images and alteration of time and space perception
        d. May be negative for people whose grasp on reality is not firm
        e. LSD can produce bad trips and flashbacks
    4. PCP
        a. **PCP (phencyclidine)** is known as angel dust
        b. Often mixed with other substances
        c. Overdoses were common and extremely toxic
        d. Behavioral toxicity refers to tendency of users to harm themselves
        e. Use has declined since later 1970s
E. Marijuana and Hashish
    1. **Marijuana** and **hashish** are classified as hallucinogens

       a.   Effects are more mild than other hallucinogens

       b.   Use of marijuana and hashish is more common

2.   Marijuana and hashish derived from cannabis and is usually smoked and eaten

3.   The active ingredient is THC, which is not physiologically addictive

       a.   Causes accelerated heart rate

       b.   Causes reddening of whites of the eye

4.   Behavioral effects studied in variety of situations

       a.   Effects on simple behavior is mild or nil

       b.   As task becomes more complex, required response speed increases, more accuracy required, impairment becomes more apparent

       c.   Reactions include a feeling of being spaced out

       d.   Reactions can also heighten unpleasant experiences

5.   Is Marijuana Dangerous?

       a.   Effect of prolonged heavy marijuana use on blood levels of male sex hormone testosterone

       b.   Chronic marijuana use impairs function of one part of immune system

       c.   Chronic marijuana use may injure the lungs

       d.   Prolonged use of marijuana may result in psychological effects

           i.   Few users make transition to narcotics

           ii.   Amotivational syndrome does exist, but may be an accentuation of preexisting behavior patterns

6.   Marijuana as a Medical Treatment

       a.   Marijuana is useful in treating certain medical disorders

       b.   Decreases nausea and increases appetite in cancer patients undergoing chemotherapy

       c.   May help glaucoma and AIDS patients

       d.   Public appears to allow physicians to weigh risks and benefits

F.   Groups at Risk for Abuse of Illegal Drugs

    1.   Illegal substance highly related to race, class, education level, gender, and socioeconomic status

    2.   Those individuals who are medically ill, with mental disorders, and with chronic pain are at greater risk

VI.   Substance Dependence: Theory and Therapy

    A.   The Psychodynamic Perspective

       1.   Perspectives focus on homeostatic function of drugs

       2.   Drugs and Conflict

           a.   Drugs can ease adaptation in the short run

           b.   Drug abuse seen as self-medication

3,   Acquiring Self-Care
    a.   Therapy aims to provide self-care skills
    b.   Goal is to build up patients' intrapsychic strength and improve their relationships with others

B.   The Behavioral Perspective
    1.   Psychological and Biochemical Rewards
        a.   Behaviorist viewed alcohol dependence as habit maintained by antecedent and consequent reinforcers
        b.   Excessive drinking creates further psychological distress which will be alleviated by more drinking
        c.   Tension-reduction hypothesis received support from animal research
        d.   Contemporary approaches view drinking as creating pleasant states
        e.   Chemical rewards are the prime reinforcers of excessive drinking
    2.   Learning Not to Abuse Drugs
        a.   Early behavioral programs used aversion conditioning
            i.   Drug was paired with unpleasant stimulus
            ii.   Programs did nothing to alter conditions that elicit and maintain behavior
        b.   Contemporary behavioral programs attempt to remedy broad adjustment problems using combination of cognitive and behavioral techniques
            i.   Taught to identify cues and situations that lead to drug taking and alternative responses
            ii.   Taught new ways to cope with stress
        c.   Contingency management techniques used and involved earning points and then redeeming points
            i.   Patients underwent therapy
            ii.   Taught how to find nondrug recreational activities
            iii.   Taught how to avoid high risk situations
            iv.   Program worked for some alcoholics with vouchers keeping patients in program

C.   The Family Systems Perspective
    1.   Behavioral Couple Therapy
        a.   Behavioral couple therapy used for treatment of alcohol dependence
        b.   May be very effective in reducing problems in relationship
            i.   Most wife-beaters meet criteria for alcohol dependence
            ii.   Behavioral couple therapy reduces violence and reductions in drinking

      c.   Behavioral couple therapy tried with other kinds of drug abusers with gain that tended to diminish during follow-up period

   2.   Family Therapy
      a.   Most drug-dependent people live with their parents or have daily contact with parents
      b.   Family therapy seems promising in teenage drug abusers

D.   The Cognitive Perspective
   1.   Thinking About Drugs
      a.   Expectations play a role in effects of alcohol
      b.   Alcohol expectations do not explain why some people become alcohol dependent

   2.   Cognitive-Behavior Therapy
      a.   Abstinence violation effect is reduced through cognitive-behavior therapy
          i.   Slips now seen as part of recovery
          ii.   Goal is to control cognitive responses to slip to prevent it from becoming a full-blown relapse
      b.   Several factors are related to relapse
          i.   Individual factors include negative emotional states
          ii.   Environmental factors include social support, interpersonal conflict
          iii. Physiological factors include withdrawal cravings
      c.   An effective treatment will combine these factors

E.   The Biological Perspective
   1.   Genetic Studies
      a.   Findings suggest that some people inherit predisposition to alcohol dependence
          i.   Japanese, Koreans, and Taiwanese show facial flushing and signs of intoxication whereas Caucasians do not to same amount of alcohol
          ii.   Sensitivity to alcohol is related to genetic factors
      b.   Sons and brothers of severely alcohol-dependent men run 25 to 50% risk of becoming alcohol-dependent themselves
      c.   Concordance rate for MZ twins is 55% compared to 28% for DZ twins
      d.   Susceptibility to alcoholism inherited in two ways
          i.   Type 1 susceptibility affects both men and women and follows diathesis-stress model
          ii.   Type 2 susceptibility is passed from father to son and is independent on environmental influences
      e.   Susceptibly types differ
          i.   Type 1 susceptibility has onset of adulthood; rarely associated with criminal behavior; individuals tend to be dependent, quiet-living

           ii.   Type 2 susceptibility has onset in adolescence; individuals tend to be impulsive and aggressive; more prone to depression and suicide

      f.   P rats - alcohol preferring rats have been bred suggesting heritability of alcoholism

2.   Biochemical Studies

      a.   Endorphins

           i.   Nerve cells in brain have opiate receptors to which opiates attach themselves

           ii.   Enkephalins are very similar to morphine and fit the opiate receptors

           iii.   Stimulation of certain parts of brain can produce endorphins

           iv.   Pain-relieving drugs may be linked with endorphin production

           v.   Endorphins may also explain dependency and withdrawal symptoms

      b.   Dopamine

           i.   Most of abused drugs stimulate dopamine-producing neurons in median forebrain bundle

           ii.   Increased dopamine production creates drug's positive effects

           iii.   Dopamine-suppressing chemical blocks stimulant effects of alcohol

      c.   Drug Treatment for Drug Dependence

           i.   Medication is prescribed to reduce craving and withdrawal symptoms

           ii.   Alcoholics receiving Revia reported fewer cravings and lower relapse rates

           iii.   Methadone, while highly addictive, does not produce extreme euphoria of heroin, but does satisfy craving and prevent withdrawal

           iv.   Methadone maintenance switches people from dependence on heroin to dependence on methadone

           v.   Methadone maintenance programs have been successful

           vi.   Methadone does not prevent user from becoming dependent on other drugs

F.   The Sociocultural Perspective

      1.   Drugs and Poverty

           a.   Drug abuse related to racism and poverty, which create breeding ground for illegal drugs

           b.   Dramatic decline in standard of living among poor

           c.   Spread of AIDS by injecting drugs intravenously

           d.   Relationship between drugs and crime

2. Harm Reduction
   a. Harm reduction is set of interventions that concentrate on controlling the harm that drug dependency does to society at large
   b. Needle-exchange programs developed out of harm reduction approach
   c. Attempts to legalize drugs based on harm reduction
      i. Opponents say that it will encourage addition
      ii. Proponents say that it is the only way to prevent addicts from doing harm to society and to themselves
   d. Harm reduction policies have been slow to catch on in United States
   e. Prevention of drug abuse is supported

Chapter Boxes

- Binge Drinking on Campus
    - A.   Binge drinking on campus common
    - B.   Most say they see nothing wrong with binge drinking
    - C.   Campus alcohol abuse creates hardships on nonabusers
    - D.   Some campuses now set up substance-free dorms
    - E.   Binge drinking associated with difficulties making transition from being family member to being independent adult
    - F.   Person's attitude toward drinking plays role in binge drinking
    - G.   Programs focus on affective approaches and social-influence approaches
    - H.   Different student bodies show different drinking patterns

- Anabolic Steroids: Not for Athletes Only
    - A.   Anabolic steroids are synthetic version of testosterone
    - B.   Popularity spread into sports and steroids were banned
    - C.   Little solid research on hazards of long-time, high-dose steroid use
    - D.   Research suggests that steroids reduce HDL cholesterol, among other side effects
    - E.   Steroid use may actually stunt growth of bones
    - F.   Behavioral effects include irritability, aggression, and recklessness

Learning Objectives (LO)

By the time you have finished studying this chapter, you should be able to do the following:

1. Define psychoactive drugs, list seven criteria used by *DSM-IV* to diagnose substance *dependence*, and four criteria used to diagnose substance *abuse* (297-298).

2. Describe the behavioral and cognitive effects of various amounts of alcohol on the individual, and summarize statistical data on the effects of alcoholism on society at large (298-301).

3. Describe the development of alcohol dependence, and summarize data on alcohol dependence and abuse according to gender, race, ethnicity, religion, and age (302-305).

4. Summarize efforts to treat alcohol dependence, making reference to multimodel treatments, support groups, inpatient and outpatient services, and relapse prevention (305-308).

5. Describe the physical and psychological effects of nicotine, summarize the major theories of nicotine dependence, and describe legal, social, and treatment-based approaches to reducing nicotine dependence (308-312).

6. Describe the effects of depressant drugs, and distinguish among opiates, barbiturates, tranquilizers, and nonbarbiturate sedatives (312-315).

7. Describe the effects of stimulant drugs, and distinguish among amphetamines and the various forms of cocaine (315-317).

8. Describe the effects of hallucinogenic drugs, and summarize current information on the effects and possible risks associated with the use of marijuana and hashish (317-320).

9. Summarize the psychodynamic view of substance dependence and relate it to the issue of why certain high-risk groups are likely to use drugs (320-322).

10. Describe tension-reduction and positive reinforcement explanations of substance dependence proposed by the behavioral perspective, and trace the evolution of behavioral treatment programs for substance dependence (322-323).

11. Explain the use of couple and family therapies in treating substance dependence from the family systems perspective (323-324).

261

12.   Summarize the role of expectancies in the cognitive view of substance dependence, and describe three factors thought to be important in cognitive-behavioral attempts to prevent relapse after treatment (324-326).

13.   Summarize data suggesting genetic and biochemical predispositions for substance dependence, making reference to Type 1 and Type 2 alcoholism, endorphins, and dopamine, and describe the use of drugs in the treatment of substance dependence (326-328).

14.   Summarize the social-environmental causes of substance dependence as seen from the sociocultural perspective, and define and give examples of harm reduction (328-330).

Lecture Leads (LL)

Development of a drinking problem (LL 11-1)
There is no doubt that drugs and alcohol constitute a major problem in this country. Kessler et al. (1993) noted that responses to a survey indicate that 25 percent of adolescents and adults have had a substance abuse problem at some point in their lives. According to Jellinek (1960) there are several progressive steps a person goes through as they pass from a social drinker to an alcohol abuser. He developed the disease model of alcoholism based on survey results from Alcoholics Anonymous. In the initial phase, a social drinker consumes alcohol to feel good and to relieve tension. During this phase, people should be cautious of dependence on alcohol if they engage in any of the following: increasing consumption, morning drinking, regretted behavior done while drunk, and blackouts. The second phase is referred to as the crucial phase. During this phase, people have some control over when and where they take the first drink, but then lose control once they start drinking. Jellinek calls the final stage the chronic phase. At this point, the person is an addict. They drink most of the time and become intoxicated on much less volume than during earlier phases. They are so preoccupied with alcohol in this phase that they "will often destroy family ties, work, and social life. Implicit in the steps is the assumption that alcoholism is a disease and that alcoholics have no control over their drinking. As the textbook describes, the effects of alcohol may be related to one's expectations. Alcoholism is a disorder that is very difficult to treat on one's own. Although many people believe they can stop drinking alcohol when they choose to, they soon find out that help is needed. Jellinek's disease model of alcoholism has been questioned.

Resources:
Fingarette, H. (1966). Alcoholism: The mythical disease. The Public Interest, 91, 3-22.

Jellinek, E. M. (1960). The disease concept of alcoholism. New Haven: Hill House, Mifflin Company.

Jellinek, E. M. (1971). The phases of alcohol addiction. In G. Shen (Ed.), Studies in abnormal behavior. Chicago: Rand McNally.

Kessler, R. C., McGonagle, Z. S., Nelson, C. B., Hughes, M., Eshelman, S., Wittchen, H. U., & Kendler, K.S. (1993). Lifetime and 12-month prevalence of DSM-111-R psychiatric disorders in the United States: Results from the National Comorbidity Survey. Archives of General Psychiatry, 51, 8-19.

Gender differences in drinking patterns (LL 11-2)
There is an indication that there are substantial differences between the drinking patterns of men and women and that in some instances alcohol may have more serious physiological effects on women. These studies show that women are more likely to drink at home and that they are more likely to attempt to hide their drinking behavior. Also,

women have a higher percentage of body fat and a lower percentage of body water than men; if a woman and a man of identical weight consume the same amount of alcohol the toxic effects of alcohol will be more severe in the woman 's body in contrast to the man's body. Not only is heavy drinking in women associated with fetal alcohol syndrome but it is also associated with gynecological problems. Gearhart et al. conclude that since women are more likely to conceal their drinking problems, and because of the effects that heavy alcohol use has on women's health, physicians are the most likely individuals to detect their drinking problems.

Resource:
Gearhart, J. G., Beebe, D. K., Milhorn, H. T., & Meeks, R. (1991). Alcoholism in women. <u>American Family Physician</u>, <u>44</u>, 907-914.

Natural history of smoking (LL 11-3)
A description of the natural history of smoking in the individual is vital in appreciating the persistence of smoking behavior. Four stages regarding the course of smoking have been proposed with two main factors (i.e., psychosocial, psychophysiological) that work alone or conjointly in each stage. The first stage, the initiation of smoking, is largely determined by psychosocial factors influencing the individual. The onset of cigarette smoking may be an attempt by the adolescent to become an adult, which could be precipitated by parental, sibling, and peer smoking. Leventhal and Cleary (1980) suggested that attitudes toward smoking and the subjectively held images of smoking (i.e., cool, macho, sexy) are other determinants of adolescent smoking. The second stage of smoking is characterized by an increasing tolerance of the negative effects of nicotine, the dependency on the immediate positive effects of nicotine, the recognition of cues to smoking, and the threat of withdrawal reactions. For the most part, psychosocial factors contribute to the initiation of the third stage, cessation of smoking, and may include specific influences such as health consequences, expense of cigarette smoking, and providing a positive example to others. These influences appear to be extremely powerful motivators; witness the fact that most smokers in the United States report that they would like to abstain. However, successful cessation is complicated by the influences alluded to in the discussion of smoking maintenance. Recently, the fourth stage of smoking, or relapse of smoking, has attracted much interest in the psychological literature and has been proposed to be the most important issue challenging researchers and practitioners today. This interest in relapse stems from accounts illustrating the recidivistic nature of smoking. Work done by Marlatt has significantly contributed to our understanding of recidivism and relapse by emphasizing cognitive and situational variables.

Resources:
Ashton, H., & Stepney, R. (1982). <u>Smoking: Psychology and pharmacology</u>. London: Tavistock Productions.

Leventhal, H., & Cleary, P. D. (1980). The smoking problem: A review of the research and theory in behavioral risk modification. <u>Psychological Bulletin</u>, <u>88</u>, 370-405.

Hearing loss and smoking (LL 11-4)

A new health hazard can be added to the long list of health consequences of smoking. Cruickshanks et al. (1998) reported that hearing loss may be associated with smoking. In their study, the hearing of adults aged 48-92 was examined by otoscopy, screening tympanometry and pure-tone air-conduction and bone-conduction audiometry. Data were also collected regarding subjects' smoking. The results show that smokers were 1.69 times more likely than nonsmokers to have hearing loss. Even nonsmokers who lived with smokers were more likely to experience hearing loss.

Resource:

Cruickshanks, K. J. Klein, R., Klein, B. E. K., Wiley, T. L., Nondahl, D. M., Tweed, T. S. (1998). Cigarette smoking and hearing loss. Journal of the American Medical Association, 279, 1715-1719.

Caffeinism (LL 11-5)

Identified as several of the most pervasively used psychoactive drugs in society, methylxanthihes (i.e., theophylline, caffeine, theobrornine) have only recently been recognized as important components in our diet. Indeed, it is difficult to escape methylxanthines because of their widespread use in colas, headache remedies, diuretics, and asthma medications, and their natural occurrence in chocolate, tea, cola, and coffee. In fact, we consume over 5,000 tons of caffeine yearly. Therefore, there is a growing concern regarding the abuse of caffeine. Caffeinism, or the chronic consumption of caffeine, is characterized by depression, agitation, delirium, and decrements in performance and has been estimated to potentially develop in one-quarter of the population of the United States. The development of caffeinism is subtle given that caffeine is a socially approved drug considered benign and in low to moderate doses it may facilitate performance and aid to modulate mood. In fact, so strong is this effect that anecdotal data reflects that many adults cannot "function" until their first cup of coffee in the morning. As tolerance and dependence increase, the intended effects of "pick me-up" and increased concentration, stamina, and mental acuity, the actual effects of caffeine intake develop into a syndrome. That is, excessive doses of caffeine cause disturbed sleep, myocardial stimulation, agitation, nervousness, fast flow of speech and thought, and performance. In fact, behavioral manifestations of caffeinism may be hard to distinguish from a psychotic. There are reports in the literature that describe caffeine-induced delirium. Stillner, Popkin, and Pierce (1978) presented a case study of a 28-year old male participating in the 1,048 mile Iditarod Dog Sled Race. After ingesting over 1000 mg of caffeine from OTC stimulants and beverages in less than three hours, the individual experienced "tremor, impaired memory, altered levels of consciousness, vertigo, pronounced anxiety, and sensory disturbances." That in diagnoses clinicians should recognize the possibility that caffeinism might mirror more severe psychopathologies seems to be a prudent suggestion. Another danger of caffeinism is acting out caused by caffeinism's effects onf irritability and restlessness. The maintenance of caffeinism follows a viscious cycle in that in the pursuit of experiencing the positive effects of caffeine, dependency, and tolerance form, requiring increasing doses of caffeine. Then, when the negative symptoms occur, the abuser might pursue abstinence. However, moderate to severe withdrawal symptoms do accompany abstinence; anxiety and muscle tension occur even in brief periods of abstention. Other caffeine withdrawal symptoms include headaches, irritability, lethargy, and drowsiness.

Resources:

Bolton, S. & Null, G. (1981). Caffeine psychological effects, use and abuse. Journal of Orthomolecular Psychiatry, 10, 202-211.

Julien, R. M. (1998). A primer of drug action (8th ed.). New York: W. H. Freeman.

McKim, W. A. (1997). Drugs and behavior: An introduction to behavioral pharmacology (3d ed.). Upper Saddle River, NJ: Prentice Hall.

Sawyer, D. A., Julia, H. L., & Turin, A. C. (1982). Caffeine and human behavior: Arousal, anxiety, and performance effects. Journal of Behavioral Medicine, 5, 415-439.

Stillner, V., Popkin, M. K., & Pierce, C. M. (1978). Caffeine-induced delirium during prolonged competitive stress. American Journal of Psychiatry, 135, 855-856.

Comorbidity: PTSD and cocaine dependence (LL 11-6)
A recent study by Najavits et al. (1998) suggests that clinicians ought to consider screening substance abusers for PTSD. In their study, 122 cocaine-dependent outpatients participated in an outpatient treatment program. The subjects were assessed on a number of measures such as the Trauma History questionnaire and the PTSD checklist. The results show that in this sample of cocaine dependent patients, a large number experienced lifetime traumatic events. Females were found to have had more physical and sexual abuse than males. About 20% of the sample met the diagnostic criteria for PTSD. The authors suggest that additional screening for PTSD might have implications for treatment among cocaine-dependent outpatients.

Resource:

Najavits, L. M. et al. (1998). Cocaine dependence with and without PTSD among subjects in the National Institute on Drug Abuse Collaborative Cocaine Treatment Study. American Journal of Psychiatry, 155, 214-219.

Relapse prevention and the AVE (LL 11-7)
The approach taken by Marlatt and his coworkers has emphasized the interaction of cognitive, behavioral, and physiological variables in relapse. Marlatt and Gordon developed a system to organize and describe the determinants of relapse. The classification scheme was constructed by tracking the relapse episodes of 35 college-age smokers after undergoing a cessation program. Intrapersonal/environmental determinants and interpersonal determinants were identified to account for 57% of all relapse episodes. Of particular interest, is the class of intrapersonal/environmental determinants, which

consists of (a) coping with negative emotional states, (b) coping with negative physical/physiological states, (c) enhancement of positive emotional states, (d) testing personal control, and (e) giving in to temptations or urges. To evaluate the classification system, the responses of 64 smokers regarding relapse episodes were analyzed (Cummings et al., 1980). Intrapersonal determinants were accountable for 50% of the relapse episodes reported by subjects. Of that 50%, negative emotional states were described as being the primary determinants in 37% of relapse occurrences. In a preliminary test of the classification system, Marlatt and Gordon found a comparable 43% of relapses occurred due to negative emotional states in a sample of 35 smokers. Along these same lines of research, Marlatt (Marlatt & Gordon, 1980) has proposed another factor that operates in relapse. He describes the factor in terms of an individual being in a high-risk environment and not able to exercise coping responses, which increases the probability of relapse. When relapse occurs, the individual experiences and reacts to the Abstinence Violation Effect (AVE). AVE consists of a cognitive dissonance component, which produces guilt, and a subjective attribution effect, which suggests dejection and a lack of willpower to the violator. To reduce the dissonance and a subjective loss of self-control, the individual returns to baseline and relapses. Shiffman (1982) used a telephone counseling hotline to collect data on the antecedents of relapse. Negative emotional states such as anxiety, anger, frustration, and depression preceded 71.2% of relapses. It is apparent that the majority of all relapses are due to the subject's inability to appropriately cope with "negative emotional reactions [due] either to noninterpersonal, environmental events or to interpersonal situations" (Cummings et al., 1980, p. 304). A subject in Cummings et al. described a relapse where rain had flooded a basement that caused $4,000 worth of damage; the individual recognized the inevitability of smoking when a pack of cigarettes was bought following the assessment of the damage. Work by Abrams, Monti, Elder, Brown, and Jacobs (1984) strengthens the reported role of intrapersonal determinants in relapse and corroborates the AVE model by suggesting the intrapersonal situations were more competently coped with by quitters than with relapsers.

Resources:

Abrams, D. B., Monti, P. M., Elder, J. P., Brown, R. A., & Jacobus, S. I. (1984, May). Assessment of psychosocial stress and coping in males and females who relapsed or quit smoking. Paper presented at the meeting of the Society of Behavioral Medicine, Philadelphia.

Cummings, C., Gordon, J. R., & Marlatt, G. A. (1980). Relapse: Prevention and prediction. In W. R. Miller (Ed.), The addictive behaviors: Treatments of alcoholism, drug abuse, smoking, and obesity. Oxford: Pergamon Press.

Marlatt, G. A., & Gordon, J. R. (1980). Determinants of relapse: Implications for the maintenance of behavior change. In P. O. Davidson & S. M. Davidson (Eds.), Behavioral medicine: Changing health lifestyle. New York: Brunner/Mazel.

Shiffman, S. (1982). Relapse following smoking cessation: A situational analysis. <u>Journal of Consulting and Clinical Psychology</u>, <u>50</u>, 71-86.

Culture and drug abuse (LL 11-8)
In our society, the abuse of drugs such as heroin, cocaine, marijuana, and LSD are clearly looked down upon by most people. In contrast, the abuse of other drugs, like caffeine and nicotine is generally not a source of great concern, and the abuse of alcohol actually falls somewhere in the middle of these two extremes. But can you imagine being accused of substance abuse for excessively consuming sweets or salty snacks? In Northern India the repeated excessive consumption of these kinds of foods is constituted as an abuse condition that is referred to as *chat* or *pan*. The belief in this culture is that people must control over their eating and should not become addicted to food. At the other extreme, the substances we view to be at the heart of addictions are in some instances a normal part of life in other cultures. Take for example the Meo people of Laos; opium-smoking behavior has long been considered a part of traditional life. Families actually grow opium for trade as a commodity.

Resource:
Triandis, H. C., & Draguns, G. (Eds.) (1980). <u>Handbook of cross-cultural psychology: Vol 6. Psychopathology</u>. Boston: Allyn & Bacon.

Talking Points (TP)

Real people (TP 11-1)

There are several famous people who have battled substance abuse and dependence. Ask students for examples. Here are some to get the list going: Jim Morrison, Dick Van Dyke, Thomas Edison, Drew Barrymore, River Phoenix, John Belushi, Betty Ford, Chris Farley, Judy Garland, Sigmund Freud, H. G. Wells, Elvis Presley, Oprah Winfrey, Janis Joplin. Ask students for illustrations of substance dependence and use portrayed on TV, soap operas, movies, and in fiction and nonfiction books.

Drug use vs. drug abuse (TP 11-2)

Before students review the chapter, ask them to discuss the difference between drug use and drug abuse. From that discussion, introduce the concept of drug dependence.

Keeping track (TP 11-3)

Ask students to keep track of the legal, nonprescription drugs they take within the next week. Students should be asked to predict their level of drug use and then to compare their prediction with the actual use. Remind students that caffeine is considered a psychoactive drug and that it appears in many foods and drinks.

Alcohol's cost (TP 11-4)

One way to underscore the personal costs of alcohol is to illustrate how it has affected us all. For instance, you may wish to ask your students if they know of anyone who was in an automobile accident where drinking was involved? Do your students know anyone who has died because of alcohol (e.g., accident, cirrhosis, suicide)? You may wish to refer back to an earlier activity in Chapter 1 on assessing the prevalence of psychological disorders.

Nicotine: The "skeleton key" (TP 11-5)

Much of nicotine's action on the body is due to its similarity in chemical structure to acetylcholine. The similarity is so remarkable that nicotine can readily fit into some acetylcholine receptors and has been described as a "skeleton key."

Preventing smoking (TP 11-6)

One approach in preventing children from beginning to smoke is to frighten them. Probably many of your students remember someone coming into their elementary class and showing a picture of a healthy lung and a picture of a diseased lung due to smoking. Do these types of approaches work?

Smoking cessation (TP 11-7)

Although the incidence of smoking had been decreasing until recently, many of your students will be smokers and will have gone through the difficulties associated with attempting to quit. Ask these students to describe their efforts to quit. What type of withdrawal symptoms did they experience? Did they experience the AVE? Next,

269

challenge them to quit for a specified time. Have them keep a diary of their feelings and cravings; encourage them to admit when they cheat. Discuss these diaries with the students' input in class, using concepts introduced in the chapter.

Drug factory in your head (TP 11-8)

As you discuss endorphins, a helpful metaphor to share with students is that we have a factory in our heads that produces drugs, in this case an analgesic. Simple, but it gets the point across.

Coca-Cola was literally coke (TP 11-9)

Many students might know this one already, but ask if they know the history of Coca-Cola. Why is Coca-Cola called that? At one point, cocaine was an ingredient, but was later replaced with caffeine.

High-risk situations (TP 11-10)

According to research, the risk of relapse greatly increases in high-risk situations. Consider telling students that relapse prevention and the AVE can be applied in other contexts where there is a desire to modify behavior such as studying and exercising. Ask your students to describe high-risk situations that increase the chance the student will fail to maintain the behavior change. For instance, Friday nights may be difficult for students to study at the library. All-you-can-eat buffets are dangerous for those trying to control their eating. A friend asking you to go to a movie puts studying at risk.

The abstinence violation effect (TP 11-11)

The AVE is sometimes referred to as "the-what-the-heck-effect" since it describes the reaction that people have to lapse. The AVE turns the lapse into a full-blown relapse.

Drug testing (TP 11-12)

In recent years, drug testing has become mandatory for certain types of employment (military, government, or security) or participation in some activities (e.g. high school, college, and professional sports). Develop a discussion on the relative merits of such policies. What are the pros and cons of each side of the argument? Does the government or your employer have a right to know what you do off the job, even when it might be illegal? Are there some careers where drug testing is not needed?

Alcohol's heritability and its implication (TP 11-13)

Recent evidence would suggest that alcoholism has a highly heritable component, especially for men. Nonalcoholic sons of alcoholic fathers show markedly different patterns of physiological arousal in response to certain stimuli than sons of nonalcoholic fathers. Discuss the implications of this research in terms of primary prevention and later intervention.

The 12 Steps of AA (TP 11-14)
The textbook makes reference to the Twelve Steps of Alcoholics Anonymous. There are a couple of interesting points in the steps. For instance, several of them are related to acceptance, belief, and reliance on God. A few of the steps refer to mending broken relationships. AA's Serenity prayer is: God grant me the serenity to accept the things that cannot change, courage to change the things I can, and wisdom to know the difference. What about the substance abuser who does not believe in God or is uncomfortable in such a setting? What effect does references to "a Power greater than ourselves" have on recovering alcoholics?

Pregnancy and drug use (TP 11-15)
There are a number of cases in state courts in which women are being prosecuted for child abuse because they took drugs while they were pregnant. Should women who intentionally abuse drugs while pregnant be imprisoned in order to prevent harm to their unborn child? This issue can also be extended to smoking tobacco: should we imprison mothers who smoke or who drink alcohol? Ask the class for some discussion of alternatives to imprisonment. Can they design a system that will allow for zero drug use in these individuals? Will pregnant women who are users simply avoid prenatal care for fear that they will be prosecuted?

necessarily the **road to destruction**.	p. 296
as anyone knows who has ever enjoyed a beer at a **ball game**.	p. 296
the problem lies not in the drug but in the **way a person uses the drug**.	p. 297
(e.g., **chain smoking**)…	p. 297
alcohol has been the traditional "**high**" of Western culture.	p. 298
Barrooms, as we know, are where brawls may occur.	p. 300
Amorous types being making **wanton** remarks to strangers…	p. 300
Another serious danger sign is morning drinking, to **get oneself "going."**	p. 301
The traders were given to binge drinking and **drunken brawls**…	p. 303
"**it's Miller time**" or that "**the night belongs to Michelob**."	p. 304
sometimes follow a "**cold-turkey**" termination of…	p. 306
For generations, the use of nicotine products was considered a "**vice**"…	p. 309
the tobacco companies have been hit by **class action suits**…	p. 310
During the **Civil War**…	p. 312
not all people have the "**honey-licking**" experience.	p. 313
the cause of well-publicized deaths of **Judy Garland** and **Marilyn Monroe**.	p. 314
only by prescription or "**on the street**"…	p. 315
They can produce a **kaleidoscope** of colors and images.	p. 318
As a result, **ballot initiatives** in some states…	p. 320
NFL guard attempts suicide after flunking drug test in 1991.	p. 321
have continued leaving the cities for **greener pastures**…	p. 328
American politicians seem wedded to a philosophy of **zero tolerance**.	p. 329

Activities and Demonstrations (ACT/DEMO)

Messages in alcohol and cigarette print ads (ACT/DEMO 11-1)
Objective: To illustrate the messages present in prints ads for alcohol and cigarettes
Materials: Alcohol and cigarette print ads from magazines and tabloid newspapers
Procedure: Have students form small groups of four to five students each. Give each group two or three print ads and have them evaluate the ads in terms of what messages are being implicitly and explicitly communicated.
Discussion: Project a copy of the ads on the overhead and ask the spokesperson from the group to describe the ad and the messages. Summarize the findings on the article and correct any incorrect notions. Are these ads directed to certain segments of the population? Did the tobacco companies create "Joe Camel" to appeal to children? What effects do these messages have on drug use and attitudes toward drug use? As an alternative, show television commercials for beer to students.

Resolved: Marijuana should be decriminalized (ACT/DEMO 11-2)
Objective: To identify the issues involved in decriminalizing marijuana
Materials: None
Procedure: Have students form small groups. Each group should come up with a list of pros (e.g., " Legalization would mean taxation, which would be an additional source of government revenue.") and cons (e.g., " Heavy marijuana use has serious side effects") about legalizing marijuana or giving marijuana through prescriptions. Have one person from each group read the list of pros and cons developed by the group. These comments can be aggregated and then discussed.
Discussion: Are there particular themes that emerged in the pros and cons? In what way, should psychology contribute to the controversy?

Support groups and self-help (LL 11-3)
Objective: To acquaint the students with individual organizations and their programs
Materials: None
Procedure: Have a small group (three to four) of students attend a local self-help group for family and friends of those recovering from addictions. Many students will be surprised at the variety of such programs in their areas. The students should consider programs designed to help people stop smoking--some are private enterprises, others are sponsored by medical groups such as HMOs, others are sponsored by religious groups such as Seventh Day Adventists.
Discussion: Explain how the family environment can reward addictive behavior and demonstrate how the addictive cycle can operate for many years. Discuss the trip with the students and have them explain their own perceptions of the best parts and worst parts of the programs.

Debate on drug testing (LL 11-4)
Objective: To explore the different perspectives of drug testing in our society.
Materials: None

Procedure: In recent years, drug testing has become mandatory for certain types of employment or participation in some activities (e.g. sports, flying airplanes, or joining the military). Have each side of the debate team debate the relative merits both for and against such enforcement policies. Pick individuals for the pro and con sides of the debate who are likely to do thorough research and a good job of debating. Many times there will be volunteers for either the pro or con side of the debate.

Discussion: It might be particularly effective to poll your students before the debate, then assign the students to research and take the *opposite* position from what they first declared. Then poll them after the debate and see if their position has changed at all. After the debate, students should discuss the pros and cons of drug testing. Discuss the debate and try to form a class conclusion on this topic.

Community resources (ACT/DEMO 11-5)

Objective: To identity community resources for substance dependence

Materials: None

Procedure: Have students research community resources that are available for persons and their family members who suffer from or are at-risk for substance abuse and dependence. Create a resource manual to help both the campus and local communities find assistance for problems they encounter for themselves or family members (or friends) who have problems with any form of substance abuse. List information such as the name of each group, contact person(s), phone numbers, the types of services they offer, and whether any fee is involved. More specifically, the resource manual could include what steps a person who thinks they or a family member has a drug problem should take to get help.

Discussion: Students will learn that there are many resources available. A resource manual would be a valuable asset to the community

Developing a drug prevention program (ACT/DEMO 11-6)

Objective: To encourage students to think about drug abuse prevention

Materials: None

Procedure: This activity can be conducted with students working individually or in small groups. Students are to take the role of policy makers. Their charge is to develop national, state, or local programs aimed at drug abuse prevention. The programs ought to incorporate what is known about drugs abuse, dependence, and treatment. Each program should include an objective and goals that describe how the objective will be reached. The goals should be explicitly linked to the literature summarized in the textbook. A good place to start is the local D.A.R.E. program

Discussion: Select several programs to be presented and discussed. The critical question is the degree to which the programs take into account the research on drug abuse and dependence. One avenue of discussion might be to compare and contrast what students developed to what is typical included in drug abuse prevention programs.

Guest speakers (ACT/DEMO 11-7)

Objective: To invite professionals involved in drug abuse, enforcement, and treatment

Materials: None

Procedure: There are several speakers you may wish to invite to your class to discuss their area of expertise. Ideas include a psychologist, psychiatrist, chemical dependency counselor specializing in the treatment of addictive disorders, a representative from MADD, SADD, Alcoholics Anonymous, Narcotics Anonymous, Al-Anon, or other self-help groups, or a drug enforcement officer, or DARE officer, or a representative from NORML or group advocating total drug abstinence. Make sure you schedule this presentation early, since many mental health professionals and others are very busy.

Discussion: Beforehand, instruct students to review this chapter and be prepared to ask questions of their guest speakers. Afterwards, ask students to discuss speakers' presentations.

Films and Videos

Addiction Caused by Mixing Medicines. FHS. Nonaddictive prescription drugs can and often do lead to addiction, and one of the primary dangers of mixing prescription drugs-individually prescribed for specific purposes, is the addictive effect. In this program, an addictionologist and a clinical pharmacist explain how mixing medicines can lead to problems, which groupings of drugs are likely to cause problems, and how dangers can be minimized.

Addiction: The Family in Crisis. FHS. This program tells the poignant story of one man's addiction to alcohol and explains the process of addiction in the brain. It shows how a person starts abusing a drug. With continued drug use, the brain's pleasure circuit is activated and behaves as if the drug is important for survival. The program explores how the family of the alcoholic is devastated by his behavior, the typical role of "enabler" that family members too often play, and why families should also seek treatment. The program follows the alcoholic through a treatment program as he learns the causes of his addiction and how to keep his alcoholism under control through abstinence.

Adult Children of Alcoholics: A Family Secret. FHS. In this program, famous adult children of alcoholics speak out about childhood nightmares and adult behavior that continues to reflect the problem of a parent's alcoholism: some chose alcoholic partners, and others developed drug, gambling, or other addictions. All speak of the difficulties of coping with the damage inflicted by an alcohol-centered childhood.

Alcohol Addiction. FHS. Access and attitudes explain why people begin to drink; genetic predisposition may explain why some people cannot stop. At the Rutgers University Alcohol Research Lab, this program explores the nature of alcohol addiction, concluding that addiction is a biochemical disease still best treated by behavioral means.

Alcohol and the Family. Breaking the Chain. FHS. This program analyzes the signs of alcoholism and shows how a family member, coworker, or friend can help break the chain; discusses the impact of alcoholism on the children of alcoholics; and evaluates the options and prognosis for alcoholism treatment.

Calling the Shots. CDF. A review of the way alcohol is advertised, with emphasis on encouragement to drink.

Can You Stop People from Drinking? FHS. This program looks at how Russia and the United States. are attacking the seemingly intractable problem of alcohol abuse by means of both old and new weapons: prohibition, hypnotism, imprisonment, surveillance, deception, aversion therapy, and such group therapy as Alcoholics Anonymous. WGBH Collection.

Cigarettes: Who Profits, Who Dies? FHS. For those who believe that the tobacco mortality statistics don't apply to them, here is a message from the folks who make cigarettes that is so grossly cynical it may finally get through. This program features former cigarette models who are now dying of cigarette-related cancer, who were once selected because of their wholesome young looks to persuade others to become addicted to cigarettes. It also shows the new international tactics devised by American tobacco companies in the face of falling demand for their products in this country.

Cocaine: The End of the Line. FHS. The program explains the origin of cocaine, how it works, and how cocaine use is dangerous; shows how cocaine kills and injures otherwise healthy young people; defines the typical coke user; explains why cocaine is so addictive and why addiction is so difficult to overcome; and provides a quiz on some of the myths about cocaine.

Cracking a Craving. FHS. This program explains the surge in cocaine use, the latest research into what cocaine does to the brain, what makes the brain seek it again and again, and how cocaine and its smokable form, crack, differ in addictive potential. The program also explores new ways to treat cocaine addiction.

Dangerous Medications and Their Effects. FHS. Medications can cause serious problems: car accidents, insomnia, Parkinsonism, and sexual dysfunction. Dr. Sidney Wolfe, author of *Worst Pills, Best Pills,* indicates how to use medications safely and suggests safer alternatives to many. This specially adapted Phil Donahue program also features people whose lives were turned around once they were diagnosed as suffering from medication-induced problems.

Drug-Taking and the Arts. FHS. This program explores how drugs have influenced artistic production in the course of the last 200 years, focusing on major European and American literary figures and visual artists. Actors portray some of the authors, others speak for themselves, and literary critics, psychiatrists, and substance abuse specialists analyze the effects of drugs on the artists. The program seeks to determine whether drugs help the artist produce better art, and if so, how; whether they give the artist insight or only the illusion of insight; whether different drugs produce different sorts of art; and how certain drugs create specific physiological effects in the brain.

Enablers. FHS. This specially-adapted Phil Donahue program investigates the role of enablers, who think they are helping a loved one by covering up his or her addiction while actually contributing to the abusive behavior.

Female Alcoholism. FHS. This program examines the changing stereotype of the female alcoholic and analyzes some case histories of alcoholic women. It explains the dangers of drinking during pregnancy, the effect of Fetal Alcohol Syndrome (FAS) on newborns, and the emotional effect on children of being raised by an alcoholic mother.

Hooked on Heroin: From Hollywood to Main Street. FHS. Heroin once seemed to attract the extremes, the young and rich of show business or the down and out. But not anymore. This program examines why some of the unlikeliest people have become junkies, like the Boy Scout who (24 years ago) "just wanted to try it," and the housewife who (seven years ago) was "just going to try it one time." It talks to Steve Tyler, lead singer of Aerosmith, who describes what it was like to be down--and to come back up, and recover; to DEA officers who warn of the growing epidemic of heroin addiction; and to a drug dealer who explains the attraction of snorting over shooting up.

Kids under the Influence. FHS. This program looks at alcohol, our number-one drug problem among kids. It examines school problems, run-ins with the law, and the long-term physical and psychological disorders caused by alcohol consumption; demonstrates the enormous influence of peer pressure and seductive advertisements; shows the wrenching process of rehabilitation; and explains why alcohol is so easily abused by young people and what can be done about it.

New Substance Misuse. FHS. There is a range of substances that, when used as intended and in the appropriate quantity, are beneficial; when misused, they are often deleterious to health and may be fatal. This program examines the most commonly misused substances, explaining the effects of each and the problems it can cause. The substances covered include: stimulants (amphetamines, caffeine, cocaine, nicotine, MDMA); depressants (alcohol, barbiturates, solvents, benzodiazephines); hallucinogens (cannabis, LSD, "magic" mushrooms); and opiates (morphine, heroin).

Smoking. Time to Quit. FHS. This program discusses various ways to stop smoking and the motivation to stop: quitting before or at the onset of pregnancy, when the motivation to protect the unborn child is very strong; a couple quitting together; stop-smoking support groups and their techniques for training ex-smokers to say "No" when a cigarette is offered; and being willing to try to quit again after relapsing.

Substance Abuse among Latinos. FHS. In the face of high unemployment and underemployment, lack of adequate housing, a failing public school system, and a shift to non-traditional families, "just saying no" is not enough. This program looks at culturally

277

specific approaches being generated within the Latino community to combat drug and alcohol abuse and examines such factors as language, religion, and family ties in reaching and teaching the Latino population at risk for AIDS and/or substance abuse.

The Addicted Brain. FHS. This documentary takes viewers on a tour of the world's most prolific manufacturer and user of drugs--the human brain. The biochemistry of the brain is responsible for joggers' highs, for the compulsion of some people to seek thrills, for certain kinds of obsessive compulsive behavior, even for the drive to achieve power and dominance. This program explores the cutting edge of developments in the biochemistry of addiction and addictive behavior.

The Broken Cord. Louise Erdrich and Michael Dorris. FHS. In this program with Bill Moyers, authors Louise Erdrich and Michael Dorris explain how traditions of spirit and memory weave through the lives of many Native Americans and how alcoholism and despair have shattered so many other lives. The devastating effect of fetal alcohol syndrome on their adopted son and on the Native American community as a whole is also discussed.

The Perfect Drug Film. IU. Reviews history of drug use and the touting of various drugs as panaceas for a variety of personal and societal ills.

The Power of addiction. FHS. The program covers both chemical and behavioral addiction, describes the signs of compulsive behavior, and analyzes such possible causes of addictive behavior as neurotransmitter imbalance and genetic and environmental factors. It also examines the physiological and psychological mechanisms of cocaine addiction and recovery from it.

Walking through the Fear. Women and Substance Abuse. FHS. Increasing numbers of women are addicted to alcohol and drugs, yet only one in five people in treatment centers is a woman. Why aren't women seeking or getting the help they need to overcome their addictions? This program investigates the problems women face when they seek such help, and four women tell what life was like before they sought help and how their life changed after recovery.

Using Movies and Mental Illness as a Teaching Tool

Many of the film vignettes in *The Lost Weekend* can be easily adapted for the classroom – for example, the hallucination in which Don Birnam sees a bat attack and kill a mouse in the wall is unforgettable.

Your students will know of many artists, actors and writers who have coped with alcoholism or drug addiction, and it may be useful to start this class simply generating a list of well known personalities who have struggled with substance abuse.

Most of your students will have seen films like *Animal House* that glamorize drinking (or at least treat substance abuse as a normal and appropriate behavior). It shouldn't be hard to come up with a list of films that tacitly condone and support the abuse of alcohol and drugs.

A stimulating class discussion can be generated by showing the murder scene from *Dead Man Walking* and asking your students to debate whether or not the intoxication of the two criminals should be extenuating factors when sentencing for the murders occurs.

Most cinematic portrayals of alcoholism have involved men. However, the different effects of alcoholism on men and women can be discussed after viewing *Days of Wine and Roses*, and the special features of alcoholism in women can be illustrated by selected scenes from *When a Man Loves a Woman*. There are dramatic group therapy scenes in *Drunks* and *Clean and Sober*. It may be useful to have someone who belongs to AA come to class to discuss the organization after excerpts from these films are shown.

There are vivid scenes in *Trainspotting* can set the stage for a classroom discussion of heroin addiction; for example, a scene in which a mother discovers her neglected baby has died and immediately copes with the situation by getting high is especially memorable.

Movie	Link to Chapter	Page Reference to Wedding and Boyd
• The Lost Weekend • Ironweed • Clean and Sober • Leaving Las Vegas • Drunks	alcohol dependence (p. 298)	p. 79 p. 86 p. 86 p. 87 p. 87
• Clean and Sober • The Seven Percent Solution • I'm Dancing As Fast As I Can • Reefer Madness • The Man with the Golden Arm • Easy Rider • The French Connection • Pulp Fiction	drug dependence (p. 312)	p. 88 p. 89 p. 89 p. 89 p. 91 p. 95 p. 97 p. 97

Classroom Assessment Techniques (CAT)

One-Sentence Summary (CAT 11-1)
Ask students to summarize a specific piece of information in this chapter by responding to the question, "Who does/did what to whom, when, where, how and why?"

Focused Listing (CAT 11-2)
Select an important point from this chapter (e.g., addiction, tolerance) and ask students to write five words or phrases that describe the point.

Directed Paraphrasing (CAT 11-3)
In two or three sentences, students should paraphrase some important idea, concept, or definition presented in Chapter 11. Consider paraphrasing dependence, abuse, and withdrawal.

Minute Paper (CAT 11-4)
Ask your students to about an important question they have that remains unanswered.

Definition Matrix (CAT 11-5)
Using the handout, students should summarize the characteristics of psychoactive drugs. Students should attempt to write only a few words or phrases.

Suggestions for Essay Questions

- Describe the concepts of addiction, tolerance, and withdrawal in the context of alcohol dependence.
- Compare the pros and cons of the legalization of marijuana. Where do you stand on the issue. Defend your position.
- If you were a clinical psychologist treating a person for nicotine dependence using the cognitive approach, how would you help him avoid the abstinence violation effect?

Definition Matrix
Classroom Assessment Technique

Drug	Classification	Effects	Dangers
alcohol			
nicotine			
opium			
morphine			
methadone			
pentobarbital			
Valium			
Dexedrine			
cocaine			
LSD			
PCP			
marijuana			

Chapter 12

Sexual Dysfunctions, Paraphilias, and Gender Identity Disorders

Chapter Map

Section	Instructor Manual Components
Defining Sexual Disorders	*Kinsey's research (LL 12-1)* *What is best? (TP 12-1)* *Reviewing the criteria for abnormal behavior (TP 12-2)* *Normal here, abnormal there (TP 12-3)* *Immorality vs. abnormality (TP 12-4)* *Defining normal and abnormal sexual behavior (ACT/DEMO 12-1)*
Sexual Dysfunctions • Forms of Sexual Dysfunction • Diagnosing Sexual Dysfunction • Groups at Risk for Sexual Dysfunction	*Viagra (LL 12-2)* *Premature ejaculation (LL 12-3)* *Test to determine cause of erectile disorder (TP 12-5)*
Sexual Dysfunction: Theory and Therapy • The Psychodynamic Perspective • The Behavioral and Cognitive Perspective • Multifaceted Treatment • The Biological Perspective	*Should Viagra be covered by health insurance? (TP 12-6)*

Paraphilias • Fetishism • Transvestism • Exhibitionism • Voyeurism • Sadism and Masochism • Frotteurism • Pedophilia • Groups at Risk for Paraphilias	*Unusual paraphilias (LL 12-4)* *Demographics of pedophilia (LL 12-5)* *Case studies (LL 12-6)* *Pedophobia? (TP 12-7)* *Mooning, streaking, and cross-dressing (TP 12-8)* *Sex and advertising (ACT/DEMO 12-2)*
Paraphilias: Theory and Therapy • The Psychodynamic Perspective • The Behavioral Perspective • The Cognitive Perspective • The Biological Perspective	*Guest speakers (ACT/DEMO 12-3)*
Gender Identity Disorders • Patterns of Gender Identity Disorders • The Psychodynamic Perspective • The Behavioral Perspective • The Biological Perspective • Gender Reassignment	*Effects of husbands' revelation of transvestism and* *transsexualism (LL 12-7)* *Illustrating gender identity disorder (TP 12-9)*

Chapter Outline

I.   Defining Sexual Disorders
    A.   Western culture's social morality influenced by religion and sexology
    B.   Definition of sexual normality helped guarantee survival of human species and the family
    C.   Direction of sex drive influenced by socialization
    D.   Human sexual behavior viewed across culture is extremely variable
    E.   Within culture, attitudes toward sexuality may change over time
        1.   Sexual behavior does not necessarily conform to declared standards of sexual morality or normality
        2.   Social climate of 1960s and 1970s questioned traditional sexual morality
            a.   American Psychiatric Association dropped homosexuality from list of psychological disorders in 1973
            b.   Research suggests that there was no justification for regarding homosexuality as pathological pattern

II. Sexual Dysfunction
    A.   Our society has had two upheavals regarding sex
        1.   Sexual revolution of 1960s and 1970s and openness about sex
        2.   Spreading of AIDS by casual sex
    B.   Forms of Sexual Dysfunction
        1.   **Sexual dysfunctions** are disorders of disruption of sexual response cycle or pain during intercourse
        2.   Research of Masters and Johnson led to better understanding of sexual dysfunction
        3.   Sexual Desire Disorders
            a.   First phase of sexual response cycle is desire phase
            b.   Hypoactive Sexual Desire Disorder
                i.   **Hypoactive sexual desire disorder** refers to lack of interest in sexual activity even in sexual fantasy
                ii.   Low desire defined within context of age, gender, and cultural norms
                iii.   Biological factors include pain, illness, and reduced testosterone
                iv.   Psychological factors include depression, stress, ambivalence about sex and conflict in relationship
                v.   Is most common complaint of couples seeking treatment for sexual dysfunction
            c.   Sexual Aversion Disorder
                i.   **Sexual aversion disorder** characterized by lack of interest in sex and disgust or fear of sex
                ii.   Related to sexual trauma, dyspareunia
        4.   Sexual Arousal Disorders

a. Arousal is second phase of sexual response cycle
b. Female Sexual Arousal Disorder
    i. **Female sexual arousal** disorder related to insufficient vaginal lubrication
    ii. Few known biological factors
    iii. Psychological factors include emotional distress, sexual trauma, and lack of trust
c. Male Erectile Disorder
    i. **Male erectile disorder** formerly known as impotence
    ii. Related to multiple causes
    iii. Age and medical conditions, substance abuse are factors
    iv. Psychological factors include performance anxiety, stress, depression

5. Orgasmic Disorders
  a. Third phase of sexual response cycle is orgasm
  b. Female Orgasmic Disorder
    i. **Female orgasmic disorder** involves woman having trouble reaching orgasm
    ii. Common causes include other sexual problems, inadequate sexual stimulation, and anxiety about sex
    iii. Antidepressant drugs becoming more frequent cause
  c. Male Orgasmic Disorder
    i. **Male orgasmic disorder** is male's inability to reach orgasm
    ii. May be caused by antidepressants and problems letting go with partner
  d. Premature Ejaculation
    i. Most common complaint is **premature ejaculation** which is reaching orgasm too soon
    ii. May be due to both psychological and biological causes

6. Sexual Pain Disorders
  a. Dyspareunia
    i. **Dyspareunia** is pain during sexual activity
    ii. Usually due to gynecological or urological problems
  b. Vaginismus
    i. Vaginismus involves contraction of muscles that surround outer part of vagina
    ii. Muscles contract causing pain during intercourse
    iii. Often related to sexual trauma

C. Diagnosing Sexual Dysfunction
  1. **Lifelong dysfunction** refers to problem existing since earliest sexual experiences
  2. **Acquired dysfunction** refers to problem that develops after normal functioning
  3. **Generalized dysfunction** refers to dysfunction present in all sexual situations
  4. **Situational dysfunction** refers to dysfunction present in some sexual situations or with some partners
  5. Term sexual dysfunction must meet criteria
     a. Dysfunction diagnosed with evidence that dysfunction causes marked distress or interpersonal difficulty
     b. Dysfunction must persist over time
  6. One failure often creates anxiety which impairs sexual responsiveness on next occasion
D. Groups at Risk for Sexual Dysfunction
  1. More education and money person has, less at risk
  2. Racial and ethnic differences
  3. Prevalence varies with gender

III. Sexual Dysfunction: Theory and Therapy
  A. The Psychodynamic Perspective
    1. Sexual dysfunction attributed to unresolved Oedipal conflict
    2. Current approach views sexual dysfunction as disturbance in object-relations
    3. Therapy involves uncovering conflict and working through it
  B. The Behavioral and Cognitive Perspectives
    1. Learned Anxiety and the Spectator Role
       a. Early respondent conditioning in which sexual feelings paired with shame, disgust, and anxiety over possible failure seen as central
       b. Painful experiences cause person to worry and assume **spectator role**
       c. Spectator role caused by several factors
    2. Assessment
       a. Assessment important for treatment and takes into account all relevant factors
       b. Sexual script developed to describe who does what to whom, and what thoughts, emotions, and sensations each associates with sex
       c. Attitudes, patterns of sexual arousal, and sexual trauma part of assessment
    3. Direct Symptomatic Treatment
       a. Couple is retrained to experience sexual excitement without performance pressure
       b. Training is in form of sensate focus exercises

                                 i.   Allow partners to rediscover sexual response without anxiety

                                 ii.   Improve communication by providing feedback

               c.   Start-stop and squeeze techniques used in premature ejaculation

               d.   Paradoxical instruction used in erectile disorder

               e.   Education and self-exploration exercises used to treat lifelong orgasmic dysfunction in women

               f.   Sexual aversion disorder treated with systematic desensitization

       4.   Cognitive Psychology and Direct Treatment

               a.   Masters and Johnson used direct treatment of sexual dysfunction with emphasis on the couple

               b.   Cognitive approach focuses on mental processes underlying sexual response and attitudes and beliefs hostile to sex

C.   Multifaceted Treatment

       1.   Kaplan: Remote Causes

               a.   Kaplan argues that sexual dysfunction caused by immediate and remote causes

                               i.   Immediate causes include performance anxiety, poor technique, and poor communication

                               ii.   Remote causes include intrapsychic conflicts

               c.   Combined direct treatment and psychodynamic treatment into psychosexual treatment

               d.   Remote causes ignore as long as patient is responding to immediate causes

               e.   Remote causes may prevent patient from responding

               f.   Direct therapy brings to surface psychological problems

       2.   Family Systems Theory: The Function of the Dysfunction

               a.   Masters and Johnson see patient as the couple

                b.   Sexual dysfunction has function in couple's total relationship

                c.   Questions about power and control may be related to sexual dysfunction

               g.   Secret payoffs may underlie sexual dysfunctions and must be dealt with

       3.   Results of Cognitive-Behavioral Direct Treatment

               a.   Outcomes may not match outcomes of Masters and Johnson's therapy

               b.   Research in early stages for many treatments of sexual dysfunction

               c.   Group therapy may be useful for some dysfunctions

               d.   Combining relationship therapy with direct treatment may be beneficial

D.   The Biological Perspective

1. Some cases of sexual dysfunctions caused by organic factors
2. Diagnostic tools used to differentiate between psychological and organic sexual dysfunctions
3. Most sexual dysfunctions involve both psychological and physiological factors
4. Biological treatments have focused on erectile disorder
   a. Vacuum pump used for enhancing erections
   b. Injecting a vascular dilation agent
   c. Using a vasodilator
   d. Drug called yohimbine stimulates secretion of norepinephrine
   e. Penile prosthesis is available
   f. Oral medications are available and they act on the tissues of penis itself
5. Trend is to integrate biological and psychological treatments

IV. Paraphilias
   A. Recognized patterns that deviate from standard are called **paraphilias**
   B. Distinction made between paraphilias that involve harm to others and those that are victimless
   C. When pattern or object becomes central focus and sine qua non of person's arousal and gratification, then pattern is considered abnormal
   D. Fetishism
      1. **Fetishism**--reliance on inanimate objects or on a body part to exclusion of person as a whole for sexual gratification
      2. Example of spectrum disorder
      3. Exclusive fascination with inanimate object known as partialism
      4. Most fetishes associated with human body such as fur, women's stockings, shoes, and underpants
   E. Transvestism
      1. **Transvestism**--sexual gratification through dressing in clothes of opposite sex
      2. After cross-dressed, transvestite masturbates or has heterosexual intercourse
      3. As a group, transvestites no more prone to psychological disturbances than general population
      4. Most lead quiet, conventional lives
      5. Transvestism confused with other forms of cross-dressing
         a. Cross-dressing for sexual pleasure in transvestism
         b. Cross-dressing to assume a female role (e.g., drag queens who are typically homosexual; entertainers as part of performance) not transvestism
         c. Often confused with transsexuals who have gender identity disorder
      6. Related disorder is **autogynephilia** in which man depends for sexual arousal on the fantasy of being a woman

F.   Exhibitionism
1.   **Exhibitionism**--sexual gratification through display of one's genitals to involuntary observer
2.   Most exhibitionist are not dangerous
3.   Typical exhibitionist is young man, sexually inhibited, and unhappily married
4.   Gratification is derived from women's shock, fear, and revulsion and then from masturbation
5.   In some cases, exhibitionism is symptom of more pervasive disturbance
6.   Most exhibitionists are shy, submissive, immature men who experience feelings of social and sexual inferiority and doubts their masculinity
7.   Exposing genitals gives them sense of masculine powers
8.   Best cure for exhibitionist is not to respond to it

G.   Voyeurism
1.   **Voyeurism**--sexual gratification through clandestine observation of other people's sexual activities or sexual anatomy
2.   Often occurs alongside normal sexual interest
3.   Must take into account invasion of person's privacy
4.   Risk involved in watching strangers is important to gratification
5.   Voyeurism provides substitute gratification and reassurance of power
6.   Most voyeurs are harmless

H.   Sadism and Masochism
1.   **Sadism**--sexual gratification through infliction of pain and/or humiliation on others
2.   **Masochism**--sexual gratification through pain and/or humiliation inflicted on oneself
3.   Terms named after literary figures who wrote about physical and psychological cruelty
4.   Degree of cruelty ranges from sticking person with pin to mutilation
5.   **Sadomasochistic** relationship seen in complementary partners
6.   Most sadists and masochists are heterosexual, well educated, affluent, and undisturbed by their sexual activities
7.   Drawing line between normal and abnormal may be difficult
     a.   DSM-IV requires evidence of distress of interpersonal difficulty
     b.   Many are satisfied with their sexual patterns

I.   Frotteurism
1.   **Frotteurism**--sexual gratification through touching and rubbing against a nonconsenting person
2.   Frotteurs operate in crowded places where they are more likely to escape

290

3. Sense of power over unsuspecting victim is important
J. Pedophilia
   1. **Pedophilia--child molesting**
   2. Involves serious violation of child's right; child may suffer serious psychological harm
   3. About 10-15% of children and adolescents are victims
   4. Most pedophiles are male
      a. Appears to be law-abiding and escapes detection
      b. Most are acquainted with victim and his/her family and may be related to victim
   5. Molestation usually does not include physical violence, but persuasion using authority
   6. Molestation occurs in repeated incidents with same child
   7. Pedophilia usually accompanied by other paraphilias
   8. Two types of molesters
      a. Situational molesters
         i. More or less normal
         ii. Have heterosexual histories and prefer adult sexual partners
         iii. Molestation is impulsive and usually response to stress
         iv. Incest offenders usually this type
      b. Preference molesters
         i. Prefer children as sexual partners, usually male children
         ii. Do not view their behavior as abnormal
         iii. Child molesting is regular sexual outlet and planned
         iv. Have a higher recidivism rate
   8. Causes of pedophilia are varied
      a. May be arrested psychological development
      b. Early experience of arousal with other children
      c. Attempt to reenact their histories of molestation
   9. Children do not report their victimization immediately
      a. Child victims report sleep and eating disorders and types of fears
      b. Adults who were victimized as children report depression, self-destructive behaviors, and distrust of others
   10. Some types of child abuse seem to be more harmful
      a. Abuse at early age
      b. Continuing over long period of time
      c. Close relationship with pedophile
      d. Violent or severe abuse
   11. **Incest** is sexual relations between family members
      a. Rate of incest is 7-17%
      b. Victims of fathers report more harm than other perpetrators

   c. Abuse by father or stepfather more damaging
     i. Typical incestuous father limits extramarital sexual contacts to daughter or several daughters
     ii. Tend to be highly moralistic
     iii. Father-daughter incest occurs in troubled marriage
     iv. Wife is often isolated from other family members
     v. Daughter may assume caretaking role in family
   d. Long-term effects on daughter are profound
  K. Groups at Risk for Paraphilias
   1. Most of paraphilias are dominated by males
   2. Masochism is exception with 20:1 male-female ratio
   3. Socialization differences, arrest records, and biological differences may account for male-female difference
V. Paraphilias: Theory and Therapy
  A. The Psychodynamic Perspective
   1. Oedipal Fixation
    a. Paraphilias are continuation into adulthood of diffuse sexual preoccupations of child
    b. Paraphilias result of fixation at pregenital state resulting in castration anxiety
    c. Transvestism seen as denial of mother's presumed castration
    d. Sadism is seen as attempt to take part of castrator to relieve anxiety
    e. Other psychodynamic theories suggest role of person's inability to disentangle and control basic id impulses
   2. Group and Individual Therapy
    a. Usual procedure is to uncover conflict by working through it
    b. Group therapy places individual in situation where they learn they are not the only one
    c. Research suggests that psychodynamic therapy to be ineffective
  B. The Behavioral Perspective
   1. Conditioning
    a. Deviation results from respondent-conditioning process where early sexual experiences associated with unconventional stimuli
    b. Sadism and masochism involve failure to learn to discriminate among types of arousal
    c. Deviations may be due to child being cuddled by parents only after being punished, pairing physical affection with punishment
   2. Unlearning Deviant Patterns

a. Multifaceted approach combines psychotherapy with techniques to change arousal patterns
b. Goal is to change sexual arousal patterns, beliefs and behaviors
c. First step is to bring deviant sexual behavior under temporary control
d. Behavioral techniques used to eliminate deviant approach
   i. Stimulus satiation
   ii. Covert sensitization
   iii. Shame aversion therapy
e. Treatment attempts to build appropriate sexual orientation and includes training in social and sexual skills
f. Trend towards relapse prevention training

C. The Cognitive Perspective
   1. Learning Deviant Attitudes
      a. Way sex drive is expressed depends on childhood attitudes
      b. Sex offenders tend to objectify their victims as sources of gratification rather than as human beings
   2. Combating Deviant Beliefs
      a. Procedures is to identify deviation-supporting beliefs, challenge them and replace them with appropriate beliefs
      b. Many programs include training in victim awareness where they are confronted with emotional damage done to victims
      c. Another technique is role reversal

D. The Biological Perspective
   1. Deviations may be related to neurological disorders
   2. Studies have inconclusive results
   3. Castration, drugs, and brain surgery have been used
   4. Changes in deviant arousal in laboratory may not generalize

VI. Gender Identity Disorders
   A. **Gender identity disorders** characterized by sense of gender is opposite of one's biological gender
   B. GID defined by two features
      1. Gender dysphoria is unhappiness with one's own gender
      2. Desire to change to other gender
   C. Cross-dressing known since ancient times
   E. **Transexual** refers to people seeking to change gender by means of hormones or surgery
   F. Patterns of Gender Identity Disorder
      1. Homosexual male-to-female transsexuals
      2. Homosexual female-to-male transsexuals
      3. Heterosexual male-to-female transsexuals
      4. GID can be of childhood and adolescent or of adulthood

293

5.   Most children who have desire to be opposite do not grow up to be transsexual adults

G.   The Psychodynamic Perspective
1.   GID seen as disturbance in parent-infant bond
2.   Males said to be in overlong, symbiotic relationships with mother, creating a female identity in infant
3.   Females identify with father instead because of mother's physical or emotional absence
4.   Some argue that psychoanalysis is not appropriate since opposite-sex parent part of core identity and cannot be changed

H.   The Behavioral Perspective
1.   GID is caused by gender role behavior being shaped toward opposite sex by caretaker
2.   Treatment involves stopping reinforcement for cross-dressing behavior and providing reinforcement for gender-appropriate behavior
3.   Another idea suggests that GID is result of imprinted gender fixation

I.   The Biological Perspective
1.   Hypothesis suggests GID due to hormone imbalance
2.   Difference in brain also believed to be involved

J.   Gender Reassignment
1.   One solution is to change the identity to fit body
2.   Alternative is to change body to fit identity in process called **gender reassignment**
3.   Process involves steps
    a.   Undergoes detailed evaluation by mental health professional
    b.   At least three months of psychotherapy
    c.   Hormone treatments to initiate physical changes
    d.   In real-life test, individual must live completely in desired gender for at least one year
    e.   Last phase is surgery
         i.   Outcomes of gender reassignment surgery is improvement or satisfaction in two-thirds to nine-tenths of patients
         iii.   Some regretted surgery having serious psychological breakdowns
    f.   Outcomes of surgery influenced by several factors
         i.   Longer patient kept in real-life test and more realistic expectations, the better the outcome
         ii.   Female-to-male reassignment yields more satisfaction
         iii.   Person's prior psychological health also predictor of success

Chapter Boxes

- Sex in America: Myths and Reality
    - A. Survey suggests that Americans are far more conservative sexually than thought
    - B. Most Americans have limited sexual histories and have less sex than might have been guessed
    - C. Homosexuality less prevalent than is often claimed
    - D. Surveys reveal ethnic and religious differences in sexual behavior
    - E. Self-report survey limited by what people choose to report

- What is Normal Sexual Response in a Woman
    - A. Some argue that definition of sexual normality is male-centered
    - B. Some women only gain orgasm through direct stimulation of clitoris and not through intercourse
    - C. No evidence that women who only achieve orgasm through stimulation of clitoris are less healthy or mature than those who do not
    - D. Female sexual response is extremely variable

Learning Objectives (LO)

By the time you have finished studying this chapter, you should be able to do the following-.

1. Discuss the difficulties involved in defining normal and abnormal sexual behavior, using historical and cultural factors and the issue of homosexuality as examples (336-339, 342).

2. Define sexual dysfunction, and describe the dysfunctions grouped under each of three phases of the sexual response cycle (338, 340-341).

3. Describe two sexual pain disorders, and discuss the issues surrounding the diagnosis of sexual dysfunctions, distinguishing among lifelong, acquired, generalized, and situational dysfunctions (341-343).

4. Summarize statistics on the distribution of sexual dysfunction by gender, education, ethnicity, and income (343-244).

5. Explain the psychodynamic perspective on sexual dysfunction, and then describe behavioral and cognitive approaches that have largely displaced the psychodynamic viewpoint (344-347).

6. Summarize multifaceted treatment of sexual dysfunction, making reference to the family systems approach, and to Kaplan's theory involving immediate and remote causes (347-349).

7. List and describe possible organic causes of sexual dysfunction, and describe treatments for dysfunction based on the biological perspective (349-350).

8. Define paraphilias according to *DSM-IV,* define fetishism, transvestism, exhibitionism, and voyeurism, describe the persons likely to engage in each, and explain how each one presents problems for the client and/or interferes with the rights of others (350-354).

9. Define sadism masochism, frotteurism, pedophilia, and incest, describe the persons likely to engage in each, and explain how each one presents problems for the client and/or interferes with the rights of others (354 357).

10. Explain the psychodynamic perspective on the paraphilias, with special emphasis on the role of Oedipal fixation (357-358).

11. Explain the behavioral and cognitive understandings of the paraphilias, and give examples of learning-based treatment strategies (358-360).

296

12. Explain the biological view of and treatment for the paraphilias (360).

13. Define gender identity disorder describe three patterns in which this disorder manifests itself, and give examples of treatment for gender identity- disorder from the psychodynamic, behavioral, and biological perspectives, including sex reassignment surgery (360-364).

Lecture Leads (LL)

Kinsey's research (LL 12-1)

Alfred Kinsey was a professor of zoology at Indiana University and later coordinated a marriage course at the university. He soon became interested in sexual behavior and started to collect data, founding the Institute for Sex Research. Kinsey's research in the 1940s and 1950s has been said to profoundly influence the way we perceive sexuality, and the curriculum and practice of sex education. Now, there is growing awareness of serious flaws in his methodology and allegations of unethical treatment of children. These flaws and charges of unethical conducted are detailed in Reisman and Eichel (1990). For instance, one problem was sampling bias. His sample was biased with nearly 25% of the so-called "normal" male sample actually being prison inmates of which a significant number were sex offenders. Moreover, he eliminated black male subjects. He discounted the possibility that this volunteer bias could have confounded his results. This alleged volunteer bias may have seriously skewed his sample, which raise, questions about Kinsey's conclusions, such as 13% of the male population was predominantly homosexual and that 70% of males have had sex with prostitutes. Even more controversial is Kinsey's research on child sexuality. His conclusions were based on interviews of pedophiles and, in one of the most shocking, grievously unethical procedures, the molestation of children. Children were sexually stimulated to achieve orgasms. Kinsey conducted sexual experiments on children from 2 months to 15 years of age. In the chapter entitled "Early Sexual Growth and Activity" in Sexual Behavior in the Human Male (1948), Kinsey reported orgasm data of these children on page 161, Table 34. He measured the length of time the child was stimulated and the number of orgasms occurring in a time period. Based on these data and others, he concluded that children are sexual beings, children haven't had orgasms because of a lack of experiences like the ones in his research (see page 178). Reisman and Eichel suggest that Kinsey's conclusions have gone unchallenged and "If the public learns the truth, the 'sexperts' in the field of human sexuality and the sex industry will be shaken to its foundation. Whole shelves of books will have to be rewritten. Both public and [even] religious schools will have to discard their sex ed courses."

Resources:

Kinsey, A. C., Pomeroy, W. B., & Martin, C. E. (1948). Sexual behavior in the human male. Philadelphia: W. B. Saunders

Reisman, J. A., & Eichel, E. W. (1990). Kinsey, sex and fraud: The indoctrination of a people. Lafayette, LA: Huntington House Publishers.

Viagra (LL 12-2)

There are about 30 million American males suffering from erectile disorder and many of them have found relief in Viagra (Sildenafil). The recent introduction of Viagra has received much attention in the media and with good reason. Viagra reverses male erectile disorder with few side effects. Viagra increases blood flow into the penis in about an hour after being taken orally and represents an improvement over other treatments such as those described in the textbook. Less than 15% of those who take Viagra report facial flushing and about 3% experience short-term problems with seeing blue. Patients who take Viagra report feeling like they did many years ago. But as of yet, many health insurance companies are reluctant to provide coverage for Viagra. One significant question is should insurance pay for someone's sexuality. If health insurance companies do ultimately cover Viagra, at what level will it be? Who will decide how many times a month a man needs an erection? In addition, Viagra is not an aphrodisiac; a man will not benefit from it if he lacks a libido. Viagra has also had the effect of bringing the topic of male sexuality out into the public forum and has started to reduce the stigma associated with male erectile disorder. Viagra will not help a man to improve sexual performance if he already has normal erections.

Premature ejaculation (LL 12-3)
The most common male sexual dysfunction is premature ejaculation. Metz et al. (1997) review the literature describing the dysfunctions's prevalence, neurophysiology, and neruropharmacology. The authors point out that poor clinical outcomes may be due to failing to recognize the two basic types of premature ejaculation. Treatment should be tailored to biogenic and psychogenic premature ejaculation.

Resource:
Metz, M. E. et al. (1997). Premature ejaculation: A psychophysiological review. Journal of Sex and Marital Therapy, 23, 3-23.

Unusual paraphilias (LL 12-4)
There are several unusual paraphilias that are described as being not otherwise specified or atypical. The breadth of these paraphilias effectively conveys the range of human sexual experience. Acrotomophilia refers to being aroused by a partner who has an amputated limb. Scatologia is a paraphilia centered on making obscene phone calls. If a person is dependent on the smell, taste, or sight of feces for sexual gratification, that person may be considered to have coprophilia. Klismaphilia is marked by a dependence on receiving an enema to experience sexual gratification. Urophilia refers to the desire to urinate on one's partner or to be urinated upon for sexual pleasure. An individual who desires sexual gratification by creating and managing a disaster such as a traffic accident may have symphorophilia. Narratophilia refers to the paraphilia that involves dependence of using dirty words or stories in the presence of one's partner. Zoophilia, or bestiality, is the use of animals to receive sexual gratification. Sexual gratification is achieved when a person with keptophilia enters and steals from a stranger or potential partner. Autogonistophilia refers to a dependency on being observed or being on stage. Finally, hybristophilia is evident if a person is dependent on being with a sexual partner known to have committed a violent crime such as rape, or murder, or who served a prison sentence. Follow up with a discussion focusing on why these disorders are abnormal, using the criterion presented in Chapter 1.

Resources:
Crooks, R., & Baur, K. (1990). Our sexuality (4th ed.). Redwood, CA: The
    Benjamin/Cumings Publishing Company.

Money, J. (1986). Lovemaps. New York: Irvington Publishing.

Solomon, P., & Patch, V. D. (1971). Handbook of psychiatry. Los Altos, CA: Lang
    Medical

Demographics of pedophilia (LL 12-5)
A number of interesting studies have suggested that certain backgrounds are associated
with pedophilia. For instance, Dhawan and Marshall (1996) found that among male
rapists, child molesters, and nonsexual offenders, 62% of the rapists, 50% of the
molesters, and only 20% of the nonsexual offenders reported a history of sexual abuse as
children. Another study examined 170 pedophiles for birth order effects (Bogaert et al.,
1997). The results indicate that homosexual pedophiles and bisexual pedophiles were
more likely to be later borns than heterosexual pedophiles. The authors discuss how
these data question some theories on pedophilia.

Resources:
Bogaert, A. F., Bezeau, S., Kuban, M., & Blanchard, R. (1997). Pedophilia, sexual
    orientation, and birth order. Journal of Abnormal Psychology, 106, 331-335.

Dhawan, S., & Marshall, W. L. (1996). Sexual abuse histories of sexual offenders.
    Sexual Abuse: Journal of Research and Treatment, 8, 7-15.

Case studies (LL 12-6)
Examining case studies can be a useful augment to the textbook descriptions of sexual
dysfunctions. Sbrocco et al. (1997) describe the cases involved three males (35, 45, and
55 years old) who experienced similar sensations during panic attacks and during sexual
arousal. Wise and Goldberg present the case of a 47-year-old with coprophagia. A 40-
year-old male with a underwear fetish is described in Klavens (1995). In this particular
case, the subject undergoes psychoanalysis and discovers that his fetish is related to a
love-hate tie to women. Potential serial killers are considered in Johnson and Becker
(1997). Several teenagers (14-18 year olds) with sexually sadistic fantasies of killing are
examined. It was noted that these teenagers hold similar fantasies as those who actually
became serial killers. Cooper and Cosgray, Hanna, Fawely, and Money describe several
cases of autoerotic asphyxiation. Collacott and Cooper document the case of a 30-year-
old learning-disabled man with a fetish for observing women urinate. Finally, Sanders
(1996) describes how a 15-year-old male, who had a fixation on diapers, feces, and older
female caregivers, received therapy and showed a successful outcome.

Resources:
Collacott, R. A., & Cooper, S. A. (1995). Urine fetish in a man with learning
    disabilities. Journal of Intellectual Disability Research, 39, 145-147.

Cooper, A. J. (1996). Auto-erotic asphyxiation: Three case reports. <u>Journal of Sex and Marital Therapy,</u> <u>22,</u> 47-53.

Cosgray, R. E., Hanna, V., Fawley, R., & Money, M. (1991). Death from auto-erotic asphyxiation in a long-term psychiatric setting. <u>Perspectives in Psychiatric Care,</u> <u>27,</u> 21-24.

Johnson, B. R., & Becker, J. V. (1997). Natural born killers? The development of the sexually sadistic serial killer. <u>Journal of the American Academy of Psychiatry and the Law,</u> <u>25,</u> 335-348.

Klavens, G. S. (1995). A fetish as a creative attempt to master trauma: A report of a psychoanalysis. <u>Journal of Clinical Psychoanalysis,</u> <u>4,</u> 223-252.

Sanders, G. L. (1996). Recovering from paraphilia: An adolescent's journey from despair to hope. <u>Journal of Child and Youth Care,</u> <u>11,</u> 43-54.

Sbrocco, T., Weisberg, R. B., Barlow, D. H., & Carter, M. M. (1997). The conceptual relationship between panic disorder and male erectile dysfunction. <u>Journal of Sex and Marital Therapy,</u> <u>23,</u> 212-220.

Wise, T. N., & Goldberg, R. L. (1995). Escalation of a fetish: Coprophagia in a nonpsychotic adult of normal intelligence. <u>Journal of Sex and Marital Therapy,</u> <u>21,</u> 272-275.

Effects of husbands' revelation of transvestism and transsexualism (LL 12-7)
Two wives of transvestites and two wives of transsexuals were studied after learning of their husbands' status. The subjects, who ranged from 35 years of age to 48 years of age, completed several open-ended questions. Their responses were analyzed with particular attention to questioning of their heterosexuality, which was how the sexual orientation confusion was operationalized. The results reveal that the two wives of the transvestites experienced sexual orientation confusion, while the two wives of the transsexuals did not. In a related article, Brown (1994) describes the typical female partner of cross-dressing men.

Resources:

Brown, G. R. (1994). Women in relationships with cross-dressing men: A descriptive study from a nonclinical setting. <u>Archives of Sexual Behavior,</u> <u>23,</u> 515-530.

Hunt, S., & Main, T. L. (1997). Sexual orientation confusion among spouses of transvestites and transsexuals following disclosures of spouse's gender dysphoria. <u>Journal of Psychology and Human Sexuality,</u> <u>9,</u> 39-51.

Talking Points (TP)

What is best? (TP 12-1)
History has shown us two extremes in how society views sexuality. On the one extreme is the view of sexuality as only for procreation, and discussion of it is strictly prohibited and morality is tied to a belief in absolute truth. On the other extreme is a culture where there is no-holds-barred sex, "whatever feels good, do it", and morality is based on relativism. Lead a discussion with students focusing on the advantages and disadvantages of each extreme as related to sexuality.

Reviewing the criteria for abnormal behavior (TP 12-2)
It is a good idea to review the criteria for abnormal behavior from Chapter 1. You may want to frame this discussion by asking how the various sexual dysfunctions, gender identity disorders, and paraphilias relate to each of the criterion (i.e., norm violation, statistical rarity, personal discomfort, maladaptive behavior).

Normal here, abnormal there (TP 12-3)
Lead a discussion on what is considered to be normal behavior in our country and other countries in terms of sexual behavior. Examples could be men holding hands in public, men kissing in European countries, women walking arm in arm in Europe. Ask for input from students from the individualistic perspective as well as the collectivist's perspective.

Immorality vs. abnormality (TP 12-4)
Have students discuss the immorality of a sexual disorder in contrast to its abnormality. It is quite clear that pedophilia will probably be considered both immoral and abnormal by students. Disorders such as foot fetishes make this distinction much more unclear. Homosexuality may be considered quite immoral by some but is not abnormal by definition. Discuss how personal biases and political correctness can cause the clinician to erroneously classify a patient.

Test to determine cause of erectile disorder (TP 12-5)
A technique to determine if a male's erectile disorder was psychological or physical involved a postage stamp. The stamp was stuck on the man's penis as he went to bed. In the morning, the stamp is examined, and if it was ripped, it indicated that during REM, the man had an erection. This would suggest a psychological cause for his erectile disorder. A more contemporary method uses a snap gauge, which is a fabric band that is placed around the penis at night.

Should Viagra be covered by health insurance? (TP 12-6)
Most students have probably heard about this successful new treatment of male erectile disorder. Many health insurance companies do not cover Viagra. Ask students to think about the pros and cons of coverage for Viagra.

Pedophobia? (TP 12-7)
Some pedophiles have begun to assert that their sexual behavior is an orientation or an alternative lifestyle and should not be consider abnormal. Some have suggested that we should start looking for the word, "pedophobia" to be used to describe people who would not support the rights of pedophiles or those who see their sexual behavior as immoral or abnormal.

Mooning, streaking, and cross-dressing (TP 12-8)
Students will no doubt have questions about the paraphilias. One common question involves the practice of mooning, which is exposing one's buttocks as an insult to someone. Ask your students if they thinking mooning matches the diagnostic criteria for exhibitionism. There is a scene in the movie *American Graffiti* that involves mooning that your students might remember. Some of your students might recall streaking from the 1970s. Ask students to think about whether streaking constitutes exhibitionism. Cross-dressing is another area that fascinates many students. There are two public figures that cross-dress. Do Dennis Rodman and Ru Paul meet the diagnostic criteria for transvestism or even a gender identity disorder? Why did Dustin Hoffman's character in *Tootsie* cross-dress?

Illustrating gender identity disorder (TP 12-9)
This is a very effective way to communicate the dysphoria experienced by those with gender identity disorders. Select a male and a female student who are able to tolerate some attention. Ask them to look at each other and say to the male student, "You have just taken a shower and have stepped out of the shower. You are naked and you look at yourself in the mirror. This is what you see." Point to the female student. Ask the male student, "How does this make you feel? You identify yourself as a male, yet you have a female's body." Reverse the roles.

Activities and Demonstrations (ACT/DEMO)

Defining normal and abnormal sexual behavior (ACT/DEMO 12-1)
Objective: To illustrate the difficulty in defining normal and abnormal sexual behavior
Materials: None
Procedure: Mary Kite has developed a classroom exercise to illustrate the obstacles in defining normal and abnormal sexual behavior. Kite has created a 30-item questionnaire that requires students to rate the normalcy of particular behaviors. Behaviors include, "watching X-rated movies several times a week," "using sex toys during sex," and "having rape fantasies." After completing the survey, students should be placed in groups of no more than three. Their task is to develop a definition of normal sexual behavior and abnormal sexual behavior. Each group, then, should share their definitions with the class.
Discussion: Keep track of the definitions. Ask your students to think about how the current DSM-IV would change if the definitions of proposed abnormal sexual behavior were accepted. Another area of exploration is to examine how the students' backgrounds have influenced their definitions.

Resource:
Kite, M. E. (1990). Defining normal sexual behavior: A classroom exercise. Teaching
    of Psychology, 17, 118-119.

Sex and advertising (ACT/DEMO 12-2)
Objective: To demonstrate the amount of sexual material in advertising
Materials: None
Procedure: Have students watch television, read popular magazines, and observe newspapers and outdoor advertising to record the number of sexual advertisements they see. For each time, students should record the type of media, the product advertised, and the implied message.
Discussion: Summarize the types of advertisements on an overhead and update it throughout the discussion. What are the most erotic advertisements? What are the most offensive? What type of product is the most common product? What is the least likely product to use sex in advertising? What is the subtlest use of sex? Do the students think that there should be more or less emphasis on sex in advertising? List as many sexually explicit advertisements in television, radio, newspapers, popular magazines, or outdoor advertising as you can that have occurred in the last 48 hours

Guest speakers (ACT/DEMO 12-3)
Objective: To illustrate the type of treatments used in clinical practice
Materials: None
Procedure: There are a number of avenues that your students can explore when you invite speakers to your class to discuss the various sexual dysfunctions and paraphilias presented in the chapter. For instance, consider inviting psychologists, sex therapists, or psychiatrists who specialize in treatment or research of sexual dysfunctions or paraphilias. Another idea is to invite a spokesperson from a local gay rights group to

305

speak to your class. Of course, to be balanced, you'll want to invite a representative that can present the opposing view.

Discussion: Beforehand, instruct students to review this chapter and be prepared to ask questions of their guest speakers. Afterwards, ask students to discuss speakers' presentations.

Films and Videos

Boys Will Be.... BAX. Looks at domestic violence by focusing on the characteristics of a successful, middle-class, intelligent, friendly, wife batterer.

Date Rape. FHS. An adaptation of a Donahue program on the subject of date rape.

Homosexuality: Nature vs. Nurture. FHS. Biological, genetic, psychological, and cultural explanations of sexual orientations.

Men Who Molest: Children Who Survive. FML. Examines four child molesters and their treatment.

My Husband Is Going to Kill Me. PBS. Looks at domestic violence and the death of one abused wife.

No More Secrets. FHS. Deals with childhood sexual abuse and the possible long-term damage it inflicts.

Normalcy--What Is It? PBS. Dr. Milton Diamond discusses issues of normalcy in human sexual behavior. On-the-street interviews emphasize the range in what average individuals experience as either normal or abnormal.

Overcoming Erection Problems. IML. Sexually explicit film depicts in-office and home treatments of males with erectile difficulties.

Sexuality--The Human Heritage. AVC. Depicts various factors affecting the development of sexual identity including biological and psychosocial.

Sexual Dysfunction. FHS. Examines the psychological causes of the sexual dysfunctions as well as their treatment, including the use of penile implants to treat erectile disorder.

The Battered Woman. PBS. Seven abused women reveal their experiences; discusses causes of this problem and responses to it.

Three Styles of Marital Conflict. RP. Shows the styles of the Hidden Agenda, the Passive Partner, and the Underadequate/Overadequate.

Using Movies and Mental Illness as a Teaching Tool

It is important to be sensitive to students' values and belief systems, and some students will be decidedly uncomfortable if suggestive vignettes (like those in *Crash*) are shown in class. However, vignettes from films like *Some Like It Hot, Tootsie* and *Victor/Victoria* provide an innocuous way of introducing a discussion of gender identity and sex roles. *To Wong Foo, Thanks for Everything, Julie Newman* and *The Adventures of Priscilla, Queen of the Desert* are two non-threatening and entertaining films that will force your students to examine their attitudes about transvestites and cross-dressing.

There are dramatic scenes from *Equus* that will be appropriate trigger vignettes for a classroom discussion of bestiality and fetishes. *The Good Mother* raises important questions about societal attitudes toward sexuality and we have found this film to be a wonderful stimulus for classroom discussion of the ways in which child rearing practices influence adult sexuality.

If you are making a deliberate attempt to include world class films in your course, it may be useful to have your students watch – and come to class prepared to discuss – the remarkable German film *The Blue Angel*. This is film making at its best, and the psychologically complex story of a German professor who becomes obsessed with a cabaret singer can be a springboard for a spirited class discussion of sexual masochism.

The lives of actors and directors are of considerable interest to most college students. It will be provocative and fun to start a class discussion of the work of directors like Roman Polanski and Woody Allen, and the ways in which life imitates art.

Movie	Link to Chapter	Page Reference to Wedding and Boyd
• La Cage aux Folles	homosexuality (p. 336)	p. 99
• La Cage aux Folles • To Wong Foo, Thanks for Everything, Julie Newmar • sex, lies, and videotape • Equus • Crash • Basic Instinct • The Good Mother • Tie Me Up! Tie Me Down! • Blue Velvet • Lolita	paraphilias(p. 350)	p. 104 p. 104 p. 105 p. 106 p. 106 p. 107 p. 107 p. 109 p. 110 p. 111
• The Christine Jorgenson Story • The Crying Game • Second Serve	gender identity disorder (p. 360)	p. 102 p. 102 p. 102

Classroom Assessment Techniques (CAT)

Memory Matrix (CAT 12-1)
Students should use the handout provided to review the purposes, functions, and importance of key terms.

Focused Listing (CAT 12-2)
Select an important point from this chapter (e.g., acquired dysfunction, gender identity disorder, paraphilias, spectator role) and ask students to write five words or phrases that describe the point.

Learning Review (CAT 12-3)
Students are to write in order five of the most important ideas they learned in this chapter.

Muddiest Point (CAT 12-4)
Instruct students to write about an issue, concept, or definition presented in Chapter 12 that they find most confusing or difficult to understand.

Suggestions for Essay Questions

- ❑ How does culture affect the way we define sexual deviance? Give examples.
- ❑ Describe the various forms of sexual dysfunction, linking each to the appropriate phase of the human sexual response cycle.
- ❑ Compare and contrast the therapeutic approaches of Masters and Johnson and Kaplan.
- ❑ Describe the essential features of the paraphilias.
- ❑ Describe the steps generally taken in gender reassignment.

Chapter 13

Schizophrenic and Delusional Disorder

Chapter Map

Section	Instructor Manual Components
Schizophrenia • The Prevalence of Schizophrenia • The History of the Diagnostic Category • The Symptoms of Schizophrenia • The Course of Schizophrenia • The Subtypes of Schizophrenia • The Dimensions of Schizophrenia • Groups at Risk for Schizophrenia	*An insider's view of schizophrenia (LL 13-1)* *Suicide risk (LL 13-2)* *Introducing schizophrenia (TP 13-1)* *Not multiple personality (TP 13-2)* *Symptoms of schizophrenia (TP 13-3)* *Art and treatment of mentally ill (TP 13-4)* *Homeless and schizophrenia (TP 13-5)* *The disordered monologue (ACT/DEMO 13-1)* *Virtual hallucinations (ACT/DEMO 13-2)* *Pseudopatients (ACT/DEMO 13-3)*
Delusional Disorder • The Symptoms of Delusional Disorder • Groups at Risk for Delusional Disorder	*Role playing schizophrenic and delusional disorders (ACT/DEMO 13-4)*
Problems in the Study of Schizophrenia	

Schizophrenia: Theory and Treatment	Saccadic eye movements (LL 13-3)
• The Biological Perspective • The Cognitive Perspective • The Family Systems Perspective • The Behavioral Perspective • The Sociocultural Perspective • Unitary Theories: Diathesis and Stress	*Working with families of schizophrenics (LL 13-4)* *Handedness and schizophrenia (LL 13-5)* *Gender differences in of schizophrenia (LL 13-6)* *The cure worse than the illness? (TP 13-6)* *Family history (TP 13-7)* *Role playing (TP 13-8)* *Community resources (ACT/DEMO 13-5) Guest speakers (ACT/DEMO 13-6)*

Chapter Outline

I.   Introduction
    A.   **Psychoses** are a class of disorders in which reality contact is radically impaired
    B.   Psychoses are most severe of all psychological disorders

II.   Schizophrenia
    A.   **Schizophrenia** describes group of psychoses
    B.   The Prevalence of Schizophrenia
        1.   About 1-2% had or will have schizophrenic episode
        2.   Rates are similar in other countries
        3.   Patients occupy half of hospital beds or are released to smaller facilities or into community
        4.   Health care cost of schizophrenia is about $19 billion
    C.   The History of the Diagnostic Category
        1.   In 1896, Kraepelin proposed type of psychosis dementia praecox
            a.   Begins in adolescence
            b.   Leads to irreversible mental breakdown
            c.   Term means premature mental deterioration
        2.   Bleuler argued dementia praecox was poor description
            a.   Disorder not necessarily premature
            b.   Most patients did not have complete mental deterioration
            c.   Proposed term schizophrenia
                i.   Term schizophrenia refers to split among different psychic functions within single personality
                ii.   Does not refer to multiple personality
    D.   The Symptoms of Schizophrenia
        1.   DSM-IV lists five characteristics symptoms
            a.   Two or more of symptoms must be shown for at least two months and disturbed for at least six months
            b.   Episodes that last less than a month, diagnosis of brief psychotic disorder is used
            c.   Episodes that last at least a month, but less than six months, diagnosis of schizophreniform disorder
        2.   Disorders of Thought and Language
            a.   Delusions
                i.   **Delusions** are firmly held beliefs that have no basis in reality
                ii.   Delusions affect at least three-quarters of schizophrenic patients
                iii.   Most schizophrenics do not realize the implausibility of their firmly held beliefs and will not abandon them

      iv.   Patterns include delusions of persecution, delusions of control, delusions of reference, delusions of grandeur, delusions of sin and guilt, hypochondriacal delusions, and nihilistic delusions

      v.   Thought delusions include thought broadcasting, thought insertion, and thought withdrawal

      vi.   Delusions may represent way schizophrenics explain to themselves their mental chaos

  b.   Loosening of Associations

      i.   **Loosening of associations** refers to characteristics of speech where ideas jump from one track to another

      ii.   Problem may lie in mind's way of dealing with associations where process of editing breaks down

      iii.   Patients with schizophrenia have particular problems with subtle secondary associations

      iv.   Research suggests that patients do not understand context well enough to process the last word of a sentence

  c.   Poverty of Content

      i.   **Poverty of content** characterizes the lack of meaning conveyed

      ii.   Speech may include many words with correct grammar

  d.   Neologisms

      i.   Some suggest schizophrenics have difficulty in finding the right words with which to say something

      ii.   **Neologisms** are new words that result from combining parts of two or more regular words or using words in a new way

  e.   Clanging

      i.   **Clanging** is the pairing of words that have no another to one relation beyond fact that they rhyme or sound alike

      ii.   Clanging speech often sounds like nonsense

  f.   Word Salad

      i.   Language may show complete breakdown on associational process

      ii.   Becomes impossible to determine any links between successive words and phrase

      iii.   **Word salad** refers to speech where words and phrases are combined into completely disorganized fashion

3.   Disorders of Perception

  a.   Breakdown of Selective Attention

        i.   Schizophrenics seem unable to focus and concentrate on important stimuli in environment

        ii.   Researchers believe that breakdown of selective attention may underlie most of the other symptoms

    b.   Hallucinations

        i.   **Hallucinations** are perceptions in the absence of any appropriate external stimulus

        ii.   Auditory hallucinations are the most common, notably hearing two or more voices

        iii.   Visual hallucinations are second most common

        iv.   Some patients do realize that hallucinations are not real; severely psychotic patients believe hallucinations are real perceptions

4.   Disorders of Mood

    a.   Some patients have deep depression or manic elation or an alternation between the two; diagnosis of schizoaffective disorder is used

    b.   Two patterns of mood disorders seen

        i.   **Blunted affect** where patient shows little emotion or **flat affect** where patient shows no emotion

        ii.   **Inappropriate affect** refers to expression of emotion unsuitable to the situation; the inappropriateness is subtle and typically involves facial expression, gestures associated with being happy

5.   Disorders of Motor Behavior

    a.   In some cases, motor behavior is normal

    b.   Motor behavior can include repetitive motor behaviors, purposeless behavior called **stereotypy**

    c.   Sometimes high levels of motor activity is seen

    d.   More common is inactivity where person is in a catatonic stupor

6.   Social Withdrawal

    a.   Emotional detachment is early sign

    b.   Withdrawal from involvement with environment and other people

    c.   May be due to social handicaps and attentional problems

E.   The Course of Schizophrenia

1.   The Prodromal Phase

    a.   Onset of schizophrenia may be sudden in some cases, occurring in a few days

    b.   Onset of schizophrenia may occur gradually over years

    c.   Downhill slide known as the **prodromal phase**

2.   The Active Phase

    a.   In **active phase**, patient shows prominent symptoms of schizophrenia

    b.   No one patient is likely to show all symptoms

3.   The Residual Phase

    a.   Active phase is followed by **residual phase** in most patients

    b.   In residual phase, patient shows behavior similar to prodromal phase

    c.   Patient may show symptoms such as blunted or flat affect

    d.   Some patients may return to normal functioning, but is usually not typical

    e.   More typical pattern is increasingly impaired functioning between episodes of residual phase

    f.   Schizophrenic tend to die about 10 years younger than other people

F.   The Subtypes of Schizophrenia

1.   Schizophrenia has been divided into subtypes based on behavior; but often problematic

2.   Subtype diagnosis may have value in research

3.   DSM-IV list five subtypes and includes undifferentiated type and residual type

4.   Disorganized Schizophrenia

    a.   **Disorganized schizophrenia** best fits the stereotype of a crazy person

    b.   Three symptoms are characteristic

        i.   Pronounced incoherence of speech (e.g., neologisms, clanging, word salad)

        ii.   Mood disturbance

        iii. Disorganized behavior or lack of goal orientation

    c.   May also show other symptoms

    d.   Onset is usually gradual and occurs at early age

5.   Catatonic Schizophrenia

    a.   **Catatonic schizophrenia** marked by disturbance in motor behavior

    b.   Disturbance can be in form of **catatonic stupor** or complete immobility, remaining in this state for weeks

    c.   May also show waxy flexibility at imes and at other times shows frenzied motor activity

    d.   Bizarre postures requires extraordinary expenditure of energy

    e.   Patients may also show catatonic ridigity and **echolalia**, parroting what is said to them; echopraxia and catatonic negativism are other symptoms

6.   Paranoid Schizophrenia

a. **Paranoid schizophrenia** involved delusions and/or hallucinations related to themes of persecution and grandeur

b. Far more common than disorganized or catatonic types

c. Paranoid schizophrenics show better functioning and are more "normal" than disorganized or catatonic types

d. Active phase appears after 25 years of age and is preceded by years of fear and suspicion

7. Dimensions of Schizophrenia

   a. Examining dimensions provides another way to study schizophrenia

   b. Dimensions allow patients to fall somewhere on the dimensions

   c. Process-Reactive, or Good-Poor Premorbid

      i. **Process-reactive dimension** describes onset of schizophrenia

      ii. Process schizophrenia describes gradual onset

      iii. Reactive schizophrenia describes sudden onset triggered by traumatic event

      iv. Biogenic psychosis focuses on process; psychological psychosis focuses on reactive

      v. Good-bad premorbid dimension refers to how well patient was functioning before onset

      vi. Process (or poor premorbid) associated with long history of poor adjustment; more likely to have long hospitalizations

      vii. Reactive (or good premorbid) associated with normal history

   d. Positive-Negative Symptoms

      i. **Positive-negative dimension** attracted attention

      ii. **Positive symptoms** characterized by presence of something that is normally absent

      iii. **Negative symptoms** characterized by absence of something that is normally present

      iv. Negative symptoms associated with poor premorbid adjustment tend to have earlier onset and worse prognosis

      v. Related to different kinds of cognitive problems

      vi. May be two biologically distinct types of schizophrenia

      vii. **Type I schizophrenia** associated with positive symptoms and tends to respond to medication

      viii. **Type II schizophrenia** associated with negative symptoms and does not respond well to medication

              ix.   Some symptoms may be in response to primary symptoms
- e.   Paranoid-Nonparanoid
  - i.   Paranoid-nonparanoid dimension refers to presence or absence of delusions of persecution and/or grandeur
  - ii.   May be related to process-reaction dimension
- 8.   Groups at Risk for Schizophrenia
  - a.   Symptoms may differ depending on culture
  - b.   There are certain known risk factors associated with schizophrenia such as socioeconomic status, age, gender

III.   Delusional Disorder
- A.   The Symptoms of Delusional Disorder
  - 1.   Delusional system is the fundamental abnormality in **delusional disorder**
    - a.   In other aspects, individual seems normal
    - b.   Does not include other characteristics symptoms of schizophrenia
  - 2.   DSM-IV lists five categories of delusional disorder
    - a.   Persecutory type involves belief that one is being threatened or maltreated by others
    - b.   Grandiose type refers to belief that person is endowed with extraordinary power or knowledge
    - c.   Jealous type is delusion that one's sexual partner is being unfaithful
    - d.   Erotomanic type refers to belief that person of high status is in love with patient
    - e.   Somatic type involves false conviction that one is suffering from physical abnormality or disorder
- B.   Groups at Risk for Delusional Disorder
  - 1.   Differs from schizophrenia
  - 2.   Strikes more women; later onset
  - 3.   Lifetime risk is .3%

IV.   Problems in the Study of Schizophrenia
- A.   Subjects available for research are hospitalized and take antipsychotic drugs
- B.   Any differences may be function of medication or hospitalization
- C.   Disagreement with what actually constitutes schizophrenia creates problem for research
- D.   Differential deficits are specific to disorder in question and presumably central to it
  - 1.   Problems faced by subjects may not lead directly to disorder

2.   To show differential deficits, research must show schizophrenics consistently showing differences

V.   Schizophrenia: Theory and Therapy
  A.   The Biological Perspective
    1.   Genetic Studies
      a.   Family Studies
        i.   Earliest genetic studies were family studies
        ii.   Children of one and two schizophrenic parent(s), has 13% and 46% chance, respectively, of becoming schizophrenic
        iii.   Compared to general population risk of 1-2%
        iv.   Person with a schizophrenic first-degree relative is 10 times likelier to develop schizophrenia
      b.   Twin Studies
        i.   Average concordance rate for MZ twins is 46% compared to 14% for DZ twins
        ii.   Concordance differences tends to be greater when index twin has more severe symptoms
        iii.   There are several problems with twin studies, such as small sample and sharing of environment
        iv.   Twins reared apart share same intrauterine environment
        v.   Research now examining offspring of MZ twins who are discordant for schizophrenia
      c.   Adoption Studies
        i.   Subjects in adoption studies are those children who are adopted away from their biological families as infants
        ii.   Several studies show that adopted children who later become schizophrenic are much more likely to have biological, rather than adoptive relatives with schizophrenia
      d.   Mode of Transmission
        i.   Researchers suspect that schizophrenia is caused by variety of genetic subtypes
        ii.   Others suggest that schizophrenia is product of many genes and their combination with environmental factors
      e.   Genetic High-Risk Studies
        i.   Genetic high-risk studies examine children who were born of schizophrenic mothers and are therefore genetically vulnerable to schizophrenia
        ii.   Research has identified factors that separate high-risk children who developed schizophrenia from

318

high-risk and low-risk children who remain normal; home life, early separation and institutionalization, school problems and criminal behavior; attention to problems; and birth complications
     iii. Studies support role of genetic inheritance
     iv. High rate of attention problems suggest that attention deficits are primary symptoms
     v. Specific types of stress may lead to schizophrenia
  f. Behavioral High-Risk Studies
     i. Behavioral high-risk studies selects high-risk people on basis of behavioral traits associated with schizophrenia
     ii. Perceptual Aberration-Magical Ideation Scale used to screen subjects
     iii. Perceptual abnormalities often show up in histories of those who are later diagnosed with schizophrenia
2. Brain Imaging Studies
  a. New brain imaging techniques include PET, CT, and MRI
  b. Chronic schizophrenics have smaller than normal brain size
  c. Brain ventricles tend to be enlarged
     i. May be result of cumulative of antipsychotic drugs
     ii. Evidence suggests similar abnormalities in first-episode schizophrenics
     iii. Abnormalities found near structures near ventricles
  d. During cognitive tests, PET scans reveal abnormally low frontal-lobe activity
  e. Frontal cortex abnormalities associated with negative symptoms
  f. Temporal lobe and limbic structure abnormalities associated with positive symptoms
  g. Abnormalities found in connections among basal ganglia, temporal lobe, and frontal lobe
3. Prenatal Brain Injury
  a. High rate of birth complications seen in many schizophrenics
  b. Evidence suggests brain schizophrenics may have suffered trauma during second trimester
  c. Disruptions may have occurred in neural migration during second trimester
  d. Twin studies found signs of problems during second trimester
4. Biochemical Research: The Dopamine Hypothesis
  a. Dopamine hypothesis suggests schizophrenia associated with excess activity in parts of brain that use dopamine

        b.   Major line of evidence from research on antipsychotic drugs

        c.   Other supporting evidence comes from studies with stimulants amphetamine and methylphenidate, which increase dopamine activity in brain

        d.   Link may exist between schizophrenia and Parkinson's disease

             i.   Drugs used for Parkinson's disease can produce schizophrenic-like symptoms

             ii.   Antipsychotic drugs can produce **tardive dyskinesia**

        e.   There is evidence against dopamine hypothesis

        f.   Biological explanation probably will involve combination of biochemical imbalance

    5.   Chemotherapy

        a.   **Antipsychotic drugs** used to relieve symptoms

        b.   Most widely used group is **phenothiazines**

        c.   Newer drugs often work better than phenothiazines for Type II, negative-symptom patients

        d.   Problems associated with antipsychotic drugs

             i.   About 20-40% get little or no relief from drugs

             ii.   Long term use can have serious side effects such as tardive dyskinesia

        e.   New drugs being developed that have lower risk for tardive dyskinesia

        f.   While drugs have reduced number of chronically hospitalized patients, some suggest it has led to revolving door admission

B.   The Cognitive Perspective

    1.   Cognitive theorists focus on the diathesis

    2.   Biological abnormality causes attention deficits that create a predisposition to schizophrenia

    3.   Overattention

        a.   Overattention related to Type I, positive-symptom schizophrenia

        b.   Symptom of Type I are product of their overattention

        c.   Information processing fucntions are overburdened and nervous system overaroused, and cannot screen out stimuli

        d.   Many studies support poor selective attention and distractibility

        e.   Inability to screen out distractions related to Type I, positive-symptom schizophrenia, but not to Type II, negative-symptom schizophrenia

    4.   Underattention

       a.   Type II schizophrenics appear to be underattentive to external stimuli

       b.   Studies using orienting response and backward-masking paradigm support theory

       c.   Underattention leads to negative symptoms

5.   Vulnerability

       a.   Cognitive abnormalities have been found in remitted schizophrenics, their biological relatives, and high-risk individuals

       b.   Longitudinal studies must be conducted for solid confirmation of attention-dysfunction hypothesis

6.   Cognitive Therapy

       a.   Cognitive therapy in earliest stages

       b.   In cognitive rehabilitation, techniques from rehabilitation therapy are used

            i.   Patients given tasks that require skills that are defective

            ii.   Defective skills are built up by instruction, prompting, and monetary rewards

       c.   Another approach focuses on hallucinations and delusions

            i.   Techniques used involve questioning patient

            ii.   Therapists suggests alternative explanations

            iii.   Therapy also teaches patient coping devices to deal with unwelcome thoughts

       d.   Gains in cognitive therapy may not generalize to other areas of cognition

C.   The Family Systems Perspective

1.   Trouble in the family is the focus in family systems perspective

2.   Expressed Emotion

       a.   **Expressed emotion (EE)** refers to what people in family say to one another

            i.   Expressed emotion based on level of criticism and level of emotional overinvolvement

            ii.   Patients who live with high-EE relatives were three to four times more likely to have been rehospitalized

       b.   Some studies have not found link between schizophrenia and EE

       c.   Many studies suggest that a negative and emotionally charged family atmosphere may be related to onset and course of schizophrenia

3.   Communication Deviance

       a.   Double-bind communication believed to characterize communication between child and parent

      i. Double-bind communication gives child mutually contradictory messages

      ii. Parent implicitly forbids child to point out contradiction

    b. Research shows that families of schizophrenics tend to have unusual communication patterns

    c. **Communication deviance (CD)** refers to number of deviant or idiosyncratic responses

    d. Communication deviance correlated with expressed emotion

      i. Communication deviance may be result of child's disorder

      ii. Family communication patterns may place individual at risk for schizophrenia

  4. Treatment for Families

    a. Treatments developed for families of schizophrenic patients

    b. Studies suggest that family therapy lowers risk of relapse

    c. Problem-solving therapy applied to groups of families may be superior

D. The Behavioral Perspective

  1. Learned Nonresponsiveness

    a. Schizophrenics have not learned to respond to social stimuli

    b. React to idiosyncratically chosen stimuli

    c. Rewarded for bizarre responses

  2. Relearning Normal Behavior

    a. Direct Reinforcement

      i. Behavior is changed by changing consequences of behavior

      ii. A number of ethical and legal questions raised by treatment

    b. The Token Economy

      i. **Token economy** refers to giving patients tokens for performing target behavior

      ii. Tokens exchanged for backup reinforcers

      iii. Token economies are very useful in improving behavior

    c. Social-Skills Training

      i. **Social-skills training** attempts to reduce inappropriate social behavior by teaching patients

      ii. Role-playing is critical component

      iii. Social-skills training can be effective, but may not generalize to patients' daily lives

      iv. Some patients do retain skills and make better adjustment to community

E.   The Sociocultural Perspective
1. Released patients required many kinds of assistance
2. Community treatment programs must maintain active involvement with patients long-term
3. Assertive community treatment provides greater range of services readily available
4. Personal therapy provides one-on-one case-management treatment and focuses on control of emotions
    a. Internal coping taught to identify signs of upcoming stress
    b. Personal therapy is long-term, lasting about three years
    c. Outcomes of personal therapy are promising

F.   Unitary Theories: Diathesis and Stress
1. Researchers are looking for both genetic and environmental causes
2. Several stresses have been identified that convert diathesis into schizophrenia
3. Relapses tend to be preceded by increase in stressful life events

Chapter Boxes

- Hallucinations: Terror of Comfort?
  A. Hallucinations are partly related to neurological dysfunction
  B. Hallucinations produce reactions, which may be positive
  C. Some hallucinations may be soothing, provide companionship, provide protection, or increase self-esteem
  D. Some hallucinations may have negative effects such as preventing earning a living, interfering with activities, and upsetting
  E. Patients who find hallucinations positive may be more resistance to treatment

- Is Schizophrenia an Infectious Disease? The Viral Hypothesis
  A. Viral hypothesis suggests that infection must interact with other causes
  B. Virus is probably a slow virus
  C. Schizophrenics more likely than other people to have been born in the winter; viral infections peak in spring and winter
  D. Evidence comes from studies examining relationship between schizophrenia and epidemics
  E. Those exposed in second trimester more likely to have developed schizophrenia
  F. All of the evidence is circumstantial

Learning Objectives (LO)

By the time you have finished studying this chapter, you should be able to do the following:

1. Define psychosis, and list three varieties of psychosis referred to in the text (370).

2. Summarize the history of the disorder now called schizophrenia, summarize population data on schizophrenia, and distinguish schizophrenia from brief psychotic disorder and schizophreniform disorder (370-371, 384-385).

3. Define and give examples of the following cognitive symptoms of schizophrenia: delusions, loosened associations, poverty of content, neologisms, clanging, word salad (371-376).

4. Define the perceptual symptoms of schizophrenia (breakdown in selective attention, hallucinations), and summarize the disorders of mood, behavior, and social interaction that can accompany schizophrenia (376-378).

5. Describe the course of schizophrenia, defining the prodromal, active, and residual phases of the disorder (378-380).

6. Describe three classic subtypes of schizophrenia and explain the process-reactive, positive-negative symptoms, and paranoid-nonparanoid dimensions of schizophrenia (380-394).

7. Define delusional disorder, distinguish it from paranoid personality disorder and paranoid schizophrenia, and describe five categories of delusional disorder contained in DSM-IV (385-386).

8. Discuss why schizophrenia is difficult to diagnose, and describe difficulties encountered in the study of a disorder like schizophrenia (386-387).

9. Summarize genetic research on schizophrenia, citing the results of family studies, twin studies, adoption studies, and high-risk research (387-392).

10. Describe brain structure abnormalities and evidence of prenatal brain injury found in some schizophrenics (392-395).

11. Explain the suspected role of neurotransmitters in schizophrenia, describe the relationship of dopamine to Type I and Type II schizophrenia, and discuss the pros and cons of chemotherapy for schizophrenia (395-396).

12. Summarize the cognitive perspective's ideas on the role of attention problems as a factor in schizophrenia, and describe cognitive treatments for this disorder (396-399).

13. Summarize the role of pathological interpersonal relationships in the development of schizophrenia according to the family systems approach, and describe family-based therapies that have been applied to this disorder (399-402).

14. Summarize the behavioral and sociocultural positions on the causes and treatment of schizophrenia (402-404).

15. Summarize the diathesis-stress theory of schizophrenia (404-405).

Lecture Leads (LL)

An insider's view of schizophrenia (LL 13-1)
Although the textbook does present some first person accounts of schizophrenia, you may wish to provide more detail. Frederick J. Frese (1993), director of psychology at Western Reserve Psychiatric Hospital, is a schizophrenic who is able to maintain his symptoms in remission with use of medication. From his own experiences with psychosis and with the psychotics he treats, he provided an insider's look at what it is like to be schizophrenic. Frese presented twelve areas of coping for schizophrenics and for the persons who interact with them. First, Frese noted that schizophrenics deny that they are 'crazy,' which winds up being a "Catch-22": "If you understand that you are insane then you are thinking properly and are therefore not insane. You can only be psychotic if, in fact, you believe that you are not" (p. 3). So, if you don't think you're crazy, why do you need to be cured? The answer, according to Frese, would be to go along with the "reality" of others who treat you as though you're mentally ill. He also suggested avoiding a "frontal assault" on the denial issue, and advised using terms such as "survivor" for the schizophrenic, in addition to establishing a relationship of trust.   Frese suggests that it is important to be sensitive to the fact that every person has his or her own area of vulnerability to stress, whether it means breaking out in hives, having an asthma attack, or activating a neurotransmitter response that leads to delusional thinking. People who interact with schizophrenics should keep in mind that social deficits, such as the difficulty of looking people directly in the eye, will distract the individual from focusing on the conversation. Locate biographies or autobiographies of people who have suffered from a mood disorders. First person descriptions seem to convey the essence of psychological disorders, especially mood disorders, so much more personally and tragically than clinical transcripts.

Resources:
Anonymous (1996). First person account: Social, economic, and medical effects of schizophrenia. Schizophrenic Bulletin, 22, 183.

Frese, F. J. (1993). Coping with schizophrenia. Innovations & Research, 2. Available: URL http://www. mentalhealth.com/story/p52-scO4.html.

Nijinsky, V. (1936). The diary of Vaslav Nijinksy. New York: Simon & Schuster.

Suicide risk (LL 13-2)
In this study, 9,156 schizophrenic patients were tracked after admission to several psychiatric hospitals in Denmark. Those patients who committed suicide (n=508) were matched to controls from the same group. Using regression, the authors report that suicide risk was significantly higher during the first five months following discharge from the psychiatric hospital. Other variables were also found to increase risk and they included multiple admissions in the previous year, being male, diagnosis of depression, and previous suicide attempts. The authors agree that patients have a great need for support and monitoring right after discharge.

Resource:

Rossau, C. D., & Mortensen, P. B. (1997). Risk factors for suicide in patients with schizophrenia: Nested case-control study. British Journal of Psychiatry, 171, 355-359.

Saccadic eye movements (LL 13-3)

A recent study by Clementz, McDowell, and Zisook involved an examination of saccadic eye movements in clients with schizophrenia and their first degree relatives. The authors used a number of tests designed to assess saccadic eye movements. One test in particular, the anti-saccade task, involved presenting the subjects with a visual target at a central fixation point. The fixation point was turned off and a peripheral visual target was illuminated either to the left or the right of the central fixation point. Subjects were instructed not to look at this peripheral target, but to direct their gaze at the peripheral stimulus' onset at the other side of the projection screen.. It was found that clients with schizophrenia made more errors on this task (i.e., looked to the targeted side of the screen) than nonpsychiatric patients. In a second study it was found that first degree relatives of clients with schizophrenia also made more errors on this task than a comparison group of nonschizophrenic psychiatric patients and a comparison group of nonpsychiatric patients. which suggests a possible genetic link. The researchers conclude that the differences in eye movements observed in schizophrenic patients could be due to brain differences.

Resource:

Clementz, B. A., McDowell, J. E., & Zisook, S. (1994). Saccadic system functioning among schizophrenia patients and their first-degree biological relatives. Journal of Abnormal Psychology, 103, 277-287.

Working with families of schizophrenics (LL 13-4)

Health Canada (1991), in cooperation with the Schizophrenia Society of Canada, and with permission from the Minister of Supply and Services Canada (1996) provided an extensive handbook for families of schizophrenics. During the early stages, it is suggested that persons who interact with the schizophrenic speak slowly and clearly, provide structure, routine, use persuasion rather than coercion, use a great deal of praise, and avoid stress-producing, overstimulating situations. After a period of adjustment, the focus moves toward empowering the schizophrenic by increasing responsibility for self-care and household chores, encouraging social interactions (if suitable), being with the person without being intrusive or critical, teaching appropriate ways to deal with stress, and understanding and respecting the schizophrenic's feelings. A particularly interesting suggestion was to "be forgetful." Say something like, "I forgot the milk. Can you get it please?" All of these steps are designed to help integrate the schizophrenic back into a social system. There are times, however, when the schizophrenic will act impulsively and inappropriately, and suggestions for dealing with those situations include firmly but never abusively stopping or redirecting the behavior; be polite and apologetic to anyone who may have been involved, and, if necessary, offer to compensate for, or clean up, for any damage caused; maintain a sense of humor, and try to see the "funny" side by sharing it with someone who will understand (p. 31). The burden of dealing with a schizophrenic and the potential for burnout was acknowledged, and appropriate suggestions (e.g., make time for yourself and for your other relationships, keep your sense of humor) are included as well.

Resources:
Health Canada. (1991). Schizophrenia: A handbook for families. (Original copies are
     available from Communications Directorate, Health Canada, Ottawa, Ontario
     KIA OK9.) From P. W. Long (1995-1997), Available: URL
     http://www.mentalhealth.com.

National Institute of Mental Health. (1986). Schizophrenia: Questions and answers.
     (DHHS Publication No. ADM 86-1457). Washington, DC: U. S. Government
     Printing Office

Handedness and schizophrenia (LL 13-5)
It has been theorized that a relationship exists between handedness and schizophrenia. Some schizophrenics show anomalous left-handedness caused by unilateral cerebral insult early in life. The effect may be strong enough to shift handedness from genetic right handedness to left handedness; this is referred to as pathological left-handedness. Some research implicates a disproportionate left-handedness among schizophrenics, although it is not a consistent finding. Tiwari and Mandal examined side bias of hand, foot, eye, and ear among 60 chronic schizophrenics who do not have any known cerebral insult. Subjects' preference for handedness, foot preference, eye preference, and ear preference were assessed. In addition, subjects actually performed the tasks that were used to assess their preferences. It was found that schizophrenic individuals had a strong right bias. The authors suggest that patients with no known unilateral cerebral damage may have the typical right side preference and performance, since these subjects did not have unilateral cerebral damage.

Resource:
Tiwari, G., & Mandal, M. K. (1998). Side bias in schizophrenia: hand, foot, eye, and
     ear. Journal of General Psychology, 125, 39-46.

Gender differences in of schizophrenia (LL 13-6)
Although schizophrenia is equally common in men and women, some researchers have noted that the manifestation of schizophrenic symptoms varies in men and women. For example, women are more likely than men to have sexual delusions. However, men are more likely to have delusions of inferiority. Cheek observed that a gender role reversal often occurs with regard to the behavior of men and women diagnosed as schizophrenic. Schizophrenic men tend to express more flat affect and symptoms more in line with the negative subtype of schizophrenia, whereas women tend to exhibit dysphoria, irritability, anger, and paranoia. Men typically become passive and withdrawn. Women become more active and dominant. It is difficult to say what accounts for these differences,

although most feminists claim these differences are due to the different gender roles society imposes on men and women. In addition, there appear to be differences in the brains of male and female schizophrenics. In a recent study, it was hypothesized that male schizophrenics would show a significant reduction in cranial and cerebral size, and larger ventricular size as compared to female schizophrenics. Both the male and female schizophrenic groups were matched to normal male and female controls and the groups were compared on the relevant brain structure variables using MRI measures. The results were actually the opposite. Because these finding are not consistent with previous findings the authors are hesitant to conclude that the development of schizophrenia in women is associated with more significant brain differences.

Resources:

Cheek, F. E. (1964). A serendipitous finding: Sex roles and schizophrenia. Journal of Abnormal and Social Psychology, 69, 392-400.

Goldstein, J. M., & Link, B. G. . (1988). Gender differences in the expression of schizophrenia. Journal of Psychiatric Research, 22, 141-155.

Nasrallah, H. A., Schwarzkopt,, S. B., Olson, S. C., & Coffman, J. A. (1990). Gender differences in schizophrenia on MRI brain scans. Schizophrenic Bulletin, 16, 205-210.

Talking Points (TP)

Introducing schizophrenia (TP 13-1)
Ask students to describe a "crazy" person. Chances are their description comes pretty close to schizophrenia. Unlike the anxiety disorders or even the mood disorders, the symptoms of schizophrenia are so unlike the experiences of most people; few of us have ever experienced hallucinations or delusions.

Not multiple personality (TP 13-2)
Once again emphasize that schizophrenia is not multiple personality.

Symptoms of schizophrenia (TP 13-3)
Students are often unclear about the difference between schizophrenia as a distinct class of disorders and more vague terminology such as "having a nervous breakdown" or a multiple personality disorder. Have students generate their own descriptions of the prototypic schizophrenic patient. Use this discussion to show the diversity of views on the subject.

Art and treatment of mentally ill (TP 13-4)
A lecture on the history of the treatment of schizophrenics could be developed. Some of the material from your lectures on Chapter 1 could augment this lecture. Try to find some photographs from the early 1900s or late 1800s to show the types of treatments given prior to the advent of the major tranquilizers of the mid 1950s.

Homeless and schizophrenia (TP 13-5)
Develop a lecture on the deinstitutionalization of the late 1960s and how it affects our understanding of mental health today. Many students assume correctly that the vast majority of the homeless are mentally ill. A recent statistic indicates that at least 50% of all homeless people in New York City are in need of mental health services. Use local and regional statistics to help bolster your lecture.

The cure worse than the illness? (TP 13-6)
The side effects of drug therapies for the treatment of schizophrenia can cause more distress to the schizophrenic than the actual symptoms of the disorder. Discuss the implications of this in terms of treatment compliance. Also discuss this in terms of the revolving-door phenomenon.

Family history (TP 13-7)
A family history of schizophrenia does not guarantee that one will develop the disorder. Reiterate what is known about concordance rates and heritability.

Role playing (TP 13-8)

Start this discussion by arriving at class dressed very differently. Try wearing old clothes and have an aluminum foil hat (aluminum protects the brain from harmful radiation from UFOs). You could wear any number of interesting outfits, from many buttons to only black; use your wardrobe and imagination. Upon arrival, play the role of a paranoid schizophrenic, engage in as many behaviors as you can in the classroom. After your introduction lead a discussion of the use of the behavioral approach and a cognitive approach to understanding your behavior. Have students note what different types of information are elicited from the "patient" when questions from different perspectives are used.

with the result that the person cannot meet the **ordinary demands of life**.	p. 370
Such delusions may **crystallize** into a stable delusional identity…	p. 372
the belief that one has committed **"the unpardonable sin"**…	p. 372
They get **"stuck"** on the first association…	p. 374
one to **pancake makeup**…	p. 374
Neither does it appear to reflect a **train** of tangential association.	p. 376
hearing voices that keep a **running commentary** …	p. 376
are confined to the **edge of consciousness**.	p. 376
For example, the patient may **giggle** while relating a painful memory…	p. 378
Rarely do schizophrenic patients engage in **small talk**.	p. 378
Speech may still **ramble**…	p. 379
most disorganized schizophrenic run the **gamut** of schizophrenic symptoms	p. 380
like those of a **rubber doll**…	p. 381
their African counterparts are more likely to think they are pursued by a **sorcerer**…	p. 384
they may **explode** in anger at complete strangers…	p. 385
radio talk show callers…	p. 386
Consider the analogy of a **leg fracture**.	p. 386
mostly **firsthand** interviews…	p. 389
they had more difficulty **"tuning out"**…	p. 391
Neurological tests and studies of **home movies**…	p. 392
Patients…are now free to **roam** hospital grounds.	p. 396
reducing the patient to a **"zombie"** -like state.	p. 396
was asked to wear heavy, industrial **earmuffs**….	p. 399
he or she is the **loser**.	p. 400
we are faced with the **chicken-and-egg problem**…	p. 401
belief that others are out to **"get"** them.	p. 402
complete them with an assigned **"buddy."**	p. 403

Activities and Demonstrations (ACT/DEMO)

The disordered monologue (ACT/DEMO 13-1)
Objective: To help students understand the language and thought disorders evident in schizophrenia
Materials: The "Disordered" Monologue (see Osberg, 1992)
Procedure: Osberg (1992) has developed a "disordered" monologue that can be read aloud in class to demonstrate the loosening of associations, clang associations, and the neologisms that characterize schizophrenic speech. The author suggests trying to commit the monologue to memory. On the day that you are to begin the unit on schizophrenia, walk into the classroom and recite or read the monologue.
Discussion: Student reactions will vary depending on how convincing you are. A few students may exhibit some concern about your behavior and it may be appropriate to have them discuss their feelings and impressions about how they would react for real. Follow up with an assignment to students to create their own disordered monologue consistent with the symptoms of schizophrenia.

Resource:
Osberg, T. M. (1992). The disordered monologue: A classroom demonstration of the symptoms of schizophrenia. Teaching of Psychology, 19, 47-48.

Virtual hallucinations (ACT/DEMO 13-2)
Objective: To demonstrate the nature of auditory hallucinations
Materials: The auditory tape, "Virtual Hallucinations (order (800) 818-9139)
Procedure: This tape simulates the type of auditory hallucinations that are experience by people with schizophrenia. The tape includes "voices" that a person, who has schizophrenia , might experience while on a job interview.
Discussion: Janssen Pharmaceutica, the same company that manufactures Risperdal, produced the tape. The idea behind the tape is to help family members, policy-makers, and others better understand schizophrenia to reduce the stigma often associated with schizophrenia.

Resource:
Virtual Hallucinations
PO Box 580
New York, NY 10013

Pseudopatients (ACT/DEMO 13-3)
Objective: To allow the students to feel what it might be like to have the disorder of schizophrenia.
Materials: None.
Procedure: Have a volunteer student role play one of Rosenhan's "pseudopatients" in front of the class. At the same time have another student play a psychologist. You and the student psychologist interview the patient. Have students observe and label the "patient's" behaviors using the DSM criteria.

Discussion: This demonstration will lead to a discussion of the role of labeling and interviewer bias. Also discuss the complexity of using the DSM in defining schizophrenia.

Role playing schizophrenic and delusional disorders (ACT/DEMO 13-4)
Objective: To identify the types of behaviors and thoughts associated with schizophrenic disorders and delusional disorders
Materials: None
Procedure: Have the students individually or in small groups select one of the schizophrenic or delusional disorders. Their task is to develop a role play to illustrate the disorder as well as other information (e.g., effect on family, demographics, suspected etiology, treatment perspectives). An example might be a psychologist interviewing a client; the interview could illustrate comorbidity issues. Another example of a role play could be an interaction of patients with paranoid schizophrenia with others at a party. Tell the students that they have at least overnight to prepare for their disorder and that they will be expected to role play the disorder in front of the class. If using groups, one person plays the role of the subject, and other group members can play family members, employers, friends, and clinician.
Discussion: Give feedback on the accuracy of the role play. Ask students to comment on the accuracy of the role play and to guess what disorder was being portrayed.

Community resources (ACT/DEMO 13-5)
Objective: To identity community resources
Materials: None
Procedure: Ask students to research the community resources that are available for persons who suffer from or are at-risk for schizophrenia. Create a resource manual categorized according to the particular disorder, including name of each group, contact person(s), phone numbers, the types of services offered, and whether any fee is involved.
Discussion: Students will learn that there are many resources available. A resource manual would be a valuable asset to the community.

Guest speakers (ACT/DEMO 13-6)
Objective: To illustrate the type of treatments used in clinical practice
Materials: None
Procedure: Invite speakers to your class to discuss the schizophrenic disorders presented in the chapter. Ideas include psychologists, psychiatrists specializing in schizophrenia research and treatment, and pharmacists. You may also wish to invite an administrator of a local private or state mental hospital. Students will be interested in the day-to-day lives of the patients and how staff deals with the daily routine of the hospital. Make sure you schedule this presentation early, since many mental health professionals are very busy. Contact a local support group to ask for help in identifying family members of schizophrenic patients to invite.
Discussion: Beforehand, instruct students to review this chapter and be prepared to ask questions of their guest speakers. Afterwards, ask students to discuss speakers' presentations.

Films and Videos

A True Madness. TLF. Causal factors implicated in schizophrenia are discussed. A schizophrenic is interviewed.

In Two Minds. The Mind Series. Concentrating on schizophrenia, this concluding episode examines the current state of knowledge of mental illness.

Psychopathology: Diagnostic Vignettes: No. 3 Schizophrenic Disorders. IURTS. Focuses on classic symptoms of schizophrenia. Specific attention is paid to aspects of formal thought disorder, hallucinations, and delusions.

Schizophrenia. FHS. Dr. E. Fuller Torrey reviews the suspected causes and symptoms of schizophrenia and the prognosis and family support of people with the disorder.

Schizophrenia. FHS. This specially-adapted Phil Donahue program is widely regarded as one of the most helpful programs on schizophrenia. The program offers basic information about this illness that affects nearly one million Americans, usually striking 17- to 25-year-olds. Dr. E. Fuller Torrey, noted author and psychiatrist, reviews the suspected causes, the symptoms, the prognosis for recovery, and the steps to be taken by supportive family members.

Schizophrenia: Captor of the Mind. MTI. Looks at schizophrenia and how medical science helps people who have the disorder.

Schizophrenia: Out of Mind. FHS. This program enters into the world of the schizophrenic, showing patients, their families, and mental health care professionals who deal with schizophrenics. Patients range from eager to please, indifferent, negative, or just not there; doctors and nurses are hopeful; and families are perplexed, hurt, and often guilt ridden.

Schizophrenia: The Voices Within, The Community Without. FHS. Discusses symptoms of schizophrenia and describes the psychotropic medications used to control them; focuses on the effects of deinstitutionalization.

Using Movies and Mental Illness as a Teaching Tool

Most of your students will not be familiar with the film *Clean, Shaven*; however, Wedding and Boyd are convinced this is the best teaching film available to help your students understand the experiential world of someone with schizophrenia. In his review of *Clean, Shaven*, Roger Ebert wrote "[This is] a film that will not appeal to most filmgoers, but will be valued by anyone with a serious interest in schizophrenia or, for that matter, in film." Although not well known, the film is available in most commercial outlets, and it should be easily accessible for your students. Alternately, professors using the film on a regular basis in the classroom may want to purchase their own copy. The scene in which Peter Winter covers the windows and rear view mirror of his car with newspaper is especially gripping and powerful. Either of the murder scenes in the film can be used as a prelude to a class discussion of violence and mental illness, or before a class debate over the conventional wisdom that people with mental illness are far more likely to be victims of violence rather than perpetrators of violent acts.

If a professor is primarily interested in the reaction of families to someone with mental illness, Jane Campion's film *Sweetie* is highly recommended. Families balancing the need to support their loved one with the need to set firm limits will especially appreciate the film. If a vignette is shown in class, the tree house scene is recommended.

When a class focuses on differential diagnosis, it may be useful to have your students watch *Sophie's Choice*, and then debate Nathan's probable diagnosis. Showing the flaming red knight hallucinations from *The Fisher King* will provide a pedagogical vehicle for discussing the kinds of hallucinations likely to be experienced by people with schizophrenia (hallucinations that would rarely be as vivid and well formed as those which were necessary for artistic purposes in the film).

Shine is a popular movie based on the life of pianist David Helfgott. Many of your students will have seen this film; most of them will have loved it. It is an inspiring film that conveys an important message: people can learn to cope with a devastating illness like schizophrenia, and they can make important contributions in spite of the limitations imposed by their illness. As a class exercise, students could be asked to research and report on the lives of David Helfgott and John Forbes Nash Jr., a Princeton mathematician and Nobel laureate in economics who had to cope with paranoid schizophrenia throughout this life.

337

Movie	Link to Chapter	Page Reference to Wedding and Boyd
The Fisher King Benny and Joon The Caine Mutiny	symptoms of schizophrenia (p. 371)	p. 121 p. 121 p. 121
Clean, Shaven Sophie's Choice	paranoid schizophrenia (p. 382)	p. 117 p. 122
Taxi Driver Misery Sleeping with Enemy The Fan Scissors Delusions of Grandeur The Entertainer	delusional disorder (p. 385)	p. 123 p. 123 p. 125 p. 125 p. 125 p. 125 p. 125
Shine David and Lisa	family systems perspective (p. 399)	p. 120 p. 121

Classroom Assessment Techniques (CAT)

Focused Listing (CAT 13-1)
Select an important point from this chapter (e.g., expressed emotion, blunted affect, diathesis-stress model, positive symptoms) and ask students to write five words or phrases that describe the point.

Learning Review (CAT 13-2)
Students are to write in order five of the most important ideas they learned in this chapter.

Muddiest Point (CAT 13-3)
Instruct students to write about an issue, concept, or definition presented in Chapter x that they find most confusing or difficult to understand.

Minute Paper (CAT 13-4)
Ask your students to write about an important question they have that remains unanswered.

Suggestions for Essay Questions

- Describe the historical perspectives of Kraepelin and Bleuler on schizophrenia and how their views have influenced contemporary perspectives on schizophrenia.
- Contrast the subtypes of schizophrenia.
- What is the relationship between positive-negative symptoms and Type I and Type II schizophrenia, and attentional processes?
- What causes schizophrenia? Make sure to provide evidence from genetic studies, attentional studies, and family systems perspective.

Chapter 14

Neuropsychological Disorders

Chapter Map

Section	Instructor Manual Components
Problems in Diagnosis • Identifying an Acquired Brain Injury • Specifying the Type of Injury • Specifying the Site of the Damage	*Case studies: neuropsychological disorders (LL 14-1)* *Biology as the basis for affect, behavior, and cognitions (TP 14-1)* *Revisiting student survey (TP 14-2)* *Brain imaging (TP 14-3)* *Field trip (ACT/DEMO 14-1)* *Neurological assessment (ACT/DEMO 14-2)* *Brain used in performing tasks (ACT/DEMO 14-3)* *Guest speakers (ACT/DEMO 14-4)*
Acquired Brain Injuries • Cerebral Infection • Brain Trauma • Cerebrovascular Accidents • Brain Tumors • Degenerative Disorders • Nutritional Deficiency • Endocrine Deficiency • Toxic Disorders	*Alzheimer's disease and smoking (LL 14-2)* *Cultural differences in prevalence of Alzheimer's disease (LL 14-3)* *Chromosome 12: Another Alzheimer's disease gene? (LL 14-4)* *Prenatal factors and risk for stroke (LL 14-5)* *Awareness of involuntary movements (LL 14-6)* *Changing demographics and degenerative disorders (TP 14-4)* *Perceptions of growing old (TP 14-5)* *President Reagan (TP 14-6)* *Caregivers stress (TP 14-7)* *Parkinson' Disease and Huntington's Chorea (TP 14-8)* *Neuropsychological disorders in the popular media (ACT/DEMO 14-5)*

The Epilepsies	Accidental injury and absence seizures (LL 14-7)
• Cause of Epilepsy • Types of Epilepsy • Psychological Factors in Epilepsy • Groups at Risk • Treatment of Epilepsy	*Accidental injury and absence seizures (LL 14-7)* *Famous people with epilepsy (TP 14-10)*

Chapter Outline

I.   Introduction

    A.   **Acquired brain injuries** are biological and traceable to destruction of brain tissue or biochemical imbalances in brain

    B.   Major effect is on cognitive processes such as memory

II.   Problems in Diagnosis

    A.   Identifying an Acquired Brain Injury

        1.   Symptoms of acquired brain injury resemble those of psychological disorders

        2.   Symptoms of brain injury complicated by emotional disturbances that develop in response to impairment

        3.   Before modern diagnostic technique, differentiation between brain injury and psychological disorders was difficult

        4.   Diagnosing psychological disorder as brain injury may also occur

        5.   Misdiagnosis can be fatal

        6.   A number of resources are available for diagnosis

    B.   Specifying the Type of Injury

        1.   Difficult to specify source of impairment in acquired brain injuries

        2.   Confusion comes from several sources

            a.   Symptoms of brain injuries overlap considerably

            b.   Same injury may produce widely different symptoms, depending on location in brain

            c.   Source of brain injury is only one of many factors that determine behavioral responses

            d.   There are many brain injuries about which very little is known

        3.   Delirium

            a.   Delirium is transient, global disorder of cognition and attention

                i.   Thinking is disorganized

                ii.   In half of cases, hallucinations and delusions are present

                iii.   Emotional lability is common

                iv.   Onset is sudden and severity fluctuates during course of day

                v.   Recovery is complete and patient is amnestic

            b.   Caused by widespread disruption of cerebral metabolism and neurotransmission

            c.   Causes included intoxication medication, surgery, withdrawal from drugs, head injury

            d.   Physical illness may cause delirium

                i.   Often mistaken for dementia

     ii. Misdiagnosis may be fatal
   e. Treatment of delirium is removal of its cause
  4. Specific Cognitive Impairments
   a. Impairment of attention and arousal
   b. Impairment of language function
   c. Impairment of learning and memory
   d. Impairment of visual-perceptual function
   e. Impairment of motor skills
   f. Impairment of executive function
   g. Impairment of higher-order intellectual functions
   h. Impairments of language function called **aphasia** are common
     i. Fluent aphasia produces streams of incoherent speech
     ii. Nonfluent aphasia involves difficulty initiating speech and responding to questions with short answers
     iii. Aphasia caused by injury to left hemisphere
   i. Impairments of ability to recognize familiar objects called **agnosia**
  5. Dementia
   a. **Dementia** involves impairment in at least two cognitive functions, which leads to decline in performance compromising occupation or social functioning
   b. Some dementias caused by infectious diseases
   c. Some dementias caused by progressive physical deterioration
 C. Specifying the Site of the Damage
  1. Damage may be diffused throughout brain as in degenerative disorders
  2. Damage may be restricted to specific area
  3. CT, PET, and MRI are primary methods to pinpoint site of brain damage

III. Types of Acquired Brain Injuries
 A. Cerebral Infection
  1. Cerebral infections caused by bacteria, viruses, protozoa, and fungi
  2. Cerebral Abscess
   a. **Cerebral abscess** is infection that becomes encapsulated by connective tissue
   b. It cannot drain and heal and it continues to grow
   c. Infection occurs in body and travels to brain
  3. Encephalitis
   a. **Encephalitis** is generic term that refers to inflammation of brain

b.   Caused by viral or nonviral agents

c.   Typically transmitted by mosquitoes, ticks, and horses

d.   Symptoms include seizures, delirium, lethargy, and brain damage

4.   Mad Cow Disease

    a.   **Mad cow disease** is type of spongiform encephalopathies that attacks brain

    b.   In humans, called Creutzfeldt-Jakob disease

    c.   Symptoms include memory impairments, behavioral change, difficulty walking, visual perception deterioration

    d.   Brain has widespread degeneration and protein deposits

5.   Meningitis

    a.   **Meningitis** is acute inflammation of the meninges

    b.   Infection may be introduced through body infection or outside agent entering skull

    c.   Drowsiness, confusion, irritability, problems with concentration, memory defects, and sensory impairments are symptoms

6.   Neurosyphilis

    a.   **Neurosyphilis** is deterioration of brain tissue due to syphilis

    b.   Degenerative disorder called general paresis linked to syphilis in late nineteenth century

    c.   Incidence of syphilis had dramatically decreased

7.   AIDS Dementia

    a.   AIDS dementia seen in 15% of those diagnosed with AIDS

    b.   Appears in late stages of AIDS

    c.   Early symptoms often go unnoticed or mistaken for other problems

    d.   First signs are cognitive changes such as forgetfulness; later confusions, disorientation, and poor coordination

    e.   AIDS dementia often caused by other infectious agents

    f.   Damage to brain is often diffused

8.   Groups at Risk

    a.   Common illness may be related to encephalitis

    b.   People at risk for herpes infection, at risk for encephalitis

    c.   Organisms that are transmitted through insect and rodent bits

    d.   People living in different locations are at risk for different disorders

9.   Treatment of Cerebral Infections

    a.   Treatment depends on type of infection

    b.   Bacterial and fungal infections are treatable

    c.   Viral infections are more challenging to treat

d.   Some argue that HIV infection may be reversible in early stages; secondary infections that may lead to AIDS dementia may be eliminated

e.   Family support and memory aids are important

B.   Brain Trauma
1.   Brain trauma is injury to brain due to jarring, bruising, or cutting
2.   Traumatic head injury is leading cause of disability and death in children and young adults
3.   Most victims show long-term disabilities
4.   Concussion
  a.   A **concussion** results from blow to head that momentarily disrupts brain function
  b.   Temporary loss of consciousness and subsequent amnesia prior to injury is usual result
  c.   Longer the unconsciousness is, the more severe the symptoms and less likely person will recover completely
  d.   Aftereffects may be experienced months or years later
5.   Contusion
  a.   A **contusion** is injury that occurs when brain is bruised
  b.   Person lapses into coma for hours or even days
  c.   Victim may experience **traumatic delirium**, which disappears within a week
  d.   More severe injury leads to permanent instability and intellectual impairment
  e.   Repeated head injuries can result in cumulative damage
  f.   Boxers may be susceptible to ementia pugilistica and other structural changes in brain
6.   Laceration
  a.   In a laceration, an object ruptures and destroys brain tissue
  b.   Most serious form of brain trauma
  c.   Damage may result in death, extreme disability, or minor disability, but depends on site of damage
  d.   Typically results in physical impairment or personality change
7.   Groups at Risk
  a.   Two-thirds of victims are males with highest risk age group 15- to 24-year-olds
  b.   Falls are second most common cause of head injury
  c.   Most common cause is automobile and motorcycle accidents
8.   Treatment of Brain Trauma
  a.   Many head injuries are devastating
  b.   Rehabilitation can range from intensive inpatient treatment to periodic outpatient treatment

C.   Cerebrovascular Accidents: Strokes

1. **Cerebrovascular accidents** are known as **strokes** and involve blockage or breaking of blood vessel in brain ,damaging tissue
2. Third leading cause of death
3. Marked by stroke syndrome, which is acute onset of specific disabilities involving the CNS
4. Many people have small CVAs that occur in less critical areas of brain; less noticeable effects on behavior occur
   a. **Infarction** occurs when supply of blood to brain is cut off leading to death of brain tissue
      i. An **embolism** is a ball of fat, air, or clot that breaks off from side of vessel and clogs vessel too narrow to let it pass
      ii. In **thrombosis** involves fatty material that gradually builds up and blocks flow of blood in vessel
   b. **Hemorrhage** occurs when blood vessel in brain ruptures causing blood to spill out into brain tissue
      i. Often caused by hypertension
      ii. In brain, hemorrhage is usually due to aneurysms
5. The Effects of a Stroke
   a. Aftereffects depend on nature of stroke, extent of damage, and location of damage
   b. Typical effects are aphasia, agnosia, apraxia, and paralysis
   c. Most common stroke is due to infarction due to thrombosis in left-middle cerebral artery causing aphasia and impairment on right side of body
   d. Emotional disturbances usually accompany CVAs either as part of injury or reaction to impairment
   e. In some patients, behavioral symptoms may disappear while others are remedied through rehabilitation
   f. In general, the younger the person and the smaller the damaged area, the better the chance of recovery
6. Groups at Risk
   a. Clearest risk factor for CVA is age
   b. Men are more vulnerable than women
   c. Other high-risk groups include those with diabetes, family history, African-Americans
   d. High cholesterol, obesity, smoking, and hypertension increase risk
7. Treatment of Stroke
   a. People often ignore first signs of stroke
   b. Important to seeking treatment at first sign of symptoms
   c. Medications can limit effects of stroke if given in a timely manner
D. Brain Tumors
   1. **Brain tumors** classified in two ways

        a.   **Metastic brain tumors** originate in different part of body and spread (metatasize) to brain

        b.   **Primary brain tumors** originate in brain; may be intracerebral and extracerebral

2.   First signs of brain tumor are subtle and insidious

3.   Progressive destruction, patient develops at least one of several symptoms

4.   Symptoms related to location of tumor in brain; as tumor grows adjacent areas of brain and their functions are affected

5.   Groups at Risk

        a.   Not much is known about risk factors

        b.   Some cancers metastasize to brain

        c.   Smoking increases risk for lung cancer

6.   Treatment of Brain Tumors

        a.   Some tumors are surgically removed

        b.   Radiation treatment may used if surgery would destroy language and major motor areas

        c.   Surgery, chemotherapy, and radiation are used in combination

E.   Degenerative Disorders

1.   **Degenerative disorders** consists of syndromes characterized by general deterioration of intellectual, emotional, and motor functioning due to progressive pathological change in brain

2.   Symptoms vary depending on site of damage

3.   Aging and Dementia

        a.   Dementia is severe mental deterioration and was believed to be a natural part of aging

        b.   Dementia is result of degenerative brain disorders

        c.   Almost all old people show some psychological changes due to normal aging

        d.   Dementias are pathological and result of organic deterioration of brain

        e.   Diagnosis of syndromes is difficult

            i.   Many other problems mimic symptoms of dementia

            ii.   Alzheimer's disease difficult to distinguish from other dementias

            iii.   There is considerable overlap of symptoms

            iv.   Symptoms often related to person's premorbid personality and psychosocial history

4.   Alzheimer's Disease

        a.   **Alzheimer's disease** is most common form of dementia

        b.   Autopsies reveal neurofibrillary tangles and senile plaques

        c.   Primary symptoms are cognitive deficits, especially loss of memory

  d. Early signs include irritability and failure of concentration and memory

  e. Symptoms create difficulties for families of Alzheimer's patients

  f. Rate of progression is highly variable

  g. Research suggests a genetic role and may involve several genetic abnormalities

    i. May be related to Down syndrome and chromosome 21

    ii. Production of amyloid may be controlled by genes on chromosome 21

    iii. Other chromosomes may be implicated as well

    iv. Buildup of beta amyloid may be caused by breakdown of several regulatory mechanisms each controlled by a different gene

  h. Research suggests that Alzheimer's may have multiple contributing factors

5. Lewy Body Disease

  a. **Lewy body disease** may be second most common degenerative brain disease

  b. Rounded structures in neurons throughout brain are found

  c. Clinicians must rely on analysis of patient's symptoms for diagnosis

  d. Symptoms of Lewy body disease are similar to those of Alzheimer's disease

  e. Fluctuations in day-to-day functioning seen in Lewy body disease

  f. Most cases involve memory impairment followed by symptoms of Parkinson's disease

6. Vascular Dementia

  a. **Vascular dementia** is cumulative effect of several CVAs

  b. Common symptoms include blackouts, heart problems, kidney failure; psychological symptoms include language and memory defects, emotional lability, and depression

7. Huntington's Chorea

  a. **Huntington's chorea** is genetically transmitted

  b. The basal ganglia is damaged; area is responsible for posture, muscle tonus, and motor coordination

  c. Early signs include vague behavioral and emotional changes

  d. Involuntary, spasmodic jerking of limbs characterize disorder

  e. Increasingly bizarre behavior is seen in patients

8. Parkinson's Disease

a. **Parkinson's disease** involves damage to basal ganglia, especially substantia nigra

b. Cause is unknown, but may be related to heredity, viruses, toxins, head trauma

c. Primary symptom is tremors that are present during rest, but diminish or cease when person is sleeping

d. Another symptom is an expressionless, masklike countenance

e. Patients walk in a distinctive slow, stiff gait

f. Many patients also experience psychological disturbances such as memory, learning, judgment and concentration problems and dementia

9. Groups at Risk

a. Since women live longer, more women will experience dementia

b. Percentage of men who will develop dementia is same

c. Age and gender related to type dementia an individual is likely to develop

d. Educational level may affect incidence or rate of diagnosis of Alzheimer's disease

e. Some stroke patients developed vascular dementia with high blood pressure a risk factor

f. A test now exists to identify defective gene that causes Huntington's chorea

10. Treatment of Degenerative Disorders

a. Drugs that increase levels of acetylcholine have been used to treat Alzheimer's disease

b. There is no cure and little treatment for Alzheimer's disease

    i. Behavioral therapy may suppress some symptoms

    ii. Most common treatment is custodial care

    iii. Many patients are able to remain at home with their families, especially if family can receive support services

c. High blood pressure, diabetes, obesity, and smoking are risk factors for vascular dementia; after damage, decline is irreversible

d. Drugs that increase amount of dopamine among Parkinson's disease patients can control tremor, but do not cure it

F. Nutritional Deficiency

1. Insufficient intake of essential vitamins can result in neurological damage and psychological disturbances

2. Beriberi and pellagra are two common syndromes in less industrial countries

3. **Korsakoff's psychosis** is related to alcoholism

349

        a.   Primary pathological is deficiency of B12 or thiamine

        b.   There are two classic behavioral signs of Korsakoff's psychosis

            i.   Anterograde amnesia is inability to incorporate new memories

            ii.   Confabulation is tendency to fill in memory gaps with invented stories

        c.   Suggests a psychotic impairment of judgment and spreads to other aspects of psychological impairment

G.   Endocrine Disorders

    1.   Endocrine glands produce hormones that affect bodily mechanisms

    2.   Thyroid Syndromes

        a.   Hyperthyroidism involves excessive secretion of thyroxin, which leads to physical and psychological difficulties

        b.   Hypothyroidism involves deficient secretion of thyroxin, which leads to physical and psychological difficulties

    3.   Adrenal Syndromes

        a.   Addison's disease refers to chronic underactivity of adrenal glands which leads to physical and psychological changes

        b.   Cushing's syndrome refers to adrenal cortex overactivty leading to physical and psychological changes

H.   Toxic Disorders

    1.   Lead

        a.   Excessive ingestion of lead causes **lead encephalopathy** leading to extreme pressure in the brain

        b.   Most common victims are children and may be related to mental retardation

        c.   There are a number of sources of lead contamination

    2.   Other Heavy-Mental Toxins

        a.   Victims of toxins typically have jobs where they come into contact with mercury and manganese

        b.   Other victims come into contact in other ways such as food or air contamination, for example, fish from water polluted by mercury wastes

        c.   Mercury poisoning causes memory loss, irritability, and difficulty in concentration

        d.   Later, it causes tunnel vision, motor problems, coma, and death

    3.   Psychoactive Drugs

        a.   Alcohol, opiates, and amphetamines can cause severe psychological disturbances

        b.   Inhalation of aerosol gases and glues has become more popular way to get high

    4.   Carbon Monoxide

      a.   Carbon monoxide combines with hemoglobin to prevent blood from absorbing oxygen

      b.   Often results in death; those who survive have a number of psychological consequences such as apathy, confusion, and memory defects

IV.   The Epilepsies

A.   **Epilepsy** is broad term for disorders that have spontaneous seizure caused by disruption of electrical and physiological activity of brain cells

B.   Abnormal activity disrupts functions controlled by affected part of brain

C.   Causes of Epilepsy

    1.   Any condition that interferes with brain function can cause epilepsy

    2.   Most common cause is brain injury

      a.   If epilepsy beings in middle age, most likely cause is brain tumor

      b.   If epilepsy begins in older age, cause is most likely to be cerebral vascular disease such as stroke or cerebral arteriosclerosis

    3.   When a cause can be identified, it is known as **symptomatic epilepsy**

    4.   When cause is unknown, it is **idiopathic epilepsy**

D.   Types of Seizures

    1.   **Partial seizures** originate in one part of brain

      a.   In **simple partial seizure**, cognitive functioning remains intact; person may have sensory changes or minor psychological changes

      b.   In **complex partial seizure**, cognitive functioning is interrupted; an aura may precede seizure; person is not able to engage in purposeful activity and does not respond normally

    2.   **Generalized seizure** involves entire brain at outset or soon spreads from one part

      a.   **Absence seizures** involve spaced-out look and sense of being absent from the surroundings

      b.   **Tonic-clonic seizures** begin with a tonic or rigid extension of limbs followed by clinic or jerking movements through body

    3.   Each type of seizure requires different kind of drug, therefore, accurate diagnosis is important

E.   Psychological Factors in Epilepsy

    1.   Most common complaint is poor memory, since most epilepsies involve temporal lobes

    2.   Once thought there was an epileptic personality, but no data support that view

351

F.   Groups at Risk
       1.   Groups at risk for other acquired brain injuries are at risk for epilepsy
       2.   Gender may also affect outcome of surgical treatment for epilepsy
G.   Treatment of Epilepsy
       1.   Most people take antiepileptic drugs, which suppress seizures in 80% of patients
       2.   Some report side effects of being drugged down
       3.   Surgery involves removal of focal epileptic area and is becoming more common

Chapter Boxes

- Concussions in Football: What City Am I In?
    - A. Concussions are not uncommon in football
    - B. Repeated concussions pose risk of lasting neurological damage
    - C. Once a player has one concussion, he is four times more likely to have a second
    - D. Some players engage in "head-hunting," aiming for the head
    - E. Rough play is rewarded by teammates
    - F. Minor concussions can easily escape notice
    - G. A new helmet will spread impact of a head blow to shoulders and harsh penalties for head-hunting

- Caregivers: The Hidden Victims of Dementia
    - A. Caring for a patient with dementia can be very taxing
    - B. For many dementia patients, the best situation is to remain with their families for as long as possible
    - C. Many patients require constant supervision that places huge burden on family
    - D. Family members often experience considerable stress and are at risk for psychological and physical disorders
    - E. Availability of professional support and support groups critical for family

Learning Objectives (LO)

By the time you have finished studying this chapter, you should be able to do the following:

1. Define acquired brain injury or neuropsychological disorder, and discuss the problems involved in identifying organic causation, and in specifying the nature and site of the damage (410-412, 414).

2. Describe seven common signs of acquired brain injury and define delirium, dementia, aphasia, apraxia, and agnosia (412-414).

3. Name and describe six disorders listed in the text under the category of cerebral infection, identify those at risk for these disorders, and describe common treatments (414-417).

4. Name and describe three types of brain trauma discussed in the text, identify, those at risk for these problems, and describe common treatments (417-419).

5. Identify, and describe the effects of two types of vascular accidents, identify, those at risk for these disorders, and describe common treatments (419-422).

6. Describe the effects of brain tumors on mental and behavioral processes, identify, risk factors associated with brain tumors', and describe common treatments (422).

7. Describe the following degenerative brain disorders: Age-related dementia, Alzheimer's disease, Levy-body disease, vascular dementia, Huntington's chorea, and Parkinson's disease, identify those at risk for these disorders, and describe common treatments (422-428).

8. Describe the causes and effects of Korsakoff s psychosis (427, 429).

9. Name and describe two thyroid syndromes and two adrenal syndromes discussed under the heading of endocrine disorders (429).

10. Name and describe the effects of five substances that can lead to toxic disorders (429-430).

11. Distinguish between symptomatic and idiopathic epilepsy, distinguish among simple partial, complex partial, absence, and tonic-clonic seizures, identify, those at risk for these disorders, and describe common treatments (430-433).

Lecture Leads (LL)

Case studies: neuropsychological disorders (LL 14-1)
Supplement the case studies that the textbook presents. Case books by Ogden and Sacks are excellent sources of neuropsychological cases. Among the most well-known are Phineas Gage and H.M. Phineas Gage suffered an accident involving a 13 point rod traveling through his head. H.M. suffered from global amnesia following a neurosurgergy to treat epileptic seizures. The neurological literature is full of very interesting cases. For example Peru and Giampietro reviewed the case of a middle-aged female who showed personal neglect following two left-hemisphere strokes.

Resources:

Ogden, J. A. (1996). Fractured minds: A case-study approach to clinical neuropsychology. New York: Oxford University Press.

Peru, A., & Giampietro, P. (1997). Right personal neglect following a left hemisphere stroke: A case report. Cortex, 33, 585-590.

Sacks, O. (1985). The man who mistook his wife for a hat and other clinical tales. New York: Harper Perennial.

Alzheimer's disease and smoking (LL 14-2)
A recent prospective study found a relationship between smoking and risk of dementia. Prior research argued that smoking actually decreases the risk of Alzheimer's. Ott et al. asked for smoking histories of 6,870 subjects who were at least 55 years old, and subjects were labeled as smokers, former smokers, and never smokers. This baseline examination included an at-home interview and medical examinations. Those subjects who had signs of dementia were excluded from the study. At a two-year follow-up, subjects were assessed or their medical records were examined. Subjects were assessed using a mini mental state examination and the geriatric mental state schedule. If subjects showed signs of dementia, further testing was done, including neuropsychological testing and MRI scan. The diagnosis of dementia was made using the Diagnostic and Statistical Manual of Mental Disorders (DSM-III-R). Out of 146 cases of dementia, 105 were diagnosed with Alzheimer's disease. The results indicate that compared with never smokers, smokers were 2.2 times more likely to develop dementia and 2.3 times more likely to develop Alzheimer's disease.

Resource:

Ott, A. et al. (1998). Smoking and risk of dementia and Alzheimer's disease in a population-based cohort study: The Rotterdam study. The Lancet, 351, 1840-1843.

Cultural differences in prevalence of Alzheimer's disease (LL 14-3)
There is good evidence to suggest that Alzheimer's disease has a genetic component. Several nongenetic risk factors have been identified as well (e.g., level of education, severe head trauma). One curious feature of Alzheimer's disease, despite the well-established genetic component, is the fact that prevalence rates for this condition are not equal throughout the world. For example, it has been observed that prevalence rates for Alzheimer's disease are much lower in Japan than in North American. Studies comparing prevalence rates have been criticized because the methods used to collect data are not consistent between studies. One study examined the prevalence rates of Alzheimer's disease in two groups of subjects with very similar ethnic backgrounds who reside in very different geographic locations. The researchers examined the rates of the disease among the Yorubas, a group of people living in Nigeria, and a group of African-Americans living in Indianapolis, Indiana. They discovered that the age-adjusted prevalence rates for dementia (2.29%) and Alzheimer's disease (1.41 %) in the Nigerian sample were significantly lower than in the Indianapolis sample (8.24% and 6.24%, respectively). Because the ethnic composition of both groups is so similar, the researchers concluded that environment must account for a significant proportion of the difference in prevalence. Moreover, Binetti et al. (1998) reported some cultural differences in how the symptoms of Alzheimer's disease are expressed. For instance, Italian patients tend to score higher than American patients on measures that assess apathy, aberrant motor behavior, and agitation.

Resources:
Binetti, G. et al. (1998). Behavioral disorders in Alzheimer's disease: A transcultural perspective. Archives of Neurology, 55, 539-544.

Hendrie, H. C., et al. (1995). Prevalence of Alzheimer's disease and dementia in two communities: Nigerian Africans and African Americans. American Journal of Psychiatry, 152, 1485-1492.

Chromosome 12: Another Alzheimer's disease gene? (LL 14-4)
Recent research suggests that several chromosomes (i.e., 4, 6, 20, 21) play a role in Alzheimer's disease. The present study isolated the genetic risk for late-onset Alzheimer's disease. DNA of sixteen families with 135 total family members of whom 32 had Alzheimer's were analyzed. For a follow-up analysis, another 38 families with 216 total family members (89 family members with Alzheimer's) were used. Results indicate that a gene located on Chromosome 12 may have potential genetic risk in late-onset Alzheimer's disease.

Resource:
Pericak-Vance, M. A. et al. (1997). Complete genomic screen in late-onset familial Alzheimer disease evidence for a new locus on chromosome 12. Journal of the American Medical Association, 278, 1237-1241.

Prenatal factors and risk for stroke (LL 14-5)
Martyn, Barker, and Osmond summarized the literature suggesting that certain diseases
have prenatal origins. The study examined the relationship between stroke in adulthood
with impaired fetal growth. The methodology involved examining cause of death in over
13,000 males and subjects' birth statistics. The authors report that stroke was more
frequent in men who had low birthweights in relation to head size and weight of placenta.
The prevalence of stroke fell significantly as birthweight increased. The authors
contended that risk for stroke may be related to poor nutrition in the mother's childhood.
This poor nutrition affects the mother's ability to provide a prenatal environment that
promotes and sustains placental and fetal growth.

Resource:
Martyn, C. N., Barker, D. J. P., & Osmond, C. (1996). Mothers' pelvic size, fetal
growth, and death from stroke and coronary heart disease in men in the UK. The Lancet,
348, 1264-1268.

Awareness of involuntary movements (LL 14-6)
Snowden et al. investigated the awareness that patients with Huntington's have of their
involuntary movements. The subjects were patients of a Huntington's clinic and self-
reported their physical symptoms, in addition, objective measures of dysfunction were
collected. The results suggest that patients are not aware of the involuntary movements.
The authors argued that this denial has a physiological basis and is not a form of a
psychological defense.

Resource:
Snowden, J. S., Crawford, D., Griffiths, H. L., & Neary, D. (1998). Awareness of
          involuntary movements in Huntington's disease. Archives of Neurology, 55, 801-
          805.

Accidental injury and absence seizures (LL 14-7)
Wirrell et al. examined the relationships between absence seizures and accidental injury.
Subjects were 59 patients with absence seizures and 76 control patients with juvenile
rheumatoid arthritis. Subjects were identified by examination of pediatric EEG and
medical records. Subjects participated in a telephone interview that assessed the type,
severity, and treatment of prior accidental injuries possibly occurring during absence
seizures. Subjects with absence seizures reported more accidental injuries than the
control group with juvenile rheumatoid arthritis, especially bicycle and car accidents.
About 27% of the patients with absence seizure reported having an accident during a
seizure, of which 13% were serious enough to warrant minor treatment. Accident risk
was highest among adolescents and lowest among children. The authors suggest that
injury prevention counseling may be an important component to the treatment program.

Resource:
Wirrell, E. C. et al. (1996). Accidental injury is a serious risk in children with typical
absence epilepsy. Archives of Neurology, 53, 929-932.

Talking Points (TP)

Biology as the basis for affect, behavior, and cognitions (TP 14-1)
It bears repeating several times that our emotions, behaviors, and thoughts are rooted in the biology of the nervous system. This is no more evident than in the neuropsychological disorders. Stress this tightly knit relationship by informing students that changes in the nervous system will affect us in profound ways, and that the disorders in Chapter 14 provide excellent examples.

Revisiting student survey (TP 14-2)
It would a good idea to revisit the student survey data from Chapter 1 with your students. Most students have direct or indirect experience with the neuropsychological disorders. You may wish to ask students for personal illustrations, anecdotes, and examples from their lives that describe the disorders of Chapter 14. Perhaps there are many students who have grandparents inflicted with Alzheimer's. Sometimes, students will approach you after class and inform you about their own neuropsychological disorder. You may wish to use their case, with their permission, in class to illustrate important material.

Brain imaging (TP 14-3)
Locate some examples of EEG, PET scans, CT scans, and MRI scans to bring to class. Present them in the context of how they revolutionized our understanding of the brain.

Changing demographics and degenerative disorders (TP 14-4)
With the population aging and the prevalence of degenerative dementia highest among the elderly, what type of impact will this have on society? Discuss the social, psychological, and economic costs.

Perceptions of growing old (TP 14-5)
Before you assign students the material on degenerative disorders, ask them to describe an old person using five words (You may wish to use a different word such as aged, elderly, retired, or grandparent). Ask students to share their list, and keep track of references to senility and Alzheimer's. This is a good jumping off point to discuss that Alzheimer's is not part of the normal aging process.

President Reagan (TP 14-6)
On November 5, 1994, former President Ronald Reagan announced that he had Alzheimer's disease. Here is an excerpt of his announcement: "Upon learning this news, Nancy and I had to decide whether as private citizens we would keep this a private matter or whether we would make this news known in a public way. In the past, Nancy suffered from breast cancer and I had my cancer surgeries. We found through our open disclosures we were able to raise public awareness. We were happy that as a result, many more people underwent testing. They were treated in early stages and able to return to normal, healthy lives. So now we feel it is important to share it with you. In opening our hearts,

we hope this might promote greater awareness of this condition. Perhaps it will encourage a clearer understanding of the individuals and families who are affected by it. At the moment I feel just fine. I intend to live the remainder of the years God gives me on this Earth doing the things I have always done. I will continue to share life's journey with my beloved Nancy and my family. I plan to enjoy the great outdoors and stay in touch with my friends and supporters. Unfortunately, as Alzheimer's disease progresses, the family often bears a heavy burden. I only wish there was some way I could spare Nancy from this painful experience. When the time comes, I am confident that with your help she will face it with faith and courage." Have students analyze Reagan's announcement with regard to its effect on public awareness of Alzheimer's and the recognition that the disease will become burdensome to his family.

Caregivers stress (TP 14-7)
A few years ago, a woman in Washington state abandoned her father, who was an Alzheimer's patients, at a racetrack. The woman was later convicted with felony kidnapping and abandonment. This is a tragic yet effective example of the degree of stress that many caregivers experience. Ask your students for other examples that describe the hardships and challenges of a caregiver for a loved one with a neuropsychological disorder.

Parkinson' Disease and Huntington's Chorea (TP 14-8)
One way to describe Parkinson's disease is that it is a disorder of "poverty of movement," whereas Huntington's chorea is a "dance of movement."

Genetic testing (TP 14-9)
Since Huntington's chorea is genetically transmitted, genetic testing can determine the risk of a person in developing the disorder before any symptoms have appeared. Ask your students to consider whether they would seek such genetic testing, and if positive, how they would change their lives. As an adjunct, lead a discussion about the ethics of genetic testing. Should life and health insurance companies receive the results of genetic testing. How about employers? Should we required genetic testing for a marriage license or require genetic counseling?

Famous people with epilepsy (TP 14-10)
The textbook lists several famous historical figures with epilepsy. According to Epilepsy International, here are a few others: Alexander the Great, Richard Burton, Lewis Caroll, Charles Dickens, Danny Glover, Joan of Arc, Napoleon, Alfred Nobel, Socrates, Edgar Allan Poe, Alfred, Lord Tennyson, and Neil Young.

Cross-Cultural Teaching

This is not to say that these disorders are "**purely**" biological.	p. 410
declared "a **perfect specimen of health**."	p. 411
the diagnostician must **ferret out**...	p. 412
Their thinking is disorganized, even **dreamlike**.	p. 412
walk out of the house in **pajamas**.	p. 413
a piece of **shrapnel** enters the brain...	p. 415
most patients must be moved to a **hospice** or nursing home.	p. 417
A familiar instance of concussion is a **knockout** in a boxing match.	p. 417
Cowboys quarterback...	p. 418
if all cars were equipped with **air bags**...	p. 419
vascular dementia involves a **stepwise** deterioration...	p. 423
went on the market...amid a **great blast** of publicity.	p. 427
Consumer advocacy groups...	p. 429

Activities and Demonstrations (ACT/DEMO)

Field trip (ACT/DEMO 14-1)
Objective: To introduce the students to brain imaging techniques.
Materials: None.
Procedure: Arrange with your local hospital or medical center for a tour of their brain imaging facilities. Instruct the students to meet at the local hospital or medical center. If the facility is a long distance away, suggest car-pooling. Many students will have some knowledge of this type of equipment but will probably never have seen it in operation. Ask the students develop a list of questions prior to the tour that they would like the personnel to answer.
Discussion: Either after the tour or during the next class period, ask for additional questions from the students. Ask what they thought was the most interesting aspect of the tour. Remind students that these brain imaging techniques are helpful in making accurate diagnoses of neuropsychological disorders.

Neurological assessment (ACT/DEMO 14-2)
Objective: To demonstrate the methods and principles of neuropsychological tests
Materials: Several neuropsychological tests that your department or other psychologists in your community have available
Procedure: Select and bring several examples of neuropsychological tests into class. (Consider the Bender Visual-Motor Gestalt Test, Halstead-Reitan Battery, or the Luria-Nebraska Neuropsychological Battery). Administer parts of these tests such as the Trial Making exam. If you do not have the expertise necessary to conduct this demonstration, a guest speaker could provide assistance.
Discussion: Discuss how neuropsychologists identify deficits by using tests that are able to relate the deficit to specific areas of the brain. Your guest speaker can be a valuable resource with the interpretation of these tests if you are not qualified.

Brain used in performing tasks (ACT/DEMO 14-3)
Objective: To review the structures and functions of the brain
Materials: None
Procedure: This activity is best done in small groups. After students are placed in groups, ask each group to list three activities (e.g., playing the piano, watching a baseball game, reading a mystery novel, listening to music, hearing bad news, drinking a cool glass of water, using a word processor). Next, the group should describe the brain areas that are being used as the activity is performed. A fun addition is to bring to class a real brain and use it to point out the various structures.
Discussion: Following the group work, review the activities and brain areas involved. This is an excellent way to illustrate the interrelationships between brain and behavior. Emphasize that in the neuropsychological disorders, brain areas are damaged affecting various physical and psychological functions.

Guest speakers (ACT/DEMO 14-4)
Objective: To illustrate the material from a real-world perspective
Materials: None
Procedure: There are several guest speakers you could invite to your class. Of course, you can invite mental health professionals, but perhaps more interesting would be other individuals who can give a different perspective on neuropsychological disorders. Consider caregivers in nursing homes or retirement facilities, home health care workers, or respite caregivers. A family member of an Alzheimer's patient can give a particularly poignant and memorable presentation. Finally, your college or university is likely to have students with neurological disorders such as brain trauma or epilepsy, and these individuals can describe their challenges first-hand.
Discussion: Beforehand, instruct students to review this chapter and be prepared to ask questions of their guest speakers. Afterwards, ask students to compare and contrast the speakers' presentations.

Neuropsychological disorders in the popular media (ACT/DEMO 14-5)
Objective: To illustrate the degree of interest of the public for neuropsychological disorders and the accuracy of media reports
Materials: None
Procedure: About one week before starting Chapter 14, instruct your students to begin collecting reports from newspapers, magazines, and other media that present information about the neuropsychological disorders. Students are to bring the articles to class and briefly present them in small groups during coverage of the chapter. The group's task is to summarize the article and to analyze the accuracy of the report.
Discussion: Bring the groups together to report their findings. Summarize the overall accuracy of media reports on neuropsychological disorders. You may also wish to locate the original research article and compare it with the media version for accuracy and misinterpretation.

Films and Videos

Aging. The Methuselah Syndrome. PSU. Biological aspects of aging and information on aging.

Alzheimer's Disease: The Long Nightmare. FSH. Current research and the effects on emotional, medical, and financial aspects of the victim.

Organic Mental Disorders. CPB. The world of abnormal psychology: discusses psychological, biological, and social factors in diagnosis and treatment.

The Two Brains. CPB. The Brain Series.

Using Movies and Mental Illness as a Teaching Tool

Two films will be especially useful in teaching this section. The first of these is *On Golden Pond,* the film exemplar selected by Wedding and Boyd. It will be ideal if students can see the entire film; however, if a vignette is used in class, it should be the scene in which Norman Thayer, the retired college professor played so brilliantly by Henry Fonda, becomes lost in the woods near his cabin. Your students will enjoy speculating about whether or not Wedding and Boyd accurately captured the ways in which this individual would perform on a mental status examination.

A second helpful film that will be well known to your students is *Driving Miss Daisy.* Jessica Tandy's performance in the final minutes of the film very accurately captures the sort of cognitive deterioration associated with Alzheimer's disease. Professors interested in the family dynamics associated with Alzheimer's may want to have students see *Memories of Me.*

The cognitive sequelae of repeated head injuries can show segments from any of several excellent films about boxers, including *Raging Bull and On the Waterfront. Awakenings* is an excellent film to start students thinking about those cases in which the body fails before the mind.

Movie	Link to Chapter	Page Reference to Wedding and Boyd
• The Lost Weekend	delirium (p. 412)	p. 138
• Raging Bull • Regarding Henry	brain trauma (p.417)	p. 131 p.137
• The Grapes of Wrath • Blue Velvet	stroke (p. 419)	p. 138 p. 138
• On Golden Pond • Do You Remember Love? • Driving Miss Daisy	Alzheimer's Disease (p. 423)	p. 127 p. 137 p. 137
• Awakenings	Parkinson's Disease (p. 426)	p. 138

Classroom Assessment Techniques (CAT)

Muddiest Point (CAT 14-1)
Instruct students to write about an issue, concept, or definition presented in Chapter 14 that they find most confusing or difficult to understand.

Directed Paraphrasing (CAT 14-2)
In two or three sentences, students should paraphrase some important idea, concept, or definition presented in Chapter 14. Consider paraphrasing Alzheimer's disease, concussion, contusion, laceration, and meningitis.

Definition Matrix (CAT 14-3)
Using the handout, students should identify each of the disorders presented. For each disorder, students should provide the type, primary symptoms, groups at risk, and treatment. Students should only attempt to write only few words or phrases.

Suggestions for Essay Questions

- Compare and contrast concussion, contusion, and laceration.
- Describe the causes of epilepsy.
- Assume that you are writing an information sheet on epilepsy for school teachers. Describe the types of epilepsy.
- If you had to have one of the neuropsychological disorders described in the chapter, which one would it be? Defend your answer.

Definition Matrix
Classroom Assessment Technique

Disorder	Type	Primary symptoms	Groups at risk	Treatment
Encephalitis				
Concussion				
CVA				
Brain Tumor				
Alzheimer's Disease				
Vascular Dementia				
Huntington's Chorea				
Parkinson's Disease				
Lead Encephalopathy				
Absence seizure				
Symptomatic Epilepsy				

Chapter 15

Disorders of Childhood and Adolescence

Chapter Map

Section	Instructor Manual Components
Issues in Child Psychopathology • Prevalence • Classification and Diagnosis • Long-term Consequences	*Revisiting student survey (TP 15-1)* *Not even children are immune (TP 15-2)* *Normal children (TP 15-3)* *Developing an information packet (ACT/DEMO 15-1)* *Guest speakers (ACT/DEMO 15-2)*
Disruptive Behavior Disorders • Attention Deficit Hyperactivity Disorder • Conduct Disorders • Groups at Risk for Disruptive Behavior Disorders	*Abusing psychoactive substances (LL 15-1)* *Ritalin (LL 15-2)* *SAD as childhood depression (LL 15-3)* *Not watching where they were going (LL 15-4)* *Ritalin as a controlled substance (TP 15-4)* *ADHD and ADA (TP 15-5)* *Increased prevalence of ADHD (TP 15-6)*
Disorders of Emotional Distress • Anxiety Disorders • Childhood Depression • Groups at Risk	
Eating Disorders • Anorexia Nervosa • Bulimia Nervosa • Childhood Obesity	*Experiencing eating disorders (LL 15-5)* *Famous people with eating disorders (TP 15-7)* *Standards of beauty and advertising (ACT/DEMO 15-3)* *Survey on eating disorders (ACT/DEMO 15-4)* *Role playing a family therapy lunch session (ACT/DEMO 15-5)*

Elimination Disorders	*Bell and pad method for enuresis (TP 15-8)*
• Enuresis • Encopresis	
Childhood Sleep Disorders	*Anecdotes on sleepwalking, sleeptalking, and night terrors (TP 15-9)*
• Insomnia • Nightmares and Night Terrors • Sleepwalking	
Learning and Communication Disorders	*Famous people with dyslexia (TP 15-10)* *Field trip (ACT/DEMO 15-6)*
• Learning Disorders • Groups at Risk for Learning Disorders • Communication Disorders	
Disorders of Childhood and Adolescence: Theory and Therapy	
• The Psychodynamic Perspective • The Behavioral Perspective • The Cognitive Perspective • The Family Systems Perspective • The Sociocultural Perspective • The Biological Perspective	

Chapter Outline

I.   Introduction
    A.   Disorders of childhood and adolescence include wide range of problems
        1.   Involve failure to pass developmental milestone on time
        2.   Involve disruption of developmentally acquired skill
        3.   Some are psychological disorders that normally have onset prior to adulthood
    B.   Disorders may have no counterpart in adult psychopathology
    C.   Deciding what is abnormal more difficult in childhood and adolescence
    D.   Disorders differ in course and outcome from adult psychological disorders
    E.   Most children do not think of themselves as having treatable psychological disorders

II.   Issues in Child Psychopathology
    A.   Prevalence
        1.   One out of every five children and adolescents has moderate or severe psychological disorder
        2.   Admission rates begin to increase at age six or seven
        3.   Psychological disturbances more common in boys than in girls
    B.   Classification and Diagnosis
        1.   Classified as syndromes
        2.   Empirical method groups together preadult problems that occur together in same children or age group
            a.   Disruptive behavior disorders
            b.   Disorders of emotional distress
            c.   Habit disorders
            d.   Learning and communication disorders
        3.   Most of DSM-IV diagnostic categories can be grouped under four headings
            a.   Disruptive behavior disorders
            b.   Disorders of emotional distress
            c.   Habit disorders
            d.   Learning and communication disorders
        4.   Children change rapidly
        5.   Children may not fit neatly into one category
    C.   Long-Term Consequences
        1.   Stability is one type of predictability; antisocial behavior is stable
        2.   Continuity of developmental adaptation leads to other different disorders
        3.   Reactivity to particular stressors relates to disorders creating stresses
        4.   Some childhood disorders do predict adult disorders often indirectly

5. Some children and adolescents respond well to treatment

III. Disruptive Behavior Disorders
   A. **Disruptive behavior disorders** involve poorly controlled, impulsive, acting-out behavior in situations where self-control is expected
   B. Attention Deficit Hyperactivity Disorder
      1. **Attention deficit hyperactivity disorder (ADHD)** involves short attention span and hyperactivity
      2. More common in boys than girls; between 3-5% of elementary school children said to have ADHD
      3. Some believe that it is too readily applied to children difficult to control
      4. Symptoms affect every area of child's functioning
         a. Behavior often distinguished less by its excessiveness than by its haphazard quality
         b. Activity seems purposeless and disorganized
         c. Affects child's academic progress
         d. ADHD children tend to have poor social adjustment
      5. DSM-IV divides syndrome into three subtypes
         a. Predominantly inattentive type
         b. Predominantly hyperactive/impulsive type
         c. Combined type; most ADHD children more likely to have wide range of problems
      6. Most ADHD children still show the disorder in adolescence
      7. Many ADHD children will develop antisocial behavior
      8. Cognitive problems tend to persist into adolescence
   C. Conduct Disorder
      1. **Conduct disorder** characterized by indifference to rights of others, reckless behavior, and cruel behavior
         a. Aggression against people or animals
         b. Destruction of property
         c. Deceitfulness or theft
         d. Serious violation of rules
      2. One of most common syndromes of childhood and adolescence; estimated prevalence 4-16%; boys outnumber girls
      3. Age of onset important
         a. Childhood-onset with at least one symptom prior to age 10; usually male; physically aggressive; have few friends; more likely to develop antisocial personality disorder
         b. Adolescent-onset with no symptoms prior to age 10; less aggressive, have friends
      4. Many with conduct disorders commit serious crimes
      5. Many children comes from disorganized and unhappy families leading to poor prognosis
   D. Groups at Risk for Disruptive Behavior Disorders

369

1. Gender is strongest risk factor for disruptive behavior disorders
   a. Boys outnumber girls nine to one in ADHD
   b. Boys outnumber girls in conduct disorders
2. Gender difference subject to recent debate
   a. May be due to artifact of reporting
   b. May be due to differential socialization
   c. May be due to difference of seriousness of crimes
3. Socioeconomic factors such as correlates of poverty play role in conduct disorders

IV. Disorders of Emotional Distress
   A. Disorders of emotional distress are internalizing disorders where conflict is turned inward
   B. Diagnosis is difficult when child lacks verbal and conceptual skills; must rely on child's behavior
   C. Anxiety Disorders
      1. Separation Anxiety Disorder
         a. Separation anxiety is intense fear and distress upon separation from parents or caregivers
         b. Seen in almost all children; peaks at about 12 months
         c. In some it persists into school years; disappears and reappears triggered by stress characterizes **separation anxiety disorder**
         d. Child may have fears of horrible things happening while separated from parents
         e. Parent-child conflicts common and exacerbate disorder
         f. Estimated prevalence is between 4 to 13% of children and adolescents
      2. Social Phobia
         a. **Social phobia** is fear of social or performance situations in which embarrassment may occur
         b. Most children grow out of fear of strangers by age two and a half; children with social phobia do not
         c. Social phobia may not generalize to all social situations
         d. Children with social phobia are often well adjusted at home and have normal relationships with parents
         e. At school, child is withdrawn, interfering with academic progress and social relationships
      3. Generalized Anxiety Disorder
         a. In **generalized anxiety disorder** child experiences anticipatory anxiety doubting their own capabilities
         b. Family dynamics may play role
         c. Anxiety tends to breed failure, which brings on the very problems child was anticipating, creating vicious cycle
      4. Childhood Depression

370

        a.   Parents and teacher often fail to notice depression in children

        b.   **Childhood depression** resembles adult depression

        c.   Symptoms of depression are often expressed differently by children than by adults

        d.   Prevalence is between 2 to 5%; adolescents may be more vulnerable than younger children

        e.   Studies suggest that depressed children are at risk for mood disorders as much as depressed adults

    5.   Groups at Risk for Disorders of Emotional Distress

        a.   Girls more likely to develop separation anxiety disorder, social phobia, and generalized anxiety disorder

        b.   Young boys more vulnerable to depression

        c.   Teenage girls more likely to develop disorders of emotional distress

V.   Eating Disorders

    A.   Anorexia Nervosa

        1.   **Anorexia nervosa** is severe restriction of food intake caused by fear of weight gain

        2.   Most cases are female between ages of 12 and 18

        3.   Anorexia nervosa is physically dangerous

        4.   Most dramatic sign of anorexia is emaciation; DSM-IV criteria is body weight less than 85% of what is normal for age and height of patient

        5.   Other criteria is intense fear of becoming fat, unrealistic body image, and amenorrhea

        6.   There are two behavioral patterns

            a.   Restricting type is refusal to eat

            b.   Binge-eating/purging type eat and then purge

        7.   Most anorexics have normal appetites, at least in early stages of disorder

            a.   May become preoccupied with food

            b.   Collect cookbooks and prepare elaborate meals for others

        8.   Fear of obesity most typical feature of anorexia

        9.   Some see disorder as way of avoiding an adult sexual role and pregnancy

        10.   Some view disorder as daughter's weapon against her parents, suggesting disturbed family relationships

    B.   Bulimia Nervosa

        1.   **Bulimia nervosa** characterized by uncontrolled binge eating plus compensation

        2.   Base their self-esteem on body shape

        3.   Binge often triggered by stress or unhappiness

4. Bulimia resembles anorexia with regard to onset and gender difference
C. Childhood Obesity
1. Prevalence of obesity in children and adolescence is 20%
2. Excess weight can contribute to physical disorders and can have psychological consequences
   a. Teasing by peers
   b. Especially acute for girls
3. Obesity due to combination of physiological and psychological factors
4. Family routine plays role in childhood obesity
   a. Balance of physical exercise versus television watching
   b. Diet
D. Groups at Risk for Eating Disorders
1. Girls at greater risk for anorexia and bulimia
2. Cultural ideals of female attractiveness has contributed to problem
3. Increase in prevalence may be due to increase awareness and reporting of disorders
4. Risk for eating disorders spreading to preteenage group
5. Many girls have only partial syndromes
6. Efforts to identify at-risk girls to prevent full syndrome eating disorders from developing

VI. Elimination Disorders
A. Enuresis
1. **Enuresis** is lack of bladder control past age at which such control is usual
2. Daytime wetting is less common and may be sign of more serious psychological problems
3. Clinician decides age that separates normal accidents from enuresis
   a. DSM-IV specifies minimum age of 5 years
   b. Wetting must occur at least twice a week
   c. Suffering serious distress or impaired functioning
4. Prevalence of enuresis at age 5 is 7% for boys and 3% for girls; at age 10, 3% for boys and 2% for girls
5. Enuresis may be of two types
   a. Primary enuresis occurs when child has never achieved bladder control and may last into middle childhood; may have organic abnormality
   b. Secondary enuresis occurs when child achieves bladder control and loses it usually due to stress
6. Most enuretic children are not emotionally disturbed; emotional problem may be result of disorder
7. Enuresis may cause social problems
8. Bed-wetting almost always clears up

B. Encopresis
1. **Encopresis** is lack of bowel control
2. May occur with enuresis which it resembles
   a. Can be classified as primary or secondary
   b. More common in boys than girls
   c. Child experiences mockery and wrath from parents
3. Encopresis has prevalence of 1%
4. Typically occurs as part of larger disorder such as disruptive behavior disorder or part of severe family problems

VII. Childhood Sleep Disorders
A. Insomnia
1. Most common response to stress in early childhood is insomnia
2. Insomnia is usually in form of difficulty falling asleep or staying asleep
3. Child does not decide if problem needs treatment; parents often see it as attention-getting behavior
4. Sleeping problem may have physiological cause, but most often related to worry
B. Nightmares and Night Terrors
1. Nightmares occur more frequently in childhood than in later years
   a. Shows no particular physiological arousal
   b. May or may not be awakened by dream
   c. Usually able to describe dream in detail
   d. Occurs during REM sleeps
2. Less prevalent, but more disturbing are **sleep terrors**
   a. Shows intense physiological arousal
   b. Very hard to comfort
   c. Has no memory of episode next morning
   d. Occurs during first few hours of sleep in non-REM sleep
C. Sleepwalking
1. **Sleepwalking** is more common in young
2. Child falls asleep, about two hours later they perform complex action
   a. Eyes are open and do not bump into things
   b. Can last 15 seconds to 30 minutes
   c. Usually returns to bed
   d. Not acting out dreams
   e. Occurs during non-REM sleep
3. Usually not a serious problem

VIII. Learning and Communication Disorders
   A. Learning Disorders
      1. **Learning disorders** involves person's skill in one of three areas substantially below what would be expected for age, education, and intelligence of person and interferes with adjustment
         a. Reading disorder
         b. Disorder of written expression
         c. Mathematics disorder
      2. Prevalence is from 5 to 15% with majority of them boys
      3. About 25% of children with conduct disorders, ADHD, and depression also have learning disorders
      4. Various medical conditions involve learning disorders
      5. Many cases of learning disorders involve distortions of visual and auditory perception
         a. Struggle to distinguish sound of different words or make associations between words they hear
         b. Perceptual problems usually occur in more than one sense system
      6. Some children also show disturbances in memory and other cognitive functions
         a. Difficulties with sequential thinking and organizing thoughts
         b. May be related to attention deficits
      7. Children often do poorly in school and experience low self-esteem and low motivation
         a. Are at risk for dropping out of school
         b. Tend to have employment problems
   B. Groups at Risk for Learning Disorders
      1. Boys are more likely than girls to develop learning disorders
      2. Reading disorder occurs at equal rates in both boys and girls
      3. Socioeconomic factors operate as well
      4. Standardized tests may discriminate against certain groups
         a. In the past, disproportionately higher numbers of white middle class children diagnosed as having learning disorder
         b. In the past, disproportionately higher numbers of African-American children diagnosed as mentally retarded
      5. There is much variability in learning disorders
         a. Children with same symptoms have different underlying disorders
         b. Same disorders may produce different symptoms in different children
         c. Learning disorders can be attributed to wide range of causes
         d. Approaches to treatment extremely varied
   C. Communication Disorders

1. Delayed Speech and other Gaps in Communication
    a. Prolonged delay in speech may be early sign of problem
    b. Problems with articulation as in enunciation
    c. Difficulties with expressive language in putting thoughts into words
    d. Difficulties with receptive language in understanding language of others
        i. Most serious and longer-lasting
        ii. Can be disastrous for a child in school
        iii. Special education usually necessary
2. Stuttering
    a. Interruption of fluent speech through blocked, prolonged, or repeated words, syllables, or sounds is called **stuttering**
    b. Hesitant speech is most common
    c. Persistent stuttering occurs in 1% of population and is more common among boys
    d. Many children outgrow stuttering
    e. Organic theories have been proposed; problem with physical articulation of sounds in mouth and larynx
    f. Stuttering is probably psychogenic with parents creating anxiety that disturbs their speech, making them more anxious

IX. Disorders of Childhood and Adolescence: Theory and Therapy
    A. Psychodynamic Perspective
        1. Conflict and Regression
            a. Childhood developmental disorders stem from id/impulses and prohibitions from parents and superego
            b. Encopresis can be interpreted as a disguised expression of hostility
            c. Enuresis interpreted as sign of regression
            d. Anorexia viewed as regression
            e. Ego psychologists view anorexia is related to adolescent's drive for autonomy
        2. Play Therapy
            a. Best treatment is one that allows patient to bring to surface and work through unconscious conflicts
            b. **Play therapy** allows child to draw and play with toys
                i. Toys used for expressing aggression
                ii. Dolls and puppets for play-acting family conflicts
            c. Therapists interact with parents as well
            d. Specific approach varies from therapist to therapist
    B. The Behavioral Perspective
        1. Inappropriate Learning

a. Childhood disorders stem from inadequate learning or inappropriate learning

b. Inadequate learning is a failure to learn relevant cues for performing desired behaviors

c. Inappropriate learning refers to reinforcement of undesirable behavior

2. Relearning

a. Behavior therapists use entire behavioral repertoire to replace child's maladaptive responses with adaptive responses

b. Classical conditioning used to treat nocturnal enuresis

c. Anxiety disorders can be treated using systematic desensitization

d. Modeling can be useful in treatment of phobias

e. Operant conditioning has been successful in treatment of ADHD

f. Token economy has been used for certain behavior disorders

C. Cognitive Perspective

1. Negative Cognitions in Children

a. Problem behaviors in children stem from negative beliefs, faulty attributions, poor problem solving, and other cognitive factors

b. Real trigger in depression is cognitive factors not event

2. Changing Children's Cognitions

a. Goal of cognitive therapy in ADHD is to teach how to modify their impulsiveness through self-control skills and reflective problem solving by using **self-instructional training**

i. Self-instructional training works well for specific tasks

ii. Skills learned from self-instructional training may not generalize if not carefully reinforced

b. Attribution retaining involves teaching children to make attributions that are less internal, less stable, and less global

c. Usefulness of cognitive therapy depends greatly on age of child

d. Cognitive therapy often combined with behavioral strategies

D. The Family Systems Perspective

1. Child plays a critical role in family, and child's disorder reflects a disturbance in family

2. Family psychopathology underlies many childhood disorders and must be addressed if child's problems are to be relieved

3. Anorexia has been treated successfully through family therapy

         a.   Girls' families tend to be overprotective, rigid, and superficially close

         b.   Family therapy lunch sessions used where girl is instructed that she has won over her parents and told that she must be eat to live

E.   The Sociocultural Perspective

    1.   Cultural patterns shape the child's disorder

    2.   There are cultural differences in expression of symptoms among American and Thai children

    3.   To identify cause of disorders, the culture as well as the individual should be considered

         a.   Risk for conduct disorders correlated strongly with poverty-related factors

         b.   To address disorders, society must address those factors

    4.   Anorexia and bulimia may be influenced by culture

F.   The Biological Perspective

    1.   Childhood and adolescent disorders may have biological component

    2.   Anorexia involves both biological and psychological causes

         a.   Anorexics are hungry

         b.   Psychological factors override hunger

    3.   ADHD seems most likely to have biological basis

         a.   Most ADHD children have paradoxical response to amphetamines

         b.   Amphetamines given to normal people cause them to act like hyperactive children;

         c.   Three-fourths of ADHD children benefit from stimulants

              i.   There are side effects of Ritalin

              ii.   Academic performance usually does not improve and child must continue to be taught skills

             iii.   Potential for abuse

         d.   Drugs must be prescribed with caution

Chapter Boxes

- Antisocial Adolescents: Are There Two Types?
  - A. Most criminal offenders are teenagers
  - B. Steep decline in offenders in early adulthood means antisocial behavior is temporary and age-specific
  - C. One type of antisocial behavior is limited to adolescence
  - D. One type of antisocial behavior persists over life course
  - E. Differences may exist in preadolescent history offenders

- Recognizing Learning Disorders: Some Signs
  - A. There are no absolute signs of learning disability
  - B. Signs vary with age and the individual
  - C. If child seems to lag in comparison with child's peers, evaluation should be considered
  - D. In preschool, learning disabled children have problems with language or concentration
  - E. In kindergarten, symptoms of learning disability show up in schoolwork
  - F. Children who may be learning disabled need to be screened for psychological problems

Learning Objectives (LO)

By the time you have finished studying this chapter, you should be able to do the following:

1. Compare and contrast disorders of childhood and adolescence with disorders of adulthood, and summarize information on the prevalence of child psychopathology (438-439).

2. Explain the classification system DSM-IV uses for childhood disorders, describe how childhood disorders predict adult disorders, and describe the degree to which treatment of childhood disorders can prevent adult disorders (439-440).

3. Define disruptive behavior disorders, and describe three subtypes of attention deficit hyperactivity, disorder (440-442).

4. Describe two types conduct disorder based on age of onset, and explain how they relate to adult antisocial behavior and antisocial personality disorder (442-444).

5. Name and describe three varieties of anxiety disorder in children, and summarize information presented in your text on childhood depression (444-447).

6. Name and describe three varieties of eating disorder in children and adolescents (447-450).

7. Name and describe two varieties of elimination disorder in children (450-451).

8. Name and describe four varieties of sleep disorder in children (451-452).

9. Summarize information presented in your text on learning disorders (452-453).

10. Summarize information presented in your text on problems with stuttering, and with language articulation, reception, and expression (453-454).

11. Summarize explanations of and recommended treatments for the disorders of childhood and adolescence from the psychodynamic, behavioral, and cognitive perspectives (454-458).

12. Summarize explanations of and recommended treatments for the disorders of childhood and adolescence from the family systems, sociocultural and biological perspectives, referring particularly to the biological treatment of attention deficit hyperactivity disorder (458-460).

Lecture Leads (LL)

Abusing psychoactive substances (LL 15-1)
Children with ADHD are more likely to develop other conditions like depression or conduct disorders, or antisocial personality disorder. As a consequence, they are also more likely to use and abuse psychoactive substances. Recent research has attempted to determine if the tendency to use psychoactive substances is the result of ADHD or conduct and antisocial personality disorders. Biederman et al. studied adults diagnosed with childhood onset ADHD and a comparison group of non-ADHD adults. Results revealed that the ADHD group had significantly higher lifetime prevalence rates for substance use/abuse difficulties than the non-ADHD group. In addition, when comorbid disorders such as mood, anxiety, and antisocial personality disorders were factored out of the analysis, ADHD was the most significant factor in predicting the development of substance use disorders.

Resource:
Biederman, J., Wilens, T., Mick, E., Milberger, S., Spencer, T. J., & Faraone, S. V. (1995). Psychoactive substance use disorders in adults with attention deficit hyperactivity disorder (ADHD): Effects of ADM and psychiatric comorbidity. American Journal of Psychiatry, 152, 1652-1658.

Ritalin (LL 15-2)
Much has been written on Ritalin in the past few years. Most of the commentary has questioned the ease with which physicians prescribe the stimulant to children with ADHD. Peter Breggin writes about how the Food and Drug Administration and National Institute of Mental Health have withheld information regarding the hazards of Ritalin. Even though there is strong evidence of the drug's short term effect in reducing hyperactivity and helping to focus attention, what is missing are long-term data. In fact, the label reads, "Long-term effects of Ritalin in children have not been well-established" despite the fact that Ritalin has been on the market for 40 years. Breggin presents evidence of the adverse drug experiences that many people have had. He argues that there have been over 2,700 of these experiences filed with the FDA between 1985 and 1997. Alternatively, the environment may play a large role in ADHD by reinforcing inappropriate behavior. He argues that studies showing brain abnormalities are, for the most part, poorly design. He concludes by positing that prescribing Ritalin is never appropriate.

Resource:
Breggin, P. (1998). Talking back to Ritalin: What doctors aren't telling you about stimulants for children. Monroe, ME: Common Courage Press.

SAD as childhood depression (LL 15-3)

It has become apparent that depression is a condition that affects children as well as adults despite conventional wisdom that views children as lacking the emotional sophistication to experience this disorder. As a consequence, researchers have also begun to examine the possibility that children may also experience seasonal affective disorder (SAD). In order to estimate rates of SAD in the childhood population, Swedo et al. had 2,267 middle and high school students in a suburb of Washington, D.C., fill out a modified version of the Seasonal Pattern Assessment Questionnaire. Of the 1,835 that were returned, 3.3% of the respondents, based on their responses, could be categorized as "probable" SADS cases. Using these data, the researchers estimate that 1.7% to 5.5% of 9 to 19-year-old children may have SADS. This study also found that the rate of SAD was positively correlated with age, with the highest rates being identified in postpubertal girls and the next highest rate occurring in postpubertal boys. The authors suggest that additional data are needed from different geographic locations to obtain a clearer picture of SAD in the child population.

Resource:
Swedo, S. E. et al. (1995). Rates of seasonal affective disorder in children and adolescents. American Journal of Psychiatry, 152, 1016-1019.

Not watching where they were going (LL 15-4)

Adolescents are particular prone to automobile accidents and traffic convictions. Anecdotally, adolescents with ADHD appear to be even more prone. Nada-Raja et al examined the relationship between ADHD and driving offenses among male and female adolescents. Of the 470 males and 446 female adolescents, 83 were identified having symptoms related to ADHD, with others having symptoms related to conduct disorder or no psychological disorder. Using driving records and self-report, the researchers examined which subjects committed traffic offenses in the teenage years. Those with ADHD symptoms and conduct disorders were more likely to have had traffic convictions. Among females, ADHD symptoms was strongly related to traffic convictions and car accidents compared to other females. Jerome and Segal report similar results in a prospective study examining cognitive measures of impulsivity and attention and driving ability.

Resources:
Jerome, L., & Segal, A. (1997). ADHD and dangerous driving. Journal of the American Academy of Child & Adolescent Psychiatry, 36, 1325.

Nada-Raja, S. et al. (1997). Inattentive and hyperactive behaviors and driving offenses in adolescence. Journal of the American Academy of Child & Adolescent Psychiatry, 36, 515-522.

Experiencing eating disorders (LL 15-5)

Although the textbook does present some accounts of eating disorders, a different dimension emerges when you study first-person descriptions of the disorders. Mary Fleming Callaghan chronicles the six-year struggle of her 15-year-old daughter with anorexia nervosa. Callaghan focuses on how the disorder creates despair in the family. Her daughter, Kathleen, was 5' 8" tall, but weighed only 69 pounds at the lowest point in the disorder. Sheila Mather provides a first-person account of her recovery from bulimia, starving and overeating. She writes that she "…would eat enough for four, go to the washroom after every meal, or starve for three days straight. For ten years, nobody knew I had a problem with food--fooled everybody. Nobody knew, not even me, that my eating disorder was never about food. I had been feeding myself love, safety, security and strength. I could conquer the world, be anybody, do anything when I was eating. When I felt I was loosing control of my eating, I starved and immediately, I regained control. Then one bright sunny spring day, the sunlight shone down on me, exposing the person I had become. Student and employee by day--binger, purger, exerciser, and starver by night. I felt revolted but couldn't run. I could no longer binge, purge, starve or overeat-- my body was utterly exhausted. My emotions were painful well beyond my control. My recovery began. For the next four years I experienced emotions I had held inside me, emotions that previously I had been too afraid to feel. Little by little, I was becoming the person I had been born to be. I felt happy, excited, and alive. I felt a vibrant inspiration to participate in life. I wanted to live--and I was--living and feeling in this beautiful world." Locate biographies or autobiographies of people who have suffered from eating disorders. First-person descriptions seem to convey the essence of psychological disorders and are so much more personal and tragic than clinical transcripts.

Resources:

Callaghan, M. G.   (1995). Wrinkles on the heart: A mother's journal of one family's
        struggle with anorexia nervosa. Grove City, OH: Alabaster Press

Mather, S. (1997). Leaving food behind. Ottawa: Mather Publications

Talking Points (TP)

Revisiting student survey (TP 15-1)

It would a good idea to revisit the student survey data from Chapter 1 with your students. Most students have direct or indirect experience with the developmental disorders. You may wish to ask students for personal illustrations, anecdotes, and examples from their lives that describe the disorders of Chapter 15. Perhaps, there are many students who have siblings with ADHD. Sometimes students will approach you after class and inform you about their own disorder or their child's disorder. You may wish to use their case with their permission in class to illustrate important material.

Not even children are immune (TP 15-2)

Some students make the assumption that children are somehow not vulnerable to psychological disorders. Of course, this not true. In some sense, these patients are the most vulnerable for reasons the textbook discusses.

Normal children (TP 15-3)

The concept of what is normal development has changed considerably over the years. At one time, children were expected to work, get married, and have children at a much younger age than what would now be considered appropriate. There are also tremendous cross-cultural differences in standards of normality. Given this, discuss why children require these unique criteria to be diagnosed with a mental disorder.

Ritalin as a controlled substance (TP 15-4)

Keep an eye on your local newspapers for articles related to the theft of Ritalin. It appears that Ritalin is becoming a popular drug for getting high. The tablets are crushed and usually snorted just like cocaine or the drug is injected. It creates a cocaine-like stimulating effect. Ritalin is a Schedule II Controlled Substance and subject to strict control. Now, Ritalin has turned into an illicit street drug commanding $3 to $15 per tablet. In many states, it is a felony for one student to give another student a tablet on school grounds.

ADHD and ADA (TP 15-5)

Many children with ADHD grow up to be adults with ADHD. Adults with ADHD are at risk in the workplace since the disorder can interfere with job performance. Ask students if they think ADHD should be covered in the Americans with Disabilities Act. The act requires employees, among others, to provide reasonable accommodation to individuals with disabilities. How far should and can employers go in providing reasonable accommodation to employees with ADHD. You may also wish to extend this Talking Point to include college students' ADHD and ask students how far the faculty and institutions should go in the accommodation.

Increased prevalence of ADHD (TP 15-6)
Discuss with your students the apparent increase in the prevalence of ADHD. Are parents, teachers, and mental health professionals just more likely to diagnose difficult children with ADHD or has there been a true increase? Ask students to think back to their elementary school years for examples.

Famous people with eating disorders (TP 15-7)
To mention famous people with eating disorders is to tell students that not even the rich and famous are immune from psychological disorders Those who suffered from eating disorders include Karen Carpenter, who died of anorexia nervosa at age 32, Jane Fonda, Princess Diana, and Tracy Gold.

Bell and pad method for enuresis (TP 15-8)
Students will find it interesting to actually see the material used in the bell and pad method for enuresis. You may be able to locate one from a clinic, hospital, or hospital supply company. Discuss the principle underlying this treatment method.

Anecdotes on sleepwalking, sleeptalking, and night terrors (TP 15-9)
Students, and perhaps you, probably have stories about experiencing sleep disorders in childhood. Ask for volunteers to recount these anecdotes to illustrate the nature and symptoms of the disorders.

Famous people with dyslexia (TP 15-10)
There is a myth regarding dyslexia Here's a list of people with dyslexia: William Butler Yeats, Charles Schwab, John Irving, George Patton, Albert Einstein, Thomas Edison, Alexander Graham Bell, Leonardo da Vinci, Walt Disney, Winston Churchill, Woodrow Wilson, Cher, Whoopi Goldberg, Greg Louganis, Bruce Jenner, and Jackie Stewart.

involve a failure to pass a developmental milestone **"on time."**	p. 438
other kinds of **"acting out"** behaviors…	p. 439
disrupt games, get into fights…throw **temper tantrums.**	p. 441
a look at the **preadolescent** history…	p. 443
running away from home, **shoplifting,** using drugs…	p. 444
blushing and **tongue-tied…**	p. 445
Older children may **sulk…**	p. 446
another instrument down the throat to stimulate the **gag reflex.**	p. 448
humiliating visits to the **"husky"** department of clothing stores…	p. 449
to change pajamas, sheets, and **rubber pad.**	p. 450
a digestive problem such as **colic.**	p. 451
cause a child to be treated **"like a baby."**	p. 453
in adolescence they **strike back** by refusing to eat.	p. 455
therapies aimed at improving the reading, writing, **penmanship…**	p. 457
he would become a **sissy** in his father's eyes.	p. 458

Activities and Demonstrations (ACT/DEMO)

Developing an information packet (ACT/DEMO 15-1)
Objective: To understand the etiology, symptoms, and treatment of childhood and adolescent disorders
Materials: None
Procedure: After students are put into small groups, inform them that their task is to develop a brochure that could be given to parents whose child has just been diagnosed with one of the disorders presented in Chapter 15. The purpose of this brochure is to educate the parents so that they can deal better with their child's disorder. The groups will want to select a particular disorder. In the brochure, information about the disorder's symptoms, etiology, and treatment should be presented. Tell students to create their brochure using desktop publishing or word processing programs and to be creative.
Discussion: After all groups have completed their brochure, collect them, and redistribute each to the rest of the groups. Next, the groups are to review the accuracy of the material and design of the brochure.

Guest speakers (ACT/DEMO 15-2)
Objective: To illustrate the material from a real-world perspective
Materials: None
Procedure: A number of information guest speakers can be invited into the classroom to talk about the disorders presented in Chapter 15. You could invite someone from a half-way house for emotionally trouble youth or a children's psychiatric hospital. A psychologist or clinical social worker will be able to give insights not only into the specific disorder but also into the daily management problems associated with children and adolescents. A special education teacher or speech therapist would also provide interesting insights into the disorders. Of course, an especially instructive perspective comes from parents who have children with these disorders. Finally, if appropriate, an individual who has successfully battled an eating disorder would provide a different perspective.
Discussion: Beforehand, instruct students to review this chapter and be prepared to ask questions of their guest speakers. Afterwards, ask students to compare and contrast the speakers' presentations.

Standards of beauty and advertising (ACT/DEMO 15-3)
Objective: To demonstrate the messages about attractiveness in advertising
Materials: None
Procedure: Have students watch television, read popular magazines, and observe newspapers and outdoor advertising. For each time, students should record the type of media, the product advertised, and the implied message about beauty. Before you assign this project, ask students to describe what is a beautiful person?
Discussion: Summarize the types of advertisements on an overhead and update it throughout the discussion. What standard of beauty are advertisements conveying? How do student descriptions of beauty relate to what is found in advertisement? Relate the

activity to eating disorders. To extend the activity, discuss with students the impact that television shows have on the culture with regard to redefining attractiveness and beauty.

Survey on eating disorders (ACT/DEMO 15-4)
Objective: To collect data on eating disorders in your class and school
Materials: Eating disorders survey
Procedure: Hand out the survey and assure the students that the information will be anonymous. The survey asks the students their sex, age, whether they have ever binged or purged, and whether they live in same-sex, with children, coed, or solitary living arrangements.
Discussion: Make an overhead of the survey and use the overhead to tabulate these results. Students are often shocked to discover how common these symptoms are, especially among females. Use the DSM criteria on these disorders to lead a discussion. As an alternative or addition, have your students anonymously state their sex and how much they feel that they are either over or under their ideal weight. Lead a discussion of sex differences in expected appearance.

Role playing a family therapy lunch session (ACT/DEMO 15-5)
Objective: To illustrate the interaction in a family therapy lunch session
Materials: None
Procedure: After reviewing family systems perspective, ask for volunteers to recreate a family therapy lunch session. The role play should have a therapist, patient, father, and mother. The interaction should be characteristic of the family dynamics believed to be operating in the families of anorexics. At several points in the role play, stop the participants and ask them to report what they are feeling.
Discussion: After the role play, ask students for their reactions to the sessions. Of course, the role play is not real, but discuss with students their views of the treatment's effectiveness.

Field trip (ACT/DEMO 15-6)
Objective: To introduce the students to special needs education
Materials: None.
Procedure: Arrange with your local school or lab school for a tour of a special needs classroom and regular mainstream classroom. You will want to divide the class into small groups otherwise large groups touring classrooms can be very disruptive. Ask the students to develop a list of questions prior to attending this tour that they would like the personnel to answer.
Discussion: Either after the tour or during the next class period, ask for additional questions from the students. Ask what they thought was the most interesting aspect of the tour.

Films and Videos

An Anorexic's Tale. The Brief Life of Catherine. FHS. This docudrama tells the story of Catherine Dunbar's seven-year battle against anorexia.

Anorexia and Bulimia. FHS. This program explains the addictive nature of anorexia and bulimia and their possible effects on the cardiovascular and central nervous systems.

Dying to be Thin. FHS. This program profiles a young woman obsessed with the desire to be thin.

Dyslexia: Diagnosis and Prognosis. FHS. This program provides an overview of the nature of the various disorders called dyslexia.

Dyslexia: Diagnosis and Therapy. FHS. This program features eight children and adults of different ages, all of whose lives have been severely affected by dyslexia. The program stresses that teachers and parents are uniquely placed to recognize the signs of dyslexia.

Dyslexia: Diagnosis and Treatment. FHS. Difficulty with reading and spelling is not necessarily dyslexia. This program explains what dyslexia means and the many ways in which it is manifested; the extensive testing necessary to make a diagnosis of dyslexia and the role of heredity.

Eating Disorders. FHS. This program covers the personality profiles of the likeliest anorexic patients; explains their inability to acknowledge that they are thin enough. Explores with some anorexics how they were cured.

Fetal Alcohol Syndrome and Other Drug Use During Pregnancy. FHS. This program profiles an eight-year-old boy born with FAS, showing how alcohol enters the bloodstream of the fetus; it describes the common characteristics of children with FAS.

Interview with a Mother of a Hyperactive Child. MG. Part of a series on abnormal behavior, provides perspectives on hyperactivity from the standpoint of the family and educators.

Learning Disabilities. FHS. This program describes the nature of learning disabilities and their warning signs, and discusses this frequently misdiagnosed and misunderstood problem.

ew Coping with Learning Disabilities. FHS. Kevin Chettle spent his childhood and youth in hospitals: he was considered "aggressive, uncommunicative, and unemployable." Now he works training doctors, social workers, and psychiatrists in the needs of people like himself--people with learning difficulties.

Using Movies and Mental Illness as a Teaching Tool

There are relatively few good films exploring childhood psychopathology, and the classroom instructor will be hard pressed to find compelling vignettes to use in the classroom. Wedding and Boyd use *Fanny and Alexander* as the major teaching film for this chapter, but it is clear that we are usually seeing examples of Bergman's fertile imagination rather than true psychopathology (e.g., Alexander's hallucinations appear to be perfectly natural in the context of the film).

Students are fascinated by stories about feral children, and it may be useful to have your students compare and contrast the presentations of feral children in *Nell, Every Man for Himself and God Against All*, and *The Wild Child*.

The complex interrelationships between poverty, violence and psychopathology can be explored if students are asked to watch *El Norte, Pixote*, or *Salaam Bombay*. The special educational and emotional needs of highly intelligent children are addressed in *Little Man Tate*. *Welcome to the Dollhouse* explores childhood sexuality and the agony of adolescence, and selected vignettes from *Shine* will provide a springboard for a classroom discussion of the influence parents have on the psychological well-being of the children.

Movie	Link to Chapter	Page Reference to Wedding and Boyd
• Fanny and Alexander •	child psychopathology (p. 438)	p. 139
• The Best Little Girl in the World	anorexia nervosa (p. 447)	p. 142

389

Classroom Assessment Techniques (CAT)

Focused Listing (CAT 15-1)
Select an important point from this chapter (e.g., learning disorder) and ask students to write five words or phrases that describe the point.

Learning Review (CAT 15-2)
Students are to write in order five of the most important ideas they learned in this chapter.

Minute Paper (CAT 15-3)
Ask your students to write about important question they have that remains unanswered.

Muddiest Point (CAT 15-4)
Instruct students to write about an issue, concept, or definition presented in Chapter 15 that they find most confusing or difficult to understand.

Directed Paraphrasing (CAT 15-5)
In two or three sentences, students should paraphrase some important idea, concept, or definition presented in Chapter 15. Consider paraphrasing Alzheimer's disease, concussion, contusion, laceration, and meningitis.

Definition Matrix (CAT 15-6)
Using the handout, students should identify each of the disorders presented. For each disorder, students should provide the type, primary symptoms, groups at risk, and treatment. Students should attempt to write only a few words or phrases.

Suggestions for Essay Questions

- Discuss some issues that influence the classification and diagnosis of child psychopathology.
- Create a fictitious case study of a young child with ADHD.
- How might teachers and parents be more accurate in recognizing children who may have a learning or communication disorder?

Definition Matrix
Classroom Assessment Technique

Disorder	Type	Primary symptoms	Groups at risk	Treatment
ADHD				
Conduct Disorder				
Anxiety Disorders				
Anorexia Nervosa				
Bulimia Nervosa				
Enuresis				
Encopresis				
Night Terrors				
Learning Disorders				

Eating Disorders Survey

Please fill out the following information as honestly as you can. This form will be anonymous and you will not be identified in any way.

Age:

Gender:

Have you ever consumed so much food in a single setting that you were uncomfortable or in pain?

    If so, what did you eat?:

    What was your emotional state after eating all that food?:

    Did you purge yourself of the food, and if so, what method did you use?:

On a 5 point scale, how important is your body image to you (1=very important)?
1   2   3   4   5

On a 5 point scale, rate the quality of your relationship with your parent(s) (1= high quality)
1   2   3   4   5

On a 5 point scale, how concerned are you of gaining weight (1= very concerned)?
1   2   3   4   5

Chapter 16

Mental Retardation and Autism

Chapter Map

Section	Instructor Manual Components
Mental Retardation • Levels of Mental Retardation • Genetic Factors • Environmental Factors • Mental Retardation in Adults • Groups at Risk for Mental Retardation	*Savant Syndrome (LL 16-1)* *Language of the eyes (LL 16-2)* *Historical labels of subaverage intelligence (TP 16-1)* *Using IQ (TP 16-2)* *Thalidomide (TP 16-3)* *Fetal alcohol effect (TP 16-4)* *Nutrasweet and PKU (TP 16-5)* *Developing an information packet (ACT/DEMO 16-1)*
Autism • Symptoms of Autism • Theories of Autism • Groups at Risk for Autism	*Asperger's syndrome (LL 16-3)* *The very behaviors of children (TP 16-6)* *Create a case study (ACT/DEMO 16-2)*
People with Developmental Disabilities • Public Policy • Community Integration • Quality of Life • Support for the Family • Employment	*Transition for individuals with mental retardation (LL 16-4)* *Guest speakers (ACT/DEMO 16-3)* *Stuck between a rock and a hard place: Which one?* * (ACT/DEMO 16-4)*

Prevention and Therapy	*Background on facilitated communication (LL 16-5)*
• Primary Prevention • Secondary Prevention • Behavior Therapy • Cognitive Therapy • Pharmacological Therapy • Psychotherapy • Controversial Treatments	*Stress in families (LL 16-6)* *Behavioral treatments (TP 16-7)* *Facilitated communication (TP 16-8)* *Field trip (ACT/DEMO 16-5)*

Chapter Outline

I. Introduction
    A.   Mental retardation has a prevalence of about 2% of general population
    B.   Mental retardation poses significant problems for society

II. Mental Retardation
    A.   Mental retardation as defined by DSM-IV, has three criteria
        1.   Significantly subaverage general intellectual functioning
        2.   Significant limitations in adaptive functioning in at least 2 or 11 adaptive skills areas
        3.   Onset before 18 years of age
    B.   Definition has several important components
        1.   Adaptive functioning is person's ability to cope with life's demands and live independently according to standards of age group, community, social class, and culture
        2.   Diagnosis requires both deficits in both intellectual and adaptive functioning
        3.   Diagnosis made in context of age-mates
        4.   Definition says nothing about cause
    C.   Levels of Mental Retardation
        1.   In intelligence tests, 100 is average with standard deviation of 15
            a.   Cutoff point is IQ of about 70
            b.   There are several levels of mental retardation
        2.   Mild Retardation includes 85% of all cases
            a.   IQ of 50-55 to 70
            b.   Need more help longer with self-care tasks
            c.   Speak fluently and function independently in most areas
            d.   Can hold job, marry, and have children
        3.   Moderate Retardation
            a.   IQ of 35-40 to 50-55
            b.   By adolescence, have good self-care skills
            c.   Carry on simple conversations, read few words, and do simple tasks
        4.   Severe Retardation
            a.   IQ of 20-25 to 35-40
            b.   Can learn some self-care skills
            c.   Can perform jobs in sheltered workshop or daytime activity center
            d.   Require considerable supervision
            e.   May have trouble speaking; reading and number skills not sufficient for normal living
        5.   Profound Retardation
            a.   IQ below 20 or 25

   b. Can carry out some self-care activities

   c. Require extensive supervision and help

   d. Language is severe problem

   e. Many remain institutionalized

   f. Susceptible to disease

  6. AAMR suggest not using IQ criterion until deficits in adaptive functioning have been established

  7. AAMR recommends classification based on levels of required support or assistance

   a. Mild retardation indicated by need for intermittent assistance

   b. Moderate retardation associated with limited assistance

   c. Severe retardation indicated by extensive assistance

   d. Profound retardation indicated by pervasive assistance

D. Genetic Factors

  1. Mechanism that produces retardation is not understood

   a. Two people may have same mediate diagnosis but be at different levels of retardation

   b. Differential diagnosis is a problem

  2. Chromosomal Abnormalities

   a. Certain forms of mental retardation are X-linked

   b. **Fragile X syndrome** involves weak spot where chromosome is bent or broken

    i. Pronounced physical characteristics

    ii. Many are hyperactive and show characteristics of autism

    iii. In men, disorder has more severe consequences

   c. **Down syndrome** includes physical characteristics

    i. IQs less than 50

    ii. Susceptible to serious cardiac and respiratory diseases

    iii. Extra chromosome pair 21 or **trisomy 21**

   d. Fragile X syndrome and Down syndrome account for one-fourth of all cases

   e. Genetic counseling can provide guidance and testing

    i. Risk for Down syndrome related to mother's age

    ii. Amniocentesis involves analyzing amniotic fluid

    iii. Routinely given to pregnant women over 35

  3. Metabolic Disturbances

   a. **Phenylketonuria (PKU)** caused by defective recessive gene

    i. Child cannot metabolize amino acid phenylalaline

    ii. Phenylalaline accumulates in body and damages CNS

    iii. Most states require PKU testing of newborns

   b. **Tay-Sachs disease** transmitted by recessive genes
     i. Characterized by progressive deterioration
     ii. Is untreatable
     iii. Death is virtually certain before age of six
E. Environmental Factors
 1. Prenatal Environment
   a. Congenital Disorders
     i. **Congenital disorders** are acquired during prenatal development but are not transmitted genetically
     ii. Until recently, three common congenital causes were rubella, syphilis, and thyroxine deficiency
     iii. Most common congenital cause today is transmission of HIV virus leading to encephalopathy, meningitis, and lymphoma leading to developmental delays
   b. Drugs
     i. Thalidomide prescribed for morning sickness, but caused mental retardation and severely malformed limbs
     ii. **Fetal alcohol syndrome (FAS)** associated with drinking during pregnancy; causes distinction facial characteristics and mental retardation with IQs between 40 and 80
     iii. Illegal drugs have profound effect on fetal brain; crack babies likely to show retarded growth and brain development affected
     iv. There is interaction of prenatal and postnatal environments
   c. Malnutrition
     i. Prenatal malnutrition affects physical and behavioral development
     ii. Iron-deficiency anemia stunts physical growth causing developmental delays and contributes to behavior problems
     iii. Combination of dietary supplements and stimulation required to overcome nutritional deficits
     iv. Malnutrition often seen with other retardation-associated factors
 2. Postnatal Environment
   a. Toxins
     i. Substances can enter child's bloodstream and cause retardation
     ii. DPT vaccination, in very small number of children, can cause brain damage

            iii.   Lead poisoning has higher risk; deposits accumulate and interfere with brain cell metabolism causing damage

      b.   Physical Trauma

            i.   Trauma to brain as result of accident or abuse can cause mental retardation

            ii.   Brain can also be harmed during birth due to compression, use of forceps, and hypoxia

      c.   The Effects of Deprivation

            i.   Disproportionately high number of children from disadvantaged backgrounds are retarded

            ii.   Some cases may be due to growing up in deprived setting

            iii.   Impoverishment called pseudo-retardation suggest it is emotionally-based, not intellectual

            iv.   What began as psychological factors may become physical factors

            v.   **Brain plasticity** suggests that experiences can alter structure and function of brain

            vi.   Brain growth and development occurs very early

            vii.   Barren, deprived environment may produce a less efficient brain

            viii.   Effects of poor environment may not be reversible and may be cumulative; children raised in poverty are at risk

      d.   Teenage Mothers

            i.   Teenage mothers rarely equipped to raise children

            ii.   Underlying competence is the mother's own adolescent struggles

            iii.   They are less sensitive to child's cues, less likely to interact with child verbally, more likely to criticize and punish them

            iv.   Children are exposed to factors associated with developmental disabilities

            v.   Average IQ of teenage mother is 85

            vi.   Mild retardation appears more often in children of teenage mothers

    3.   Institutionalization

      a.   A lack of stimulation interaction with children who are institutionalized may be related to retardation

      b.   Study suggests that institutionalized child showed significant average loss in developmental quotient

      c.   Effects dependent on kind and quality of institutional care

F.   Mental Retardation in Adults

    1.   Down's Syndrome and Alzheimer's Disease

        a.   In past, people with Down's syndrome didn't live past middle age

        b.   More and more people with Down's Syndrome are surviving into old age

        c.   There is a link between Down's syndrome and Alzheimer's disease

              a.   Alzheimer's disease strikes early

              b.   Onset is marked by behavioral regression

    2.   Mental Retardation and Other Mental Disorders

        1.   Mentally retarded people at risk for other mental disorders

              a.   When IQ is over 50, symptoms of emotional disturbance are like those of normal intelligence

              b.   When IQ is lower, emotional disturbance is harder to detect

        2.   Social position may put mentally retarded at risk

        3.   Most people with mental retardation do not get treatment since emotional dysfunction is often ignored

  G.   Groups at Risk for Mental Retardation

    1.   Gender is risk factor for mental retardation with males outnumbering females

    2.   Age is risk factor; mental retardation peaks at age five or six years

    3.   Socioeconomic status related to parental intelligence and amount of stimulation child receives

        a.   Mild retardation more prevalent in families with low incomes

        b.   Severe retardation does not seem to be related to socioeconomic status

        c.   Minority group status also related factor

    4.   Prenatal and perinatal variables are major risk factors

III.   Autism

  A.   Kanner argued that autism was distinct syndrome different from schizophrenia

    1.   Kanner called syndrome **early infantile autism**

    2.   Believed autism was inborn and appeared by age two and a half years

  B.   Most psychotic disorders of children considered instances of autism

  C.   Symptoms of Autism

    1.   Social Isolation

        a.   People with autism have impaired social behavior, sometimes called extreme autistic aloneness

              i.   They do not demand attention

              ii.   Difficult to hold and cuddle

              iii.   Recoil from personal contact

              iv.   Behave as if others do not exist

b.   Degree of social isolation varies

c.   Children with autism do show emotions such as rage, panic, or crying

d.   Appears to be three types of autism based on social behavior

    i.   Aloof type where child rarely makes spontaneous social approach

    ii.   Passive type where child does not initiate contact, but does respond to someone else's initiation of contact

    iii.   Active-but-odd type where child approaches others in peculiar, naïve, or one-sided way

e.   Autism may be several disorders, instead of just one

2.   Mental Retardation

a.   Most children with autism are mentally retarded with 76 to 89% of children having IQ of less than 70

b.   There are differences in the nature of cognitive deficits of autistic and mentally retarded children

    i.   Autistic children do better on finding hidden figures than on social understanding and language

    ii.   Mentally retarded perform more evenly on all such tests

c.   Mental retardation in autism is primary cognitive problem, not result of social withdrawal

d.   Some autistic children do show signs of above-average intelligence in one limited area; these are called savants

3.   Language Deficits

a.   More than half of all children with autism do not speak at all

b.   Others babble, whine, scream, or show **echolalia**

c.   Those who do speak, use language in limited ways

    i.   Strange use of pronouns

    ii.   Some speak extremely literally

    iii.   Some cannot communicate reciprocally

d.   Severity of language problem is excellent indicator of prognosis with children most likely to benefit from treatment have developed some meaningful speech by age of five years

e.   Intellectual development is also excellent indicator of prognosis

4.   Stereotyped Behavior

a.   Many autistic children show movements that are endlessly and ritualistically done without any clear goal

b.   Twirling, tiptoeing, flapping hands, rocking, tensing part of face are common stereotyped behavior

c. Some movements can cause physical harm
d. Children engage in these behaviors to communicate desires and to obtain certain kinds of reinforcement such as sensory reinforcement, attention, and positive tangible reinforcement
e. Many children also show intense and narrow focus with toys, objects
f. Children with autism also resist any change in surroundings and routines
g. Some autistic people grow up to hold down jobs and live alone, but experience language problems and social adjustment problems

D. Theories of Autism
1. Explanations of autism have changed radically in past decades; in 50s and 60s focus was on cold, rejecting parents
2. The Biological Perspective
    a. Genetic Research
        i. Twin studies suggest genetic basis of autism; more MZ than DZ twins are concordant
        ii. Other studies show relationships between siblings with mental retardation and autism
    h. Chromosome Studies
        i. Fragile X syndrome associated with autism
        ii. Other abnormalities such as tuberose sclerosis and chromosomal abnormalities on 15 associated with autism
    i. Biochemical Studies
        i. Study suggests that children with autism do not have abnormally high levels of serotonin and dopamine
        ii. Drugs that increase dopamine worsen symptoms
        iii. Drugs that inhibit dopamine mitigate many of the symptoms, but less effective than with schizophrenia
    e. Congenital Disorders and Birth Complications
        i. Several birth complications appear to be related to autism
        ii. Relationship may not be cause-and-effect
        iii. Congenital disorders may be related to genetic factors
    f. Neurological Research
        i. Autism probably results from range of deficits in brain
        ii. Symptoms are related to functioning of CNS
        iii. Many autistic children develop seizure disorders

            iv.   Half of persons with autism display abnormal EEGs

            v.   Autistic children show reduced EEG activity in frontal and temporal regions of brain

            vi.   Autopsies reveal certain abnormalities in cerebellum and limbic system such as neuronal and dendrite abnormalities and megalencephaly

            vii.   Brain-imaging techniques have identified differences such as enlarged ventricles

3. The Cognitive Perspective

    a. Cognitive problems of autistic children are primary and cause their social problems

    b. People with autism have problems associated with executive functioning such as problem solving, controlling impulses, and inhibiting inappropriate behavior

    c. Research on categorization and memory show that autistic people have difficulty forming new concepts and understanding new information based on those concepts, in particular, forming prototypes to categorize objects leading to over-reliance on rules

    d. Social understanding is impaired, for example, comprehending gestures and understanding others' emotions and facial expressions

    e. Some argue that autistic people have no **theory of mind**

        i.   Autistic people cannot appreciate existence of purely mental states

        ii.   Cannot predict or understand behavior based on such states

4. Groups at Risk for Autism

    a. Socioeconomic status and ethnocultural background are not major risk factors

    b. Gender is a significant risk factor and may be related to risk factors for mental retardation

    c. Presence of autism in sibling is another risk factor suggesting genetic influences

IV. Society and People with Developmental Disabilities

A. Public Policy

1. Parent groups have vigorously lobbied governments for increased funding and legislation regarding the rights to free education

2. Groups have taken their grievances to federal and state courts; decisions have altered treatment of people with retardation

3. Number of professionals in field of mental retardation has expanded greatly

4. There are five basic principles regarding the rights of mentally retarded people

        a.   Free and appropriate education

        b.   Individualization

        c.   Timely progress reviews

        d.   Community integration

        e.   Human rights

    5.   Public Law 94-142 guarantees every citizen under 21 years a free and appropriate public education

        a.   Programs are tailored to individual's needs in individualized education program (IEP)

        b.   Multidisciplinary conferences used to review progress of special education student

    6.   Innovative programs such as the cascade system have been developed

B.   Community Integration

    1.   Segregation of services deprived people with mental retardation of participation in society

    2.   Community integration provides services for the mentally retarded than are integrated with same services for people without mental retardation; example is mainstreaming

    3.   Assisted-living arrangements are available, including supported living arrangements, community living facilities, and to intermediate-care facilities; designed for care of people who function on different levels

    4.   Large scale institutions are for individuals who cannot function satisfactorily in community settings; more and more individuals are being moved out of large institutions

C.   Quality of Life

    1.   Quality of life is a multidimensional concept that includes physical, material, social, emotional well-being, personal development, and activity

    2.   Research has focused on providing choices to people with developmental disabilities; choice appears to correlate with adaptive and maladaptive behavior

D.   Support for the Family

    1.   Most family are given recommendation for child to be cared for at home

    2.   Families need supportive training and counseling

    3.   Retarded children have same needs as normal children, but also have special needs

        a.   Home training can help parents deal with special needs

        b.   Training also improves parent-child bond

    4.   Adolescents with mental retardation presents additional concerns

        a.   Parents must balance child's need for independence and child's lack of maturity

b. Concerns are greatest when child has mild and moderate mental retardation

5. As person enters adulthood, family must consider extent to which individual can live independently

6. A more human approach to sex and marriage among the mental retarded has emerged
   a. People with mental retardation have right to sexual development and education about AIDS and HIV
   b. Sterilization is the last resort

E. Employment
   1. People with mental retardation must have opportunities for useful employment according to federal and state law
      a. People with mental retardation must be given planned daytime programs or supported employment
      b. Severely or profoundly mentally retarded individuals placed in **sheltered workshops** for employment tailored to their needs
      c. Most people with mental retardation want to work and can become good employees
      d. When people with mental retardation are fired it is usually for lack of social skills

V. Prevention and Therapy
   A. Primary Prevention
      1. Couples at risk for genetic factors related to mental retardation can be identified, informed of the risk, and advised
      2. A simple blood test can identify carriers of Tay-Sachs disease and genetic analysis can identify abnormalities in developing fetus

   B. Secondary Prevention
      1. When child poses risk for condition that could lead to mental retardation, secondary prevention attempts to reduce risk
      2. Medical procedures can be attempts at secondary prevention
      3. Psychological therapies such as providing stimulation and teaching parents are used to reduce risk
      4. Programs have been developed to provide stimulation for infants whose only apparent risk factor is poverty

   C. Behavior Therapy
      1. Behavioral techniques used extensively and with good success
      2. There are three basic techniques for behavior therapy
         a. Shaping--reinforcing successive approximations of desirable behavior
         b. Chaining--teaching person to finish task and gradually expand number of steps to finish
         c. Stimulus control--teaching that a behavior should occur in some situations but not in others

404

3. Self-Help and Adaptive Skills
    a. Training in self-help and adaptive skills teaches daily living skills
    b. Type of training involves several steps
        i. Breaking down of task into small steps
        ii. Backward or forward chaining
        iii. Substantial feedback and reinforcement
    c. Token economies have been especially successful in vocational training programs and social behavior
    d. Behavior therapy is most appropriate and effective technique for teaching self-help skills to those with severe mental retardation
    e. Toilet training, using behavioral techniques, improves hygiene and promotes social interaction
4. Language and Communication Skills
    a. One of most important applications of behavior therapy has been in language acquisition
    b. Step-by-step behavioral sequences appear to be useful
    c. Shaping and verbal imitation typically used to train people who are mute; sign language and picture books also used
    d. Training in communication improves prognosis and reduces behavior problems
5. Leisure and Community Skills
    a. Modeling, prompting, providing feedback, and reinforcement used to improve quality of life
    b. Children's insensitivity to social reinforcement must be conquered
6. Replacement of Maladaptive Behaviors
    a. Aggression and self-injury treated with time-outs, differential reinforcement of other behavior, and differential reinforcement of incompatible behavior
    b. Effectiveness depends on what behavior is being eliminated as the function of the behavior
    c. Any change in behavior must be supported by the environment
    d. Aim of behavior therapy is to provide these children with enough adaptive responses so they can move to a more useful and fulfilling existence
    e. Critics suggest that children become like robots
D. Cognitive Therapy
    1. Self-instructional training refers to development of self-regulatory speech that is useful in academic, leisure, and vocational skills
    2. Correspondence training involves use of rewards for action-oriented verbal statements

3.   Self-management and self-monitoring teaches individuals to regulate own behavior, evaluate performance, and to reward themselves accordingly

4.   Training in self-control involves delayed gratification of impulses

5.   Problem solving training focuses on defining problem, developing solutions, and choosing best solutions

E.   Pharmacological Therapy

1.   Pharmacology is commonly used for people with developmental disabilities

2.   Psychotropic drugs and anticonvulsive medications are common

3.   Serotonin-reducing drugs have been used to treat autism, but may not be helpful in treating core social and language deficits

F.   Psychotherapy

1.   It has been assumed that people with mental retardation could not benefit from psychotherapy

2.   There are now many forms of psychological treatment such as supportive psychotherapy, group psychotherapy, family therapy, and client-centered therapy that can help

3.   Marital counseling and parent training may be useful for those planning to marry and raise a family

G.   Controversial Treatments

1.   Facilitated communication involves a facilitator who helps individual guide their hands by typing letters on keyboard or pointing to letters on letter board

        a.   No evidence supports claims

        b.   Subjects were responded to demand characteristics of facilitators

2.   Auditory training involves a training machine that plays music, helping people to retrain person's attention and altering structure of left hemisphere

3.   Megavitamin therapy involves ingestion of high doses of B6 and magnesium

Chapter Box

- Savant Syndrome
  - A. **Savant syndrome** occurs when a person with greatly diminished mental skills shows extraordinary proficiency in one isolated skill
  - B. Skill may develop by compensation or because of biological factors
  - C. Skill is based on memory or calculation
  - D. Nadia showed extraordinary drawing skill
  - E. Skill sometimes declines as symptoms of autism improve

Learning Objectives (LO)

By the time you have finished studying this chapter, you should be able to do the following-.

1. Define mental retardation according to the *DSM-IV* and describe four levels of retardation, giving IQ scores and representative behaviors for each (464-465).

2. Summarize the research findings on the genetic causes of retardation (466-467).

3. Describe prenatal environmental factors that can result in retardation (467-469).

4. Describe postnatal environmental factors that can result in retardation making reference to pseudo-retardation and the effects of institutionalization (469-472).

5. Discuss physical and psychological comorbidity issues related to retardation in adults, making specific reference Alzheimer's disease (472-473).

6. Define autism, describe four symptom categories characteristic of this disorder, and relate autism to savant syndrome (473-476).

7. Summarize research on genetic, congenital, biochemical, and neurological problems related to autism (476-478).

8. Summarize the cognitive perspective's position on the role of sensory and attention deficits in autism (478-479).

9. Summarize five basic principles of public policy toward the mentally retarded that have evolved over the past 30 years (479-482).

10. Summarize changes in attitudes and public policy relating to family support and employment opportunities for retarded and/or autistic individuals (482-483).

11. Describe primary and secondary prevention, and outline behavioral techniques for improving the adaptive skills of retarded persons and for minimizing maladaptive behavior (483-486).

12. Describe cognitive, pharmacological, and psychotherapeutic measures that have been useful in the treatment of autistic and retarded persons (486-487).

13. Describe three controversial approaches to the treatment of autism, and discuss the degree to which they, have been effective (487-489).

Lecture Leads (LL)

Savant Syndrome (LL 16-1)
Students are typically very interested in the savant syndrome, made popular by the movie *Rainman*, with Dustin Hoffman. This is an example of a very unusual form of intelligence. The first recorded case of a savant was cited in a German magazine in 1751. Savants are individuals who score on the low end of intelligence tests, yet have one particular area of brilliance. For example, some savants can listen to a complex piece of music one time and replicate it flawlessly, whereas others can draw nearly exact duplicates of pictures seen for only a few seconds. Some savants have incredible mathematical abilities, such as multiplying 4- and 5-digit numbers in their heads at amazing speeds. Hurst and Mulhall describe an individual who can give the day of the week for any date in the 20th century. People with this syndrome were originally called "idiot savants," as most of the individuals have Intelligence Quotients of around 40 to 70. Now the common term is either "autistic savant," or simply "savant." Savant syndrome is also much more common in males than females (a ratio of 6 to 1). Savants are autistic, meaning that they do not communicate well with people and typically have very little social interaction with others.

Resources:
Foerstl, J. (1989). Early interest in the idiot savant. American Journal of Psychiatry, 146, 156.
Hurst, L. C., & Mulhall, D. J. (1988). Another calendar savant. British Journal of Psychiatry, 152, 274-277.

Language of the eyes (LL 16-2)
In a very interesting study, researchers examined whether subjects could identify mental states using various components of facial expressions. College students were able to identify mental states (e.g., interest) when presented with whole face, eye, or mouth photographs of an actress displaying mental states. When presented with photographs of the actress protraying emotions (e.g., happy, sad), the whole face provided more clues regarding the emotion than eye or mouth photographs. Moreover, photographs of the eyes were more helpful than photographs of the mouth. Next, groups of adults with autism and Asperger syndrome, following the same procedure, were impaired at identifying emotions and mental states.

Resource:
Baron-Cohen, S., Wheelwright, S., & Jolliffe, T. (1997). Is there a "language of the eyes"? Evidence from normal adults, and adults with autism or Asperger syndrome. Visual Cognition, 4, 311-331.

Asperger's syndrome (LL 16-3)
The DSM-IV classifies autism as a pervasive developmental disorder. This category includes a number of other autism-like syndromes that make up what is sometimes called the autism spectrum.   One of the more interesting ones is Asperger's syndrome, also known as Asperger's Disorder or Autistic Psychopathy. It was recognized in the 1940s, but only officially included in the DSM-IV. It is similar to autism in that Asperger's syndrome includes impairment in social interaction, language, and idiosyncratic behaviors, but is considered to be on the highest functioning end of the spectrum. It is unclear if Asperger's syndrome is just a mild form of autism or a completely different disorder. The characteristic that differentiates the two disorders is higher cognitive functioning in Asperger's; in fact, IQ is normal and may even be in the above average range with more relatively normal language ability.   Many children who do not meet the diagnostic criteria for Asperger's syndrome are often seen as "odd" or "different" and may be misdiagnosed with ADHD, Tourette's syndrome, or Obsessive-Compulsive Disorder. One of the more interesting features of Asperger's is the child's idiosyncratic interest in a specific intellectual area; this differs from the preoccupation seen in autism of extreme interest and focus on objects. Children with Asperger's often have an extreme interest in math, reading, history, weather, planes, or rockets. Finally the impairment in social interaction appears to be different than that in autism. Asperger children do not seem as aloof or out of it as autistic children and may wish for social interaction but do not know how to effectively interact.

Resources:

Bonnet, K. A., & Gao, X. (1996). Asperger syndrome in neurologic perspective. Journal of Child Neurology, 11, 483-489.

Gillberg, C. (1998). Asperger syndrome and high-functioning autism. British Journal of Psychiatry, 172, 200-209.

Williams, K. (1995). Understanding the student with Asperger syndrome: Guidelines for teachers. Focus on Autistic Behavior, 10, 9-16.

Wolf-Schein, E. G. (1996). The autistic spectrum disorder: A current review. Developmental Disabilities Bulletin, 24, 33-55.

Transition for individuals with mental retardation (LL 16-4)
An important part of the education of students with mental retardation is their preparation for life after school. The Individuals with Disabilities Education Act (IDEA) requires that transition planning be a part of the Individualized Education Plan (IEP) for students 16 years or older. Transition planning was incorporated because many mentally retarded students were unable to find employment, to develop social and interpersonal competencies, or to use available community support services. In transition planning, the family, school, and community come together to plan opportunities for the student after graduating or otherwise leaving school. The Individualized Transition Plan (ITP) is integrated into the IEP and includes goals and objectives and identification of required

services; these services are needed by the student to reach post-school outcomes set forth by the IEP team. Examples of activities developed for the student include adult services, independent living, post-secondary education, and vocational training.

Resources:

DeFur, S., Getzel, E.E., & Kregel, J. (1994). Individualized transition plans a work in progress. Journal of Vocational Rehabilitation, 4, 139-145.

Everson, J.M. (1996). Using person-centered planning concepts to enhance school to adult life transition planning. Journal of Vocational Rehabilitation. 6, 7-13.

Individuals with Disabilities Education Act of 1990 (October 10, 1990), Public Law 101-476. Title 20, U.S.C. 1400-1485. U. S. Statutes at Large 104, 1103-1151.

Wehman, P. (1992). Life beyond the classroom: Transition strategies for young people with disabilities. Baltimore, MD: Paul H. Brookes.

Background on facilitated communication (LL 16-5)

The textbook describes facilitated communication as a questionable treatment. The genesis of the treatment can be traced to educators' frustration that children with autism have communication difficulties that make it nearly impossible to assess their intelligence in a fair manner. Biklen and Schubert relate the case of Mark, a 7-year-old boy with autism who exhibited poor muscle tone and social withdrawal. Mark, despite repeated efforts on the part of his teachers, only communicated using two signs in sign language--"cat" and "more". Mark was introduced to facilitated communication through his teachers. After about two months of training, Mark allegedly began typing phrases like, "YOU TELL MOM IM SAD MISSING DAD" (in response to the fact his father was away on business) and "I FEEL LONELY WHEN I HAVE NO KIDS AT MY HOUSE" (in response to not having any playmates). At the end of the school year, Mark started having toiletting accidents; it was discovered that he felt anxious about losing his current speech therapist during the next academic year. He typed, "I AM WETTING BECAUSE I DON'T WANT TO LEAVE YOU." Biklen and Schubert studied 21 children using this method and the outcomes. They noted that children with autism don't sit down and start typing. In many instances they need physical support to keep their hands on the keyboard, they need training to use the hardware, and they may also need someone to prompt them to pay attention, which may be the demand characteristics noted in the textbook. The optimism in this article is clearly evident, and raised hopes that autistic children could indeed effectively communicate. Extend this background lecture with a task for students. Ask them to describe a research methodology to test the validity of facilitated communication.

Resource:

Biklen, D., & Schubert, A. (1991). New words: The communication of students with autism. Remedial and Special Education, 12, 46-57.

Stress in families (LL 16-6)
Which type of family experiences the most stress was the focus of a recent study. Families with an autistic child, Down syndrome, and only developmentally normal children were analyzed with regard to parental stress and adjustment. The results suggest that stress and adjustment difficulties were highest among parents with autistic children, followed by parents of Down's syndrome children and parents of developmental normal children. Specifically, parents of autistic and Down syndrome children reported stress linked to child care. However, the authors point out that these parents show resilience and coping.

Resource:

Sanders, J. L., & Morgan, S. B. (1997). Family stress and adjustment as perceived by parents of children with autism or Down Syndrome: Implications for intervention. Child and Family Behavior Therapy, 19, 15-32.

Talking Points (TP)

Historical labels of subaverage intelligence (TP 16-1)
The textbook describes the labels applied to the various levels of intelligence. These labels, which are still controversial, have not always been used. Historically, more objectionable labels have been used to describe intelligence. For instance, the term "idiot" was used to label a person with an IQ of 25 or less. With an IQ between 25 and 40, the term "imbecile" was used. A person with an IQ between 40 and 55 would be labeled "moron." Ask your students to discuss the pejorative nature of these labels. Will the currently used labels (e.g., mild, moderate, severe, profound) meet with the same reactions in the future?

Using IQ (TP 16-2)
Some critics suggest that we ignore the concept of IQ all together. They point to the fact that the demarcation line for the label of "retarded" has changed as we learn more about functional abilities. Ask students what the label serves. Should we use it at all? Ask the students to try and develop an alternative method of defining this disorder.

Thalidomide (TP 16-3)
Thalidomide was sold over the counter to relieve women of morning sickness. As the textbook describes, thalidomide caused serious teratological effects on humans. The timing of administration was critical. If a pregnant woman took thalidomide within a certain time period of five days, her child would have deformed ears. If it was consumed in another period, the child would have phocomelia, where all of parts of the hands and feet are missing, or where the hands and feet would have a flipper-like appearance. Thalidomide is making something of a comeback, but only for the treatment of leprosy in Brazil. Will we see a new generation of thalidomide babies in Brazil?

Fetal alcohol effect (TP 16-4)
A less serious version of fetal alcohol syndrome is fetal alcohol effect (FAE). Subaverage intelligence, lower birth weight, poor responsiveness, and respiratory abnormalities are among the symptoms. Although it is difficult to attach a particular dosage level with either FAS or FAE, children with fetal alcohol effect more than likely had mothers who engaged in social drinking.

Nutrasweet and PKU (TP 16-5)
Individuals with PKU are advised not drink diet soda drinks. Most of these drinks contain the artificial sweetener Nutrasweet, which contains the very same amino acid that people with PKU cannot metabolize.

The very behaviors of children (TP 16-6)
Here's a teaching moment: A college psychology instructor had just had a lunch of spaghetti at home with his family. As he left for his office, his 3-year old daughter gave him a kiss and hug and inadvertently left some spaghetti sauce on her father's shirt

413

unbeknownst to him. His suit coat covered the unfortunate deposit. But during his abnormal psychology class and a lecture on autism he took off his suit coat exposing his daughter's spaghetti sauce stain. As he mentioned the aberrant social interaction of autistic children he noticed the spaghetti sauce his daughter left for him and said, "An autistic child would never do that" referring to his daughter's display of affection. Ask students to consider that some of the very behaviors they associat with children (e.g., hugs and kisses) are absent in autistic children. Ask them for more examples.

Behavioral treatments (TP 16-7)

There has been a great deal of controversy over behavioral treatment for both autism and mental retardation. Critics argue that it is cruel and inhumane to use aversive techniques on young children. However, these techniques have been proven highly effective. Have students argue the merits of both pro and con viewpoints. Include in the discussion extinction and generalization of behavior change techniques used with these types of behaviors.

Facilitated communication (TP 16-8)

Discuss the recent failure of facilitated communication with autistic individuals. In the beginning this technique had great promise, but with scientific investigation the techniques proved to be totally ineffective. Discuss the ramifications of selling this procedure to the public in terms of hurting not only the affected individuals but also their families. A quick perusal of websites shows that there are some die-hard advocates who still support its use. Discuss with your students why "treatments" like these disappear so slowly.

with regard to **money management**.	p. 465
Thanks to widespread **immunization**...	p. 467
Even women who are only "**social drinkers**"...	p. 468
a combination of **food supplements** and home visitation...	p. 469
in the period after birth, this mass is "**sculpted**."	p. 470
they were moved from an overcrowded **orphanage**...	p. 472
sees his younger brother come home with a **driver's license**...	p. 472
are difficult to hold and **cuddle**...	p. 474
poor muscle tone, poor coordination, **drooling**, and hyperactivity.	p. 478
With respect to **executive function**...	p. 478
fill out an **income tax form**.	p. 479
One concept, for example, is the "**cascade system**."	p. 481
Many "**graduates**" of early intervention programs...	p. 483
Most behavior therapist have no **illusion**...	p. 485

Activities and Demonstrations (ACT/DEMO)

Developing an information packet (ACT/DEMO 16-1)
Objective: To understand the etiology, symptoms, and treatment of childhood and adolescent disorders
Materials: None
Procedure: After students are put into small groups, inform them that their task is to develop a brochure that could be given to parents whose child has just been diagnosed with autism The purpose of this brochure is to educate the parents so that they can deal better with their child's disorder. In the brochure, information about the disorder's symptoms, etiology, and treatment should be presented. Tell students to create their brochure using desktop publishing or word processing programs and to be creative
Discussion: After all groups have completed their brochure, collect them, and redistribute each to the rest of the groups. Next, the groups are to review the accuracy of the material and thr design of the brochure.

Create a case study (ACT/DEMO 16-2)
Objective: To demonstrate the nature of autism
Materials: None
Procedure: After reviewing autism, students are to create a case study of a child diagnosed with autism. In the case study the student should describe the child's background, interaction with others, language development, intelligence, and other pertinent background information. The content of the case study should be consistent with the material presented in the chapter. Next have students pair up and summarize their case study to their partner.
Discussion: Select several case studies to be presented to the entire class. As the cases are presented keep track of the salient content with regard to demographics and behaviors.

Guest speakers (ACT/DEMO 16-3)
Objective: To illustrate the material from a real-world perspective
Materials: None
Procedure: A number of information guest speakers can be invited into the classroom to talk about the disorders presented in Chapter 16. You could invite someone from sheltered workshop. A psychologist or clinical social worker will be able to give insights into the specific disorder and into the daily management problems associated with the children and adolescents. A special education teacher or speech therapist would also provide interesting insights into the disorders. Of course, an especially instructive perspective comes from parents who have children with these disorders. Finally, if appropriate, an individual who has successfully coped with their retardation would provide a different perspective.
Discussion: Beforehand, instruct students to review this chapter and be prepared to ask questions of their guest speakers. Afterwards, ask students to compare and contrast the speakers' presentations.

Stuck between a rock and a hard place: Which one? (ACT/DEMO 16-4)
Objective: To encourage students to think critically about the developmental disabilities
Materials: None
Procedure: After presenting the disorders in Chapter 16, place your students into groups. While in groups, students are to discuss a particular scenario: If their child had to have one of the developmental disorders, which one would each student pick and why.
Discussion: Next, select several students to present their selection and the rationale for their selection. Check to see if the evidence used in the rationale is sound and consistent with the material in the chapters.

Field trip (ACT/DEMO 16-5)
Objective: To introduce the students to special needs education
Materials: None.
Procedure: Arrange with your local school or lab school for a tour of a special needs classroom and regular mainstreamed classroom. You will want to divide the class into small groups otherwise large groups touring classrooms can be very disruptive. Prior to the tour, ask the students to develop a list of questions prior to attending this tour that they would like the personnel to answer. Another venue to visit would be a group home or hospital.
Discussion: Either after the tour or during the next class period ask for additional questions from the students. Ask what they thought was the most interesting aspect of the tour.

Films and Videos

A Is for Autism. FHS. This program offers a short but profound glimpse into the condition of autism with words, drawings, and music all contributed by autistic people.

An Autistic Child. FHS. Debra was like any other child until she was two. She had just started speaking when, for no apparent reason, she stopped talking and started screaming for days on end. Her mental development came to a halt, and for the next seven years she remained at the same developmental level.

Autism. FHS. The world of autism is shown through the experiences of a 44-year-old woman who grew up autistic.

Autism. Breaking Through. FHS. This program examines the causes and symptoms of autism and the various treatment options available, including the use of fenfluramine, behavior modification, and the treatment program developed by Dr. Kiyo Kitahara of Japan, which relies heavily on physical exercise and group interaction with normal children.

Education for All Children. RP. The Right to Education Movement is discussed. Attitudes toward handicapped children are examined.

Harry. RP. A behavioral treatment for self-injurious behavior is illustrated.

Intelligence: A Complex Concept. MGH. This film reviews the concept of intelligence and intelligence tests. Interviews with prominent experts as well as laypeople serve to highlight the complex nature of definition and assessment.

New Autism: A World Apart. FHS. This documentary features two children, age four and six, and 18-year-old Lee, who are all autistic. The program shows the strain placed on their families and how each family has learned to cope.

Special Needs Students in Regular Classroom: Sean's Story. FHS. This is the story of an eight-year-old boy with Down Syndrome who was part of a battle over "inclusion," the practice of placing mentally or physically challenged students in regular classrooms. The program chronicles Sean's first year in a regular classroom setting.

The Autistic Child. MG. This film documents characteristics of the autistic child from a number of perspectives; including psychiatric, parental, and educational. Diagnostic and intervention issues are highlighted.

The Special Child. Maximizing Limited Potential FHS. When there is doubt about a child's mental and physical coordination, screening for developmental problems should begin at three to four months to determine whether the underlying cause is behavioral, neurological, or emotional. The program covers Down syndrome, autism, problems of neurological control, speech problems, and the avoidance behavior that can result in crib death.

Who Will Teach the Water to Swim? FES. The discovery that the autistic child learns best in an environment with as few stimuli as possible resulted in the effort to teach autistic children individually. The camera follows two teachers who work at different schools in the Netherlands and shows dramatically the problems inherent in teaching the autistic.

Using Movies and Mental Illness as a Teaching Tool

While there are few films exploring childhood psychopathology, there are numerous movies that very effectively portray mental retardation and autism.

Wedding and Boyd use *Rain Man* as the primary teaching film for this chapter, but there are other equally compelling films. One of these, *Best Boy*, is highly recommended for those classes in which professors want to explore the problem of adults with mental retardation who are facing the death of their parents.

This is also a chapter that lends itself to a serious examination of eugenics and mercy killing. Students with strong feelings about the sanctity of life will find themselves challenged by movies like *A Day in the Life of Joe Egg*. Any of the multiple versions of *Of Mice and Men* will lend themselves to a classroom discussion of culpability in people with mental illness who commit serious crimes (but the recent adaptation with John Malkovich playing Lenny is especially recommended). It may be pedagogically useful to show the barn scene in which Lenny murders his young friend as a prelude to this discussion.

Any of your students enamored with Leonardo DiCaprio will enjoy his excellent presentation of a child with retardation in *What's Eating Gilbert Grape*.

Movie	Link to Chapter	Page Reference to Wedding and Boyd
• Best Boy • Forrest Gump • Of Mice and Men	mental retardation (p. 464)	p. 148 p. 150 p. 150
• Rain Man	autism (p. 473)	p. 143

Classroom Assessment Techniques (CAT)

One-Sentence Summary (CAT 16-1)
Ask student to summarize a specific piece of information in this chapter by responding to the question, "Who does/did what to whom, when, where, how and why?"

Learning Review (CAT 16-2)
Students are to write in order five of the most important ideas they learned in this chapter.

Muddiest Point (CAT 16-3)
Instruct students to write about an issue, concept, or definition presented in Chapter 16 that they find most confusing or difficult to understand.

Suggestions for Essay Questions

- Develop a proposal to minimize the environmental factors in mental retardation.
- Discuss the hallmark characteristics of autism.
- Why were so many individuals deceived into believing the efficacy of facilitated communication?

Chapter 17

Antisocial and Violent Behavior

Chapter Map

Section	Instructor Manual Components
Antisocial Personality Disorder • Characteristics of the Antisocial Personality • Antisocial Behavior and Psychopathy • Antisocial Behavior in Juveniles	*FBI Behavioral Science Unit (LL 17-1)* *Examples of APD (TP 17-1)* *APD and con men (TP 17-2)* *Creating a case study of APD (ACT/DEMO 17-1)*
Antisocial Personality Disorder: Theory and Therapy • The Sociocultural Perspective • The Behavioral Perspective • The Cognitive Perspective • The Biological Perspective • Therapy	*Treating APD with drugs (LL 17-2)* *APD and their impact (TP 17-3)* *Jeffery Dahmer (TP 17-4)*
Rape • Acquaintance Rape • The Sociocultural Perspective • The Cognitive and Behavioral Perspectives • Can Rapists Be Treated?	*Perception: Dress of rape victim and length of relationships (LL 17-3)* *The date rape drugs: Rohypnol and Liquid X (LL 17-4)* *Castration as treatment for rapists (TP 17-5)* *Men as socialized to become sexual predators (TP 17-6)* *Sex and advertising (ACT/DEMO 17-2* *Survey on date rape (ACT/DEMO 17-3)*

Domestic Violence • Types of Batterers • Role of Alcohol Abuse in Battering • Emotional Abuse • How Battered Women Escape	*Treatment for batterers may not be helpful (LL 17-5)* *Battered women who killed or seriously injured their abuser* *(LL 17-6)* *Segment of domestic violence on "COPS" (TP 17-7)* *Recounting the O.J. Simpson case (TP 17-8)* *Developing an information packet (ACT/DEMO 17-4)*
Domestic Violence: Theory and Therapy • The Sociocultural Perspective • The Cognitive and Behavioral Perspectives • The Biological Perspective • Is Therapy Effective	*Guest speakers (ACT/DEMO 17-5)*
Groups at Risk for Antisocial and Violent Behavior	

Chapter Outline

I. Introduction
   A. There are strong sociocultural correlates for violent behaviors
   B. Not all violence is associated with DSM-IV disorders

II. Antisocial Personality Disorder
   A. A predatory attitude toward people defines antisocial personality disorder (APD)
      1. Affects about 1% of females and 4 to 6% of males
      2. Antisocial behavior often involves criminal behavior
   B. Characteristics of the Antisocial Personality
      1. History of illegal or socially disapproved activity beginning before 15 and continuing into adulthood
      2. Failure to show constancy and responsibility in work, sexual relationships, parenthood, or financial obligations
      3. Irritability and aggressiveness
      4. Reckless and impulsive behavior
      5. Disregard for the truth
   C. Antisocial Behavior and Psychopathy
      1. Until about 200 years ago, psychological well-being in criminals was not considered
         a. Pinel, Rush, and Prichard speculated about some immoral and criminal behavior due to mental illness
         b. In late nineteenth century, psychopath was used to describe these individuals and assumed to be biological
         c. Later, individuals were labeled sociopaths and assumed to be due to social conditions
      2. DSM-IV bases diagnosis of APD on behavior common among criminals
         a. Fails to include interpersonal and emotional characteristics associated with psychopathy
         b. When psychopathic characteristics included, 28% of prison inmates qualified as psychopaths
         c. Diagnosis of APD moved closer to reliably identifying criminals, but further away from notion of psychopathy
      3. Psychopaths differ from normal criminals
         a. Misdeeds are not just impulsive, but also unmotivated so behavior has perverse or irrational quality
         b. Have only the shallowest emotions
         c. Show poor judgment and failure to learn from experience; poor at **passive avoidance learning**
         d. Most are able to maintain pleasant and convincing exterior
      4. There is considerable overlap between APD and psychopathy

5.   Decision to ignore term psychopathy in DSM-IV motivated to increase reliability of diagnosis

6.   Division of APD and psychopathy facilitates research and treatment

    a.   Psychopaths prone to **instrumental aggression**; remain calm, focused, and controlled when attacked; typical profile of serial killers

    b.   Criminals and APDs are prone to acts of rage and motivated by revenge

    c.   Psychopaths more likely to lie and be deceptive

7.   At least 50% of those who are diagnosed with substance abuse also have antisocial personalities

D.   Antisocial Behavior in Juvenile

1.   Most antisocial adults were delinquents during preadolescent and adolescent years

2.   Violence has been increasing among children and adolescents

3.   Juvenile delinquency under conduct disorders in DSM-IV

4.   Conduct disorders related to antisocial personality and adult antisocial behavior in general

    a.   Antisocial behavior in childhood good predicator of adult antisocial personality

    b.   Training in delinquency occurs in friendships between adolescent males

5.   All people with antisocial personality were once teenagers with conduct disorders; but reverse is not true

6.   Those who overcome own criminal history may have higher levels of physiological arousal and strong orienting response

III.   Antisocial Personality Disorder: Theory and Therapy

A.   The Sociocultural Perspective

1.   Injustices foster antisocial personalities

2.   Often people resort to antisocial behavior to acquire goals that include money and prestige

    a.   Children model their parents' behavior

    b.   Gangs become training grounds for acquiring APD

3.   Poverty, unemployment, racism, and oppression increase probability of APD

B.   The Behavioral Perspective

1.   Focus is on individual's specific environments such as one's family

2.   Media influences children

3.   Parental reinforcement also plays role in development of antisocial personality

    a.   Children who seldom engage in antisocial behavior have parents who reinforce **prosocial behavior** in children

b. Children with conduct disorders have parents who show different pattern
    i. Response tends to be punishing
    ii. Positive reinforcement given is generally not related to prosocial behavior
c. Antisocial behavior reinforced by parental reciprocity of children's negative behavior which leads to coercion followed by withdrawal of coercion
4. Parents teach children there is no connection between their positive behavior and the treatment they receive
    a. Children become desensitized to social stimuli
    b. Children believe that outcome of positive behavior determined by arbitrary force, not by their actions
    c. Negative behavior unwittingly reinforced by coercive family cycles
5. Antisocial behavior also learned through direct positive reinforcement

C. The Cognitive Perspective
1. Focus is on social information processing
2. Antisocial children not good at reading social cues, deciding on appropriate responses, and problem solving effectively in social situations
3. Child abuse may cause antisocial behavior by causing impairments in social information processing mechanisms
4. Faulty thinking is acquired through learning and may be response to developmental conditions

D. The Biological Perspective
1. Genetic Factors
    a. Twin and adoption studies support role heredity plays in criminal behavior
    b. MZ twins more likely to be concordant for criminal behavior than DZ
    c. Genetic research suggests that overlap among APD, alcoholism, and other addictions part of same heritability factor
    d. General vulnerability toward antisocial behavior, not specific vulnerability toward violence is inherited
    e. Environment may play greater role in APD among poor and working classes than genetics
2. Physiological Abnormalities
    a. People with antisocial personalities may have defect in brain functioning
    b. Abnormalities include EEG readings and increased activity in left hemisphere of frontal lobe

     i. Suggests that impaired functioning in prefrontal lobe may be link between APD and substance abuse

     ii. APD may be product of delayed development of cerebral cortex

   c. Capacity of fear is mental function that is impaired in cortical immaturity

     i. Prevents individual from responding normally to fear-inducing stimuli

     ii. Leads to inability to inhibit responses that will result in punishment

   d. Alternative explanation suggests that people with APD are underaroused stimulus-seekers

   e. People with antisocial personalities have information-processing problems that make it hard for them to switch attention from cues for reward to cues for punishment

   f. Underarousal at an early age predicts subsequent antisocial behavior

   g. Biological markers may be due to birth complications, bad parenting may make it more likely person will be violent

 E. Therapy

  1. No therapy has demonstrated efficiency with APD

  2. There has been isolated success with cognitive behavior therapy

  3. Criminals and noncriminals with APD seldom seek therapy, tend not to be motivated to change, and limited in capacity to change

  4. Medications may have promise for subgroup of men with APD with mood disorders who abuse alcohol

  5. Treatment programs for psychopaths may actually backfire and make them more dangerous

  6. Many experts say that only real way to stop ADP is to prevent it from starting

   a. Reducing stress in the environment

   b. Better health care for poor women

IV. Rape

 A. **Rape**, sexual intercourse with a nonconsenting partner, is common crime

 B. Most rapes go unreported

 C. Men rape women for several reasons

  1. Some men rape because they cannot find a willing sex partner

  2. Other rapists have antisocial personalities

  3. Element of force may be necessary for sexual arousal

  4. Some rape because of aggression rather than sexual motives

   a. Related to culture's emphasis on sex and violence

   b. To some extent, men are socialized to become sexual predators

   c. Sexual aggression related to confluence of two factors

                    i.   Related to hostile masculinity
                    ii.   Related to impersonal sex
        5.   Psychological damage suffered by rape victims is enormous
                a.   Victims are at risk for number of psychological disorders
                b.   Search for justice often leads to humiliation
                    i.   Most reported rape cases do not go to trial
                    ii.   Women is left open to retaliation
                    iii.   Often victim feels she is on trial, not rapist
                    iv.   Changes are being made; counseling centers
                            established, special training for police officers, state
                            laws revised
D.   Acquaintance Rape
        1.   Date rape became serious issue on American college campuses in
                1980s
        2.   Date rape is very common
        3.   Coercive tactics used by men include using their greater physical
                strength, preventing women from leaving enclosed space,
                continuing to touch them despite women's saying no, lying to
                women about their intentions
        4.   There are no differences between victims of assault by stranger and
                victims of date rape on measures of postassault depression,
                anxiety, relationship quality, or sexual adjustment
        5.   Psychological consequences similar to those of incest and child
                molestation
                a.   May be related to presumption of collusion on part of
                        victim
                b.   Rape victims tend to blame themselves for rape
        6.   Presumption of female responsibility based on notion of boys will
                be boys
                a.   Those men who hold such attitudes more likely to commit
                        date rape
                b.   Sexually coercive men more aggressive, more tolerant of
                        aggression, more sexually experienced, less sexually
                        satisfied, and more sexually aroused by use of force
E.   The Sociocultural Perspective
        1.   Theories state that sexual aggression toward women tolerated by
                culture and even accepted and sometimes rewarded by it
        2.   Men are all socialized to be potential rapists
        3.   There are sociocultural risk factors that exist at community level
                a.   Restricting information about sex that perpetuates rape
                        myth
                b.   Some ethnic groups are patriarchal when it comes to sex
        4.   Poverty better predicts sexual aggression than does either race or
                ethnicity
                a.   Climate of poverty increases risk of sexual aggression

   b. The same sociocultural variables that predict antisocial and violent behavior predict rape

  5. Psychologists can't entirely explain why United States is so violent or why rape is more common than in other industrial countries

F. The Cognitive and Behavioral Perspectives

  1. There is connection between alcohol use and rape
    a. Causal connections are unclear
    b. Probably alcohol removes inhibitions

  2. Rapists are lonely men with little intimacy in their lives
    a. Tend to have extremely hostile attitude toward women
    b. Subscribe to the rape myth
    c. Tend to lack empathy especially for victims or prospective victims

  3. Many rapists are also psychopaths and differ greatly from those who are not
    a. Typically part of larger pattern of criminal behavior going back to early age
    b. Less likely to stalk victims and see rape as an end in itself
    c. Rape more likely to be associated with general disregard for others and indifference to standards for moral conduct

G. Can Rapists Be Treated?

  1. Therapies for rapists have mixed results
  2. Therapy designed to unlearn deviant pattern and to change sexual arousal patterns, behavior, and beliefs
  3. **Relapse prevention** focuses on training rapists how to avoid situations that place them at risk for repeating crime and how to resist impulse to commit the offense
  4. Alternatives developed to involve criminal justice system
  5. Rapists are most likely of all sex offenders to reoffend
    a. Reoffense is the norm, not exception
    b. Most likely among psychopaths, especially those who show strong physiological arousal to rape films
  6. Prevention may be only hope such as socialization for more androgynous gender identify and placing sex with context of relationship

V. Domestic Violence

A. DSM-IV uses **partner abuse** to label violence between people who are romantically involved

  1. Women most always are victims, men the perpetrators when violence is serious
  2. National surveys suggest that women and men are equally violent
    a. Majority of aggressive acts in national surveys are pushing and shoving

        b.   When more serious acts are considered, husbands are more likely to kill their wives

        c.   Frequency counts do not consider either the impact on function of violence of the act

              i.   Violent acts done by men against female partners are much more severe

              ii.   Women are more likely to be killed and injured enough to require medical attention

3.   Battering includes physical aggression, but also intimidation subjugating, and control of intimate partner

        a.   Requires physical strength to use violence as method of control

        b.   Requires learning history that justified use of violence against intimate partners

B.   When woman leaves, there is period of terrorism that includes stalking, threats, rape and violence, which generally subsides

    1.   Deterrents to leaving include poverty and lack of social support network

    2.   Some women who leave abusive relationship suffer from posttraumatic stress disorder or depression

    3.   Leaving on the part of the women may actually increase violence and may become emotional abuse

C.   Battering is illegal in all states

    1.   Most severe battering episodes never get reported

    2.   Most states have mandatory arrest laws, but are unevenly enforced by police officers

    3.   Prosecutors must decided whether to indict arrested batterer, but may not due to full docket, changes not pressed, personal bias

    4.   Conviction may lead to probation, small fine, referral to outpatient rehabilitation program

    5.   Only real protection is to hold batterers accountable through punishment

    6.   Arrest may actually increase likelihood of further violent episodes among working-class or those in poverty

D.   Types of Batterers

    1.   Batterers were once thought to be homogenous group

    2.   Batterers differ with regard to family history and other characteristics

        a.   Those resembling men with APD

        b.   Those who combined depression with borderline personality disorder

        c.   Men who appear not to have disorders but batter their wives

    3.   Batterers can differ with regard to their physiological arousal

        a.   Type I batterers--those who calm down when they become aggressive

        b.   Type II batterers--those who become physiologically aroused when they become aggressive

    4.   Type I and II batterers differ

        a.   Type I batterers are more severely violent, use more verbal and emotional abuse, come from chaotic and violent family backgrounds, and other differences

        b.   There is higher rate of separation and divorce among Type II over a two-year period

E.   Role of Alcohol Abuse in Battering

    1.   Alcohol intoxication causes battering by removing inhibitions that normally curtail male aggression

    2.   Recent studies suggest that alcohol use probably does not explain battering episodes, even among alcoholics

        a.   Men who batter may be more likely to abuse alcohol than nonviolent men

        b.   More likely this is illusory correlation suggesting other variables

        c.   Alcohol may provide rationalization for batterers to be violent thereby reducing significance of their battering problems

        d.   In some cases, alcohol abuse can be one of the causes of violent episodes

F.   Emotional Abuse

    1.   Sometimes called verbal aggression, it is more generic and defines all forms of power and control that do not involve use of violence or threats of violence

    2.   There are several varieties of emotional abuse

        a.   Damage to pets or property

        b.   Sexual coercion involving belittling wife's' appearance or taunting her with other sexual relationships

        c.   Degradation is most common category of emotional abuse

        d.   Isolation is most serious category of emotional abuse

    3.   Emotional abuse can become effective tool for power and control

        a.   High levels of emotional abuse more likely to lead to divorce than high rates of physical abuse

        b.   In cases where husband's physical abuse declines in frequency and severity, emotional abuse tends to increase

        c.   Batterers are reinforced for emotional abuse more powerfully than they are for physical abuse

G.   How Battered Women Escape

    1.   By time of first episode, woman is often attached, in love, and may be married with children

        a.   Easy to explain episode away as isolated experience

    b. Often followed by showering of partner with love, aplogies, and promises

  2. During first and second episode, fear, economic dependency, and children make it difficult to leave

    a. Wives of Type I batterers have harder time escaping

    b. Wives of Type II batterers appear to find ways to get out

  3. There are four factors that drive women married to Type II batterers to leave

    a. Emotional abuse, especially degradation and isolation

    b. Physiological arousal in the form of alarm from men

    c. Emotional stance shifts from fear to contempt

    d. Wife's overall marital satisfaction

VI. Domestic Violence: Theory and Therapy

 A. The Sociocultural Perspective

  1. Patriarchy root of domestic violence

    a. Marriage created by men for benefit of men

    b. Women and children were seen as property

    c. Laws have changed, values continue

  2. Some evidence supports role of patriarchy in battering

 B. The Cognitive and Behavioral Perspectives

  1. Batterers grow up fearing abandonment and having markedly ambivalent attitudes toward women

  2. Batterers often experience dissociation during battering episodes

  3. **Gaslighting** is where husband attempts to drive wife insane to deny her perception of reality

  4. Cognitive-behavioral theories see battering as result of deficits in social skills and social information processing such as poor impulse control

 C. The Biological Perspective

  1. There are no biological theories to explain domestic violence

  2. Literature on APD may be relevant for Type I batterers and for some Type I baterers

  3. There may be biological differences between Type I and Type II batterers, but may not be causal

 D. Is Therapy Effective?

  1. One strategy to deal with batterers is to arrest them

    a. Not typically effective in preventing recurrences

    b. Of all police interventions, arrest is most effective

  2. Shelters for battered women provide temporary housing, assistance with employment, day care, and educational training

    a. Also offer **safety planning** that involves helping women to handle potentially violent altercation without harm

    b. Safety planning may involve friends and ways of signaling to them that danger is imminent

3.   Psychological interventions take the form of separate group therapy for batterers and victims
4.   Social support may be most beneficial for battered women
     a.   Support important for achieving self-sufficiency and overcoming feelings of isolation and powerlessness
     b.   Many programs are underfunded and services may stop when woman is physically safe
5.   Group therapy for batterers focuses on cognitive restructuring, anger management, and alternatives to violence
     a.   Education programs attempt to change abuser's attitudes toward women
     b.   Education programs have become primary method of treatment
6.   Programs for batterers are not especially effective
     a.   Many avoid treatment
     b.   It is doubtful that any treatment will help Type I batterers
7.   Treatment programs may have to tailor program to individual batterer
     a.   Batterers with APD may benefit from cognitive behavior therapy
     b.   More dependent the batter is, the more likely that psychodynamic therapy will be indicated
8.   Treatment is not just an individual problem, but also social problem
     a.   Gender inequality leads to violence
     b.   Marital violence better understood as technique of control and dominance than expression of anger
9.   Efforts at prevention need to begin early in life when children are in preschool
10. Children are victimized by battering almost as much as women are
     a.   Battering is child abuse
     b.   Many batterers abuse their children
     c.   Removal may be only treatment

VII.   Groups at Risk for Antisocial and Violent Behavior
     A.   APD diagnosed in men and men commit most of violent crimes
     B.   Poverty is significant risk factors, especially in combination with other factors such as medical problems, drug use, and bad parenting
     C.   Many of the risk factors related to APD are also related to rape
          1.   Rapists are no different psychologically from other men
          2.   Men at risk for committing rape have hostile attitudes toward women and view male-female relationships as adversarial
     D.   Location is a risk factor since it is related to attitudes toward women
     E.   Some batterers resemble men with APD, though others appear normal
     F.   All Americans are at risk for violence

432

Chapter Boxes

- Serial Killers
    - A. Groups of psychopaths commit violence for joy of killing
    - B. Most serial killers are psychopathic, but not typically psychotic
    - C. Serial killings more common than most people think
    - D. Many unsolved and motiveless murders committed by serial killers
    - E. Victims are usually strangers and symbolically related to killer
    - F. Most serial killers are sexual sadists
    - G. Many serial killers who remain in one geographic area maintain good reputations
    - H. There may be four types of serial killers: visionary, mission-oriented, hedonistic, power/control
    - I. Most are white males 25 to 34 years; tend to be charming, charismatic, intelligent, and psychopathic
    - J. Tend to choose one type of victim, someone who is vulnerable and easy to control
    - K. Plan to gain access to victim becomes less sophisticated and less elaborate over time
    - L. Many serial killers were abused as children and as adults, are dependent on drugs or alcohol
    - M. Catching serial killers poses major problems for law enforcement
    - N. Explanations suggest victims of serial killers bring back memories of people who humiliated them early in life; humiliation turns into rage

- Rape and its Aftermath
    - A. Rape is likely to have lasting psychological consequences
    - B. Victims more likely to develop major depression, alcoholism, drug abuse, phobia, panic disorder, and obsessive-compulsive disorder
    - C. Sexual dysfunction is a problem for many rape victims
    - D. Most likely disorder is posttraumatic stress disorder and is unlike other causes of the disorder
    - E. Women with most distress and most intrusion symptoms were those least likely to improve spontaneously
    - F. Feelings of guilt, feelings of threat, anger, and bodily injury during assault important factors for likelihood and severity of posttraumatic stress disorder
    - G. Rape shatters many fundamental and comforting beliefs of victims
    - H. Key to relieving posttraumatic stress disorder is to reverse cognitive process where memories trigger anxiety
    - I. Most treatment, such as systematic desensitization and cognitive therapy, have been effective for rape victims
    - J. Group therapy may be best treatment for rape victims

- Child Abuse: Causes and Effects
    A. Problem of child abuse is due to multiple, interrelated factors
    B. Majority of child abusers were themselves abused as children
    C. Other factors play role
    D. Social factors also increase risk of child abuse and include poverty and unemployment
    E. Large-scale cultural factors probably account for high rate of child abuse in United States
    F. Even after report, child abuse tends to be repeated
    G. Abuse can cause death and physical injuries such as neurological injuries
    H. Psychological effects include aggressiveness, impulsiveness, destructiveness, and low self-esteem, which are likely to impact on abusive parent

Learning Objectives (LO)

By the time you have finished studying this chapter, you should be able to do the following:

1.   Distinguish between adult antisocial behavior and antisocial personality disorder , and list the five criteria to diagnose antisocial personality disorder (494-496).

2.   List four characteristics that are typical of psychopaths as described by Cleckley, and why psychopathy is an important concept even though it is not included in the *DSM-IV* (496-497).

3.   Describe four types of serial killers, and efforts by mental health professionals and law enforcement agencies to come to grips with these perpetrators (498-499).

4.   Describe the relationship between juvenile conduct disorder and antisocial personality disorder in adults (498-500).

5.   Summarize the sociocultural, behavioral, and cognitive perspectives on the causes and treatment of antisocial personality disorder (500-502).

6.   Summarize the biological perspective on the causes and treatment of antisocial personality disorder (502-504).

7.   Summarize text information on cultural factors related to the occurrence of rape, the mentality of rapists, and the psychological effects of rape on rape victims (504-507).

8.   Summarize the sociocultural, behavioral, and cognitive perspectives on rape and discuss current thinking on the effectiveness of treatment for rapists (507-509).

9.   Summarize text information on the prevalence of domestic violence, trace the evolution of our culture's attitude toward this problem. and describe the difficulties women have in dealing with it (509-511).

10. Describe the behavior patterns of two types of domestic batterers, and list possible causal factors and victim response patterns associated with each type (511-513).

11. Summarize the sociocultural, cognitive, behavioral, and biological perspectives on the causes of domestic violence, including child abuse (513-515).

12. Describe the various treatments for domestic violence victims and domestic violence perpetrators, and discuss the effectiveness of these treatments (515-518).

Lecture Leads (LL)

FBI Behavioral Science Unit (LL 17-1)

One of the most interesting units of the FBI is the Behavioral Science Unit, which is charged with training and research for the FBI and other law enforcement agencies with regard to understanding violent crime. The unit provides courses at the FBI's Training Division at Quantico, Virginia, for example, on Violence in America, Interpersonal Violence, Applied Criminal Psychology, and Gangs and Gang Behavior. The agents that make up the Behavioral Science Unit are Special Agents and experienced veteran police officers with advanced degrees in the behavioral sciences; also included are forensic psychologists. The unit also conducts research on violent crime by detailed studies of violent offenders, and their motives, behaviors, and backgrounds. Sometimes referred to as profiling, the unit is able to create a profile of the suspects of violent crime. In fact, Robert Ressler, a former profile for the Unit, has created a profiler of JonBenet Ramsey's likely killer. He says that the killer was not a stranger and had access to the family home. Ressler was part of the unit for 16 years and interviewed Ted Bundy and John Wayne Gacy. Often the Behavioral Science Unit works closely with other FBI units to investigate child abductions and serial killers.

Resources:

Franks, L. (July 22, 1996). Don't shoot: The work of former FBI agent C. Van Zandt. The New Yorker, 72, 26-31.

R. Hazelwood, R. (1983). The behavior-oriented interview of rape victims: The key to profiling. FBI Law Enforcement Bulletin, 52, 8-15.

Hazelwood, R. R. (1987). Analyzing the rape and profiling the offender. In R. R. Hazelwood and A. W. Burgess (Eds.). Practical aspects of rape investigations: A multi-disciplinary approach. New York: Elsevier Science Publishing.

Hazelwood, R. R., & Warren, J. (1989). The serial rapist: His characteristics and victims. FBI Law Enforcement Bulletin, 58, 10-17.

Treating APD with drugs (LL 17-2)

Mulder reviews the literature regarding pharmacological treatment approaches for APD. Research has found that drugs that attempt to treat the personality disorder itself are largely ineffective. More successful approaches focus on the underlying biological correlates of APD, especially impulsivity and violent behavior. Mulder points out the lack of well-design placebo-controlled studies prevents specific recommendations, but argues that limited evidence suggests antipsychotics, mood stabilizers, and antidepressants may be useful in antisocial personality disorder.

Resource:

Mulder, R. T. (1996). Antisocial personality disorder: Current drug treatment
    recommendations. CNS Drugs, 5, 257-263.

Perception: Dress of rape victim and length of relationships (LL 17-3)
High school seniors (N=352) reacted to a narrative describing a date rape. The narrative
included a photograph of the victim. Subjects either saw a photograph of the victim
wearing provocative clothing, conservative clothing, or no photograph. The results
indicated that those subjects who viewed the victim dressed in provocative clothing were
most likely to believe that the victim was responsible for the rape; these same subjects
were the least likely to perceive the incident as rape. In another study, college students
read a vignette describing either a first date or a date of a couple dating for three months.
The vignette included a rape. Students were equally likely to perceive the incident in
both first and later date as rape. Female students were more likely to perceive the
incident as rape.

Resources:

Cassidy, L., & Hurrell, R. M. (1995). The influence of victim's attire on adolescents'
    judgements of date rape. Adolescence, 30, 319-323.

McLendon, K. et al. (1994). Male and female perceptions of date rape. Journal of
    Social Behavior and Personality, 9, 421-428.

The date rape drugs: Rohypnol and Liquid X (LL 17-4)
Many college campuses are reporting rapes involving Rohypnol, and probably many
more incidences are not reported. Rohypnol (flunitrazepam; street names include
"circles," "roofies," "roopies," "rope," "ropies," and "Ruffies") is a Schedule IV
benzodiazepine and acts much like Valium, but is much more potent. It is often used
with alcohol or other drugs and has its first effects within 30 minutes, peaking in about
two hours. The user typically experiences memory impairment, dizziness, and
drowsiness. It is legally available in Europe where it is the most widely prescribed
sedative/hypnotic. Rohypnol is smuggled into United States where it has not received
approval for medical use. The larger seizures of it typically take place in Texas and
Florida, where the drug is usually smuggled in from Mexico. In the last couple of years
there have been several cases on college campuses in which women have been drugged
with Rohypnol and then raped. The rapist typically slips Rohypnol into the woman's
drink. A recent court trial in California involved a pair of 42-year-old Romanian twin
brothers who were accused of a rape involving the drug. In a recent trail, a jury found
Matthew Morris guilty of raping of 15-year old after he drugged her with Rohypnol.
Colleges and universities have instituted date-rape drug seminars to warn college
students. Rohypnol is not the only date-rape drug used. A new club drug called gamma
hydroxybutyrate, or GHB, has been implicated in several rapes. The drug, sometimes
called "Liquid X" or "Easy Lay," may be replacing Rohypnol since it can be easily made
in a home chemistry lab with instructions available on the Internet.

Resources:

Baldas, T. (December 12, 1997). Warning sent on dangers of date-rape drugs. <u>Chicago Tribune</u>. 2L, 1:2.

Condor, B. (February 1, 1998). The Unseen invader: Undetectable drugs can leave you wondering what you did until it's too late to find out. <u>Chicago Tribune</u>, <u>13</u>, 1:2.

Gorman, C. (September 30, 1996). Liquid X. <u>Time</u>, <u>148</u>, 64.

Scheeres, J. (May 31, 1998). Trial offers look at date-rape drug; Court: Twins are accused of assaulting five women, who tell of nightmarish events; Defense has said accusers were willing or are seeking revenge. <u>Los Angeles Times</u>, B, 1:4.

Smith, L. (May 30, 1998). Trial evade is sentenced. Washington Post. 6:1.

Treatment for batterers may not be helpful (LL 17-5)
The authors review treatment programs for batterers. They suggest that many of these programs use methods that could be describe as confrontational. These methods are often delivered in a consistent, direct, and intense way. Murphy and Baxter point out that this hostile approach may actually strengthen the perpetrators' belief that healthy, desirable relationships are based on hostile confrontation. This characteristic may reduce the effectiveness of these programs. The suggestion is made that a more "supportive and collaborative working alliance" is more likely to increase the motivation on the part of batterers to change.

Resource:

Murphy, C. M., & Baxter, V. A. (1997). Motivating batterers to change in the treatment context. <u>Journal of Interpersonal Violence</u>, <u>12</u>, 607-619.

Battered women who killed or seriously injured their abuser (LL 17-6)
In a retrospective study, O'Keefe examined battered women incarcerated for killing or seriously injuring their abuser. As a comparison, battered women who were incarcerated for other offenses were also examined on a number of variables (e.g., demographics, relationship characteristics, perceived social support, and prior criminal behavior). The results showed a number of differences between these two subject groups. For example, the former group was older, experienced more frequent and severe abuse leading to more injuries, and was more likely to believe their lives were in danger.

Resource:

O'Keefe, M. (1997). Incarcerated battered women: A comparison of battered women who killed their abusers and those incarcerated for other offenses. <u>Journal of Family Violence</u>, <u>12</u>, 1-19.

Talking Points (TP)

Examples of APD (TP 17-1)
As you lecture on the diagnostic criteria for APD, ask students to give examples from fiction or nonfiction books, television, and movies.

APD and con men (TP 17-2)
After you present the characteristics of APD, ask students if they have ever had interactions with people that resemble those characteristics. Mention that the stereotypical con man fits the profile of APD. Point out that the term "con man" really is shorthand for confidence man, which says much about the behaviors of these individuals, that they gain your confidence, often by being articulate and charming.

APD and their impact (TP 17-3)
Someone once describe people with APD as causing the most damage to relationships than any other psychological disorders. Ask student to discuss whether that statement appears to be true.

Jeffery Dahmer (TP 17-4)
As the textbook describes, Jeffery Dahmer was found sane and guilty of murder. Dahmer was ultimately murdered himself in prison. Did Dahmer deserve the death penalty? Do all serial killers deserve to be executed? Are they insane?

Castration as treatment for rapists (TP 17-5)
Discuss with your students the ethics of castrating chronic rapists. If treatments for rapists are negligible, what are the alternatives for dealing with the habitual criminals?

Men as socialized to become sexual predators (TP 17-6)
Try to engage some discussion about this statement from page 504. Ask students to provide some evidence that supports it as well as evidence that contradicts it.

Segment of domestic violence on "COPS" (TP 17-7)
Locate a segment on the FOX-TV show "COPS" that illustrates mandatory arrest laws in action. Show the segment to the class and ask for reactions. Was the police officer's action justified by the available evidence inasmuch as it was depicted on the video?

Recounting the O.J. Simpson case (TP 17-8)
It might be more effective if you could located some of the media stories about the Simpson case. If you can, locate the transcripts of the various 911 emergency calls Nicole Brown Simpson made involving domestic violence. Find commentaries that appeared in newspapers and magazines following his criminal trial in which he was found not guilty and analyze the impact of the not guilty verdict on the country's views on domestic violence.

Activities and Demonstrations (ACT/DEMO)

Creating a case study of APD (ACT/DEMO 17-1)
Objective: To understand the etiology, demographics, and symptoms of antisocial personality disorder
Materials: None
Procedure: Students should familiarize themselves with APD. The activity involves each student creating a fictitious case study of the disorder. In this case study, students should provide the salient background information on the "subject."
Discussion: Divide the class into groups. Each student is to share their case study with the group. The group should provide feedback. Next, select a couple of case studies to present to the entire class.

Sex and advertising (ACT/DEMO 17-2
Objective: To demonstrate the messages in advertising that relates to sex and women
Materials: None
Procedure: Have students watch television, read popular magazines, and observe newspapers and outdoor advertising to record the number of sexual advertisements they see. For each time, students should record the type of media, the product advertised, the implied message, and the role of women.
Discussion: Summarize the types of advertisements on an overhead and update it throughout the discussion. What type of attitude toward women is being advanced in these advertisements? What role do women have in these advertisements? What are the most offensive? What type of product is the most common product? What is the least likely product to use sex in advertising? What is the subtlest use of sex? Do the students think that there should be more or less emphasis on sex in advertising? List as many sexually explicit advertisements in television, radio, newspapers, popular magazines, or outdoor advertising as you can that have occurred in the last 48 hours. As an extension, ask students to think about the role and behavior of women in slasher movies and television sitcoms. Have the roles and behaviors of women changed in the last 30 years?

Survey on date rape (ACT/DEMO 17-3)
Objective: To determine frequency of date rape on your campus
Materials: Date Rape Survey
Procedure: After reviewing date rape, handout the survey. Stress that the survey is to be completed anonymously. Collect the surveys and analyze the results.
Discussion: Before you share the results of the survey, review the questions with your students and ask students to predict the aggregate frequencies. In addition, remind them that the survey was not given to a random sample and that generalizations are to be made cautiously.

441

Developing an information packet (ACT/DEMO 17-4)
Objective: To identify community resources available for battered women
Materials: None
Procedure: After students are put into small groups, inform them that their task is to develop a brochure that would summarize the community resources available for battered women. Tell students to create their brochure using desktop publishing or word processing programs and to be creative. Alternatively, students could create websites summarizing local resources.
Discussion: After all groups have completed their brochures, collect them and redistribute each to the rest of the groups. Next, the groups are to review the accuracy of the material and the design of the brochures. Community organizations may be interested in reviewing the material for adoption and distribution.

Guest speakers (ACT/DEMO 17-5)
Objective: To illustrate the material from a real-world perspective
Materials: None
Procedure: A number of information guest speakers can be invited into the classroom to talk about the disorders presented in Chapter 17. You could invite someone from law enforcement to talk about issues related to rape and domestic violence. A corrections officer may be able to talk about the justice system in your state as it relates to youthful offenders. Somebody from the local battered women's shelter could give a presentation on the shelter and its services. Finally, if appropriate, an individual who has successfully coped with domestic violence could provide a different perspective.
Discussion: Beforehand, instruct students to review this chapter and be prepared to ask questions of their guest speakers. Afterwards, ask students to compare and contrast the speakers' presentations.

Films and Videos

Boys Will Be... BAX. Looks at domestic violence by focusing on the characteristics of a successful, middle-class, intelligent, friendly, wife batterer.

Date Rape. FHS. An adaptation of a Donahue program on the subject of date rape.

Education for All Children. RP. The Right to Education Movement is discussed. Attitudes toward handicapped children are examined.

Harry. RP. A behavioral treatment for self-injurious behavior is illustrated.

Intelligence: A Complex Concept. MGH. This film reviews the concept of intelligence and intelligence tests. Interviews with prominent experts, as well as laypeople, serve to highlight the complex nature of definition and assessment.

My Husband Is Going to Kill Me. PBS. Looks at domestic violence and the death of one abused wife.

No More Secrets. FHS. Deals with childhood sexual abuse and the possible long-term damage it inflicts.

Special Needs Students in Regular Classroom: Sean's Story. FHS. This is the story of an eight-year-old boy with Down Syndrome who was part of a battle over "inclusion," the practice of placing mentally or physically challenged students in regular classrooms. The program chronicles Sean's first year in a regular classroom setting.

The Battered Woman. PBS. Seven abused women reveal their experiences; discusses causes of this problem and responses to it.

The Psychopath/Antisocial Personality. Nature or Nurture. PBS. One of the Mind Video Modules.

The Special Child. Maximizing Limited Potential. FHS. When there is doubt about a child's mental and physical coordination, screening for developmental problems should begin at three to four months to determine whether the underlying cause is behavioral, neurological, or emotional. The program covers Down syndrome, autism, problems of neurological control, speech problems, and the avoidance behavior that can result in crib death.

Using Movies and Mental Illness as a Teaching Tool

Wedding and Boyd select *The Accused* because it is a provocative film about rape likely to generate strong feelings and lively classroom debate. However, other films will work just as well. For example, *Casualties of War* examines rape in time of war and explores the issue of situational determinants for aberrant behavior. Alcohol and drug abuse is routinely associated with violence, and *Once Were Warriors* is the best cinematic exploration of the relationship between culture, substance abuse, and violent behavior. Your students will not forget this remarkable film, and they will be eager to use the movie as the starting place for a discussion of the role of culture in modeling and sanctioning violence. This is also the right place in the course to examine the roles of women in society and societal expectations about women's behavior.

There is an active professional controversy about whether or not pornography is a harmless outlet for sexual energy or a portal of entry leading to devaluation of women and sexual violence. It may be useful to have your students use data to argue these two positions, perhaps having the males and females debate in the class. Students will be more likely to scrutinize their own belief systems if you assign women the task of defending pornography while men have to challenge it. Having students watch *The People vs. Larry Flint* before coming to class would be an excellent way to start.

Students are also fascinated by serial killers, and a class discussion of a few of the films dealing with serial killers will be worth the time devoted to this task. Some of the films that can be discussed include *Silence of the Lambs*, *Henry: Portrait* of a *Serial Killer, In Cold Blood, The Boston Strangler, Copycat, The Executioner's Song*, and *Natural Born Killers*. In the context of this discussion, it will be useful to examine the predictive validity of the psychological profiles developed by the police and FBI in these cases.

Movie	Link to Chapter	Page Reference to Wedding and Boyd
• Henry: Portrait of a Serial Killer • In Cold Blood • Silence of the Lambs • Helter Skelter • Strangers on a Train	antisocial personality disorder (p. 494)	p. 157 p. 158 p. 72 p. 72 p. 72
• The Accused • Thelma and Louise • Higher Learning	rape (p. 504)	p. 153 p. 156 p. 156
• Once Were Warriors	domestic violence (p. 509)	p. 157

Classroom Assessment Techniques (CAT)

Focused Listing (CAT 17-1)
Select an important point from this chapter (e.g., degradation, psychopath, gaslighting) and ask students to write five words or phrases that describe the point.

Muddiest Point (CAT 17-2)
Instruct students to write about an issue, concept, or definition presented in Chapter 17 that they find most confusing or difficult to understand.

Definition Matrix (CAT 17-3)
Using the handout, students should list the differences between Type I and Type II batterers.

Minute Paper (CAT 17-4)
Ask your students to write about an important question they have that remains unanswered.

Suggestions for Essay Questions

- Why should society be concerned about individuals with antisocial personality disorder?
- Discuss the psychological damage often experienced by victims of rape.
- What should a college or university do to combat the problem of acquaintance rape?
- Compare Type I and Type II batterers.

Definition Matrix
Classroom Assessment Technique

Type I Batterers	Type II Batterers

Date Rape Survey
Handout

Please fill out the following information as honestly as you can. This form will be anonymous and you will not be identified in any way.

Age:

Gender:

Do have a friend or acquaintance who was the victim of date rape?

Do have a friend or acquaintance who was a perpetrator of date rape?

Have you ever lied to a person in order to have sex with that person?

If you are a female, have you ever had sex against your will?

If you are a male, have you ever had sex with someone against their will?

Do you know of any incidences on campus that involved the drug Rohypnol and subsequent nonconsenting sex?

Chapter 18

==

Legal Issues in Abnormal Psychology

Chapter Map

Section	Instructor Manual Components
Psychological Disturbances and Criminal Law • The Insanity Defense • Competency to Stand Trial	*Not guilty by reason of insanity (LL 18-1)* *Sex offenders' rights? (LL 18-2)* *Notable cases involving insanity defense (TP 18-1)* *Who is crazy? (TP 18-2)* *Perceptions of the insanity defense (TP 18-3)* *The O. J. Simpson criminal and civil cases (TP 18-4)* *Culture and insanity (TP 18-5)* *It's society that is insane (TP 18-6)* *Analyzing a case study: Competency to stand trial (ACT/DEMO 18-1)* *Role playing abnormal behavior in the courts (ACT/DEMO 18-2)*
Civil Commitment • Procedures for Commitment • Standards for Commitment	*Predicting dangerousness (LL 18-3)* *Involuntary commitment procedures (LL 18-4)*
Patients' Rights • The Right to Treatment • The Right to Refuse Treatment • The Right to a Human Environment • Behavior Therapy and Patients Rights	*Mental health bill of rights (LL 18-5)* *Are "normal" people entitled to receive treatment? (LL 18-6)* *Ethical dilemmas (TP 18-7)* *Class debate: Confidentiality (ACT/DEMO 18-3)* *Guest speakers (ACT/DEMO 18-4)*
• Power and the Mental Health Profession	*Using mental health as a political tool (LL 18-7)* *Other important legal issues in psychology (TP 18-8)*

Chapter Outline

I. Introduction
    A. There is overlap between mental health and law
    B. Decisions about people's mental health have important legal ramifications
        1. People who are judged insane may not be legally responsible for their crime
        2. People who are judged insane may be relieved of many constitutional rights
    C. Mental health law has been changing at a rapid pace

II. Psychological Disturbance and Criminal Law
    A. Many social norms are not just standards of behavior but legal requirements
    B. Abnormal behavior may also be illegal behavior
    C. Insanity Defense
        1. Law assumes humans freely choose their actions
        2. A guilty verdict refers to a judgment of fact while a moral judgment means that person is morally punished and should be punished for it
        3. Some people commit crimes not out of free choice, but because mental disturbance deprives them of free choice
            a. In an **insanity defense** the defendant admits to committing crime, but pleads not guilty and is not morally responsible because of mental disturbance
            b. Person claims to be innocent in moral terms
            c. Designed to protect mentally disturbed from penalties given to mentally sound
    D. Legal Tests of Insanity
        1. First important ruling was irresistible-impulse decision in 1834 by an Ohio court
            a. Defendants are acquitted if they could not resist the impulse to do wrong because of mental illness
            b. Difficult to distinguish between resistible and irresistible impulses
        2. Second important test was M'Naghten ruling handed down in 1843 by a British court
            a. Case involved defendant claiming he had been commanded by God to kill English prime minister
            b. Court ruled in M'Naghten's acquittal that defendants are legally insane and not criminally responsible if by disease of the mind and consequent impairment of reason, they meet one of two criteria
                i. Did not know what they were doing
                ii. Did not know that what they were doing was wrong

        c.   Critics suggest that cognitive activity cannot be separated from emotion or from any other mental activity; legal scholars suggest that mind is not undifferentiated blob

        d.   Test serves purpose of excusing truly excusable and preserving moral authority of law

3.   Third test is Durham test

        a.   Test states defendant is not criminally responsible if unlawful act was product of mental disease or mental defect

        b.   Forces jury to rely on expert testimony

        c.   Defendants are supposed to be tried by peers not by mental health professionals

4.   Most recent test is American Law Institute's Model Penal Code of 1962

        a.   Person is not responsible if at time of conduct person lacks substantial capacity either to appreciate criminality of conduct or to conform conduct to requirements of law

        b.   Mental disease or defect does not include abnormality manifested only by repeated criminal or otherwise antisocial conduct

        c.   Code incorporates irresistible-impulse criterion and M'Naghten criterion and Durham criterion

        d.   Test can be applied without expert knowledge

        e.   ALI test adopted by many states

5.   A New Verdict--Guilty but Mentally Ill

        a.   Many defendants may escape responsibility for their crimes

            i.   Case often cited is that of John Hinckley after 1982 assassination attempt on President Reagan

            ii.   Trial focused on whether he had committed crime and whether he was sane at the time

            iii.   Defense witnesses portrayed Hinckley as suffering from schizophrenia and other mental problems

            iv.   Prosecution witnesses argued that Hinckley made conscious choice to shoot Reagan and had no compelling drive to do so

            v.   Hinckley was found not guilty by reason of insanity

            vi.   Case led to consideration of verdict of guilty but mentally ill

        b.   Guilty but mentally ill is intermediate between guilty and not guilty by reason of insanity

        c.   Defendant convicted would serve time in penal system and receive psychological treatment

        d.   Michigan first state to adopt guilty but mentally ill verdict in 1975

        e.   New verdict has not reduced number of insanity acquittals and some legal scholars question it

6. Procedural Aspects of the Insanity Defense
   a. Prosecution must prove beyond reasonable doubt all elements of a criminal offense, including the physical act and requisite mental state
   b. Before Hinckley verdict, states placed burden on prosecution to prove sanity after defense presented evidence suggesting insanity
   c. Federal rules change to place burden of proving insanity on defendant and many states have followed
      i. Has reduced number of insanity acquittals
      ii. Most insanity acquittals involved people with serious mental illnesses
   f. Prior to 1970s, defendants acquitted by reason of insanity were confined to mental hospitals
      i. After 1970s, acquittals no longer followed automatically by commitment
      ii. Long-term hospitalization permitted only under standards of ordinary civil commitment
   g. In *Jones v. United States* (1983), U.S. Supreme Court ruled that is permissible to commit insanity acquittes automatically
      i. Acquittes hospitalized until proven either no longer mentally ill or no longer dangerous
      ii. Acquittes could be hospitalized for longer than they could have been imprisoned, had they been convicted
   h. Most states have tightened up postacquittal procedures so as to make release more difficult
7. Criticism of the Insanity Defense
   a. Insanity defense poses practical and moral problems
   b. To rule on person's sanity, jury must make subjective judgment that is difficult to make and is made retrospectively
      i. Jury must rely on testimony of psychological professionals who often make diametrically opposed diagnoses
      ii. Experts called by same side often contradict each other
      iii. Court must make legal judgment, not scientific judgment
      iv. Jury is empowered to do so, not the mental health professional
   c. Szasz argues that insanity defense is difficult for jury since insanity does not exist
      i. Mental illness is a myth perpetuated by an arrogant profession

451

ii.   All behavior is of a purposeful and responsible nature

iii.   To label behavior as insane is to deny the behavior any meaning and to deny that there is conflict between the individual and society

iv.   Suggests courts do not judge other people's intentions, but instead judges them on their behavior

d.   Those who plead insane often end up in worse situation than if convicted of their crimes

    i.   People who are found not guilty by reason of insanity usually not set free

    ii.   Often committed to mental hospitals and kept there until judged not dangerous

    v.   Many people acquitted by reason of insanity are given **indeterminate sentences**, sentences with no limit

e.   Three states have abolished insanity defense

f.   Insanity defense is much less important than other issues linking law and psychology, but receives great deal of publish attention

    i.   Insanity defense used in less than 1 percent of felony cases

    ii.   Successful in less than one-quarter of cases in which it is raised

E.   Competency to Stand Trial

1.   In order to stand trial, defendant must understand nature of proceedings against them and be able to assist counsel in their own defense

2.   If defendant does not meet requirements, trial is delayed and person sent to mental health facility until competent

3.   Incompetency to stand trial is different from legal insanity

a.   Insanity defense refers to defendant's mental state at time of crime

b.   Competency to stand trials refers to defendant's mental state at time of trial

c.   Person who asserts insanity defense may be competent to stand trial and vice versa

4.   Rule of competence to stand trial often applied loosely

5.   Consequences of incompetency to stand trial can be significant

a.   May be confined to hospital for years since no means to restore competence

b.   U.S. Supreme Court rule in *Jackson v. Indiana* (1972) ruled that if person is not likely to become competent to stand trial after determining if person is likely to be competent in foreseeable future, person must be released or committed using state's ordinary civil commitment procedures

c. There is catch-22 regarding antipsychotic medication that allows defendant to fulfill competency requirement
  i. Drugs may allow person to be tried if they are lucid enough
  ii. Drugs often leave person groggy and passive
  iii. Antipsychotic medication might affect defendant's chance of successfully pleading insanity defense
  iv. U.S. Supreme Court (1992) ruled in *Riggins v. Nevada* that people being tried for a crime could not be forced to take psychotropic drugs unless trial court specifically found it necessary to a fair trial

III. Civil Commitment
  A. In **civil commitment** person has been committed not because they were charged with crime, but because the state has determined that they were disturbed enough to require hospitalization
  B. About 55% of admissions to public mental hospitals are involuntary
  C. Procedures for Commitment
    1. Involuntary commitment to mental hospital is deprivation of liberty
    2. Should person faced with involuntary civil commitment have same rights as defendant in criminal trial
      a. A jury trial
      b. Assistance of counsel
      c. Right not to be compelled to incriminate themselves
      d. Requirement that guilt be proved beyond a reasonable doubt
    3. The Right to a Jury Trial
      a. Formal judicial hearing before commitment required
      b. Some states allow for a jury at hearing, other states leave decision to judge
      c. Reasons not to include jury include expense, time-consuming, not in best interest of person whose condition is debated before jury
      d. Reason to include jury includes best protection against oppression
      e. It is unlikely that Supreme Court will require jury trials in commitment cases
    4. The Right to the Assistance of Counsel
      a. Persons facing involuntary commitment are provided with lawyers to protect their rights
      b. Lawyers do not have clear role
        i. Should lawyers act as advocates for clients' wishes
        ii. Should lawyers act as guardians pursuing clients' best interests

              iii.   Most lawyers take position to argue for clients' best interests that may well be in opposition to clients' wishes

5.   The Right Against Self-Incrimination

      a.   In criminal trials, defendants have right to remain silent, and that silence cannot be used against them

      b.   Some argue that people facing involuntary commitment should have same protection

      c.   Others argue that silence may be symptom of mental disturbance and it would be inappropriate to exclude it from evidence

6.   The Standard of Proof

      a.   Degree of certainty is called **standard of proof**

      b.   Beyond-a-reasonable-doubt standard is very difficult, 90 to 95 percent certainty

      c.   In most civil cases, the standard of proof is a preponderance of evidence, at least 51 percent certainty

      d.   In medical diagnoses, a lower standard of proof is used, 5 to 10 percent certainty

      e.   The standard of proof in involuntary commitment based on seriousness of two possible errors

              i.   **False positive**, or an unjustified commitment

              ii.   **False negative**, or failure to commit when commitment is justified and necessary

      f.   In criminal trial, a false positive is far more serious error than a false negative

      g.   In civil proceedings, false positive is considered as serious as false negative

      h.   In medical diagnosis, false negative is extremely serious mistake

      i.   When commitment is for good of society, criminal standard of proof should be used

      j.   When commitment is for good of the patient, medical standard of proof should be used

      k.   Critics argue that civil commitment is not the same as medical diagnoses

              i.   So-called good-of-the-patient commitments are often undertaken more for sake of others

              ii.   Diagnosis to commit cannot be disproved, deprives patient of liberty, stigmatizes patient, and does not necessarily lead to treatment

              iii.   No matter what reason for commitment, the beyond-a-reasonable-doubt standard should be used

      l.   U.S. Supreme Court ruling in *Addington v. Texas* (1979) adopted clear and convincing evidence as proper standard for commitment hearings

<ol type="i">
<li>Provides intermediate standard of proof</li>
<li>Corresponds to about 75 percent sure, higher than ordinary civil standard but lower than the criminal one</li>
</ol>

D.   Standards for Commitment

1. Until early 1970s mental illness and need for treatment were sufficient grounds for involuntary commitment in many states
2. Throughout 1970s reform was changing laws to require evidence not just of mental illness, but also of dangerousness to self and others as grounds

    a.   The Definition of Dangerousness
<ol type="i">
<li>Various courts and legislatures have taken different positions</li>
<li>Some states consider a threat of harm to property sufficient for commitment</li>
</ol>

    b.   The Determination of Dangerousness
<ol type="i">
<li>Determining dangerousness is difficult and involves prediction of future behavior, which may include rare events</li>
<li>Murder is a statistically rare event probably less than 1 percent; standard of proof may not be accepted by society</li>
<li>There are other factors to be consider in determination of dangerousness that encourage mental health professionals to err in direction of overpredicting dangerousness</li>
<li>Studies of predictions of dangerousness have yielded more false positive than false negatives</li>
<li>Because behavior is often situation-specific, predictions of real-world behavior based on institutional behavior have turned out to have poor validity</li>
<li>It is difficult to determine validity of predictions that are based on patient's prior real-world behavior and interviews</li>
<li>Some experts question tying commitment criteria to predictions of dangerousness</li>
</ol>

    c.   The "Thank-You" Proposition
<ol type="i">
<li>The "thank you" proposition refers to involuntary commitment when person refuses treatment on grossly irrational grounds</li>
<li>After treatment, person will be grateful that wishes were disregard</li>
<li>Large portion of involuntary patients ultimately agree that they needed the treatment that was forced upon them</li>
</ol>

    iv. Stresses patient's welfare
   d. Expert Testimony in Civil Commitment
    i. Expert testimony is called for
    ii. Some legal scholars argue that courts rely too much on opinions of mental health professionals
    iii. Moral and legal questions should not be asked of mental health professionals
   e. Making Commitment Easier
    i. In 1980s several states amended laws to make commitments easier
    ii. Research reveals few long-term effects of changes
   f. The Case Against Involuntary Commitment
    i. Critics argue that people who commit criminal acts should be dealt with by the criminal justice system
    ii. The criminal justice system would provide greater procedural safeguards
    iii. Widespread practice of plea bargaining often negates legal safeguards
    iv. Modern commitment statutes often limit indeterminate sentences

IV. Patients' Rights
  A. The Right to Treatment
   1. Since 1960s courts have suggested that involuntary mental patients have constitutional right to treatment
   2. *Wyatt v. Stickney* (1972) spelled out right to treatment
    a. Violates due process to deny people their liberty on grounds that they needed treatment and then to provide no treatment
    b. Must provide individualized treatment program for each patient
    c. Must provide skilled staff in sufficient numbers to administer such treatment
    d. Must provide human psychological and physical environment
    e. *Wyatt v. Stickney* has influenced mental health procedures in many states
   3. US Supreme Court ruled in *O'Connor v. Donaldson* (1975) that a finding of mental illness cannot alone justify commitment in simple custodial confinement
   4. In *Youngberg v. Romeo* (1982), U.S. Supreme Court found that involuntarily committed people have constitutional right to conditions of reasonable care and safety and reasonable non-restrictive environment and required training

B.   The Right to Refuse Treatment
1.   In *Washington v. Harper* (1990), U.S. Supreme Court ruled that prison's policy regarding necessity of medication should be made by doctors, not judges, and was constitutional
   a.   Lower courts usually take a more limited view of the authority of doctors
   b.   The "thank you" proposition assumes that treatment will be effective and will not have harmful side effects
2.   State statutes and regulations on right to refuse treatment vary considerably
   a.   General rule is that involuntary patients may be required to undergo "routine" treatment
   b.   More controversial forms of treatment are regulated more closely and require consent from patient or next of kin, or a court order
C.   The Right to a Human Environment
1.   The case of *Wyatt v. Stickney* affirmed right to humane environment
2.   There are several requirements of a human environment
3.   Wyatt case declared work requirements unconstitutional; patients may voluntary do work, but must be paid at least minimum wage
D.   Behavior Therapy and Patient's Rights
1.   Guarantee of patient rights may conflict with behavior therapy, which is proven to be most effective therapy with long-term institutionalized patients
2.   The reinforcers used in token economy are same that court decisions have affirmed are absolute rights
3.   Aversive techniques now carefully restricted; electric shock only allowable in extraordinary circumstances
4.   There have been several notorious cases where patients were abused in programs masquerading as behavioral aversion therapy
   a.   Use of punishment to terrify mental patients into cooperating with rules
   b.   Courts are extremely suspicious about behavioral techniques in general
5.   Behavior therapy focus of decisions regarding patient rights
   a.   Techniques relatively new and are under close scrutiny
   b.   Behavior therapy is highly specific and concrete
   c.   Behavior therapy may cause patients' distress
6.   Limiting behavior therapy may work against patients' best interest
7.   Superior effectiveness of behavior therapy may eventually encourage courts to ease some restrictions

V. Power and the Mental Health Profession
   A. Despite recent court decisions, mental health professionals have immense power
      1. Mental health professionals can declare abnormality in form of DSM
      2. Deciding abnormality includes deciding who and what needs changing in society
      3. Mental health professionals determine whether mentally disturbed people should be institutionalized or released from an institution
   B. Power of mental health profession being disputed
      1. Mental health profession is paternalistic
      2. Consumer movement makes demands on mental health profession
         a. Informed consent requires sharing of information
         b. Alternative treatments need to be discussed

Chapter Boxes

- Evolution, Misfortune, and Criminal Responsibility
  - A. Moral intuitions that underlie insanity defense have roots in evolutionary history
  - B. Those who are not conspicuously crazy may undermine effectiveness of law
  - C. Meehl suggests that criminal statutes be revised to list specific psychiatric diagnoses that would have to be established in order for insanity defense to succeed
  - D. Abuse excuse defenses are increasingly being used

- The Limits of Confidentiality
  - A. *Tarasoff* case says that psychotherapists have obligations to society that override obligations to their own patients
  - B. Therapist must divulge information to police and family of threatened victim if patient is dangerous
  - C. Prediction of dangerousness is difficult
  - D. Some believe that patient may be less inclined to confide to therapist
  - E. Therapist might be encouraged to report all threats of violence to avoid law suits
  - F. *Tarasoff* case may have positive impact on treatment

- Sex, Lives, and Mental Patients: The Hospital's Dilemma in the Age of AIDS
  - A. Mental patients have right to interact with opposite sex
  - B. Question about competency of mental patients involving risk of HIV infection
  - C. Some court decisions have found a high degree of understanding for competence is satisfied

Learning Objectives (LO)

By the time you have finished studying this chapter, you should be able to do the following-.

1. Explain the purpose of the insanity defense, describe four tests for legal insanity, and explain why one of them is now preferred over the others (525-526).

2. Summarize the procedural and ethical controversies surrounding the insanity defense, making reference to the case of John Hinckley, and discuss the concept of "guilty but mentally ill" as an alternative to "not guilty by reason of insanity" (526-530).

3. Define the purpose of competency proceedings in criminal cases, and discuss the controversies surrounding these proceedings, particularly the use of antipsychotic medications to produce competence (530-531).

4. List four rights guaranteed to persons accused of a crime, and discuss how these rights either apply or do not apply in civil commitment proceedings (531-532). ☐

5. Describe four "standards of proof' that could be used in civil commitment proceedings, and explain why one of them may be more appropriate than the others (532-533).

6. Explain "dangerousness" and the "Thank You" proposition as standards for civil commitment, and discuss the controversy surrounding these standards (533-536).

7. Discuss the role of expert testimony in civil commitment, the issue of whether commitment should be made easier or more difficult, and the argument over whether civil commitment should be used at all (536-537).

8. Summarize the cases of *Wyatt v. Stickney, O'C'onnor v. Donaldson, Youngberg v . Romeo, and Washington v. Harper* and discuss their impact on a patient's right to treatment and on the right to refuse treatment (537-539).

9. List ten rights of mental patients relating to a humane treatment environment, and discuss the potential conflict between the desire to protect patients' rights and the need to provide effective treatment (539-541).

10. Describe how recent legal decisions relating to abnormal psychology have affected client-therapist confidentiality and the power of the mental health profession (535, 541-542).

Lecture Leads (LL)

Not guilty by reason of insanity (LL 18-1)
This study examined a group of patients ages 20 to52 who committed murder and later were involuntarily committed.   For purposes of comparison the sample was divided into two groups--those found not guilty by reasons of insanity and those simply found guilty. Clinical status, neuropsychological functioning, and relationship data were analyzed. A number of differences were found. For example, those subjects found not guilty by reason of insanity were more likely perceived as psychotic at the time of the murder. They were also more likely to have killed a parent, compared to convicted murders who were more likely to have killed a spouse or lover. Convicted murders were also more likely to have substance abuse disorder. There were no differences in neuropsychological functioning.

Resource:

Nestor, P. G., & Haycock, J. (1997). Not guilty by reason of insanity of murder: Clinical and neuropsychological characteristics. Journal of the American Academy of Psychiatry and the Law, 25, 161-171.

Sex offenders' rights? (LL 18-2)
The state of Washington has been wrestling with the rights of individuals who have been labeled sexual predators. Typically, the individual has committed a sex-related criminal offense and been sentenced. After serving the sentence, the individual is released. Upon release he/she is immediately taken into custody and placed in a mental health setting within a prison, even though the individual has not committed another crime and is not insane according to legal definitions. The American Civil Liberties Union maintains that the state has no right to imprison or otherwise detain someone who has not committed a crime or who is not a danger to oneself or others, and compares the detention to that of the detention of political dissidents in the USSR. Moreover, a fundamental question in the discussion is "How is someone determined to be a sexual predator?" There is no *DSM-IV* reference to sexual predator, yet being diagnosed as one is grounds for detention in a mental health facility, with a follow-up question of how it is determined that the person is no longer a sexual predator. Lastly, how do you deliver psychological services to someone against his/her will, in that the detainees are typically uncooperative because they are being held against their will? Obviously these issues are weighted against the backdrop of a society intent on protecting itself from people who are chronic in their sexual offenses.

Resource:

Diagnostic and statistical manual of mental disorders,(4th ed) (1994). The American Psychiatric Association, Washington, D.C.

Predicting dangerousness (LL 18-3)

The hindsight bias, or the I-knew-it-all-along phenomenon, is the tendency to have known an outcome after the outcome occurs. It can operate as clinicians attempt to explain violent behavior in mentally disturbed people. After believing that a patient's dangerousness was obvious but only after the fact, clinicians come to believe in their ability to predict future behavior.

Resource:

Myers, D. (1993). Social psychology. New York: McGraw-Hill.

Involuntary commitment procedures (LL 18-4)

The exact procedures required for involuntary commitment vary from state to state. Prepare a brief presentation of your state's statutes and procedures. A good source is your local community health agency. Also examine how your state determines the competency of an individual to stand trial.

Mental health bill of rights (LL 18-5)

The American Psychological Association has published "A Mental Health Bill of Rights," which was compiled by representatives from nine mental health organizations. The basic principles for providing mental health services outline the consumer's right to know about benefits, professional expertise, contractual limitations, appeals and grievances, confidentiality, choice, determination of treatment, parity (the right to receive mental health benefits on the same basis as for physical illnesses), discrimination, benefit usage and design, treatment review, and accountability. Of particular importance are seven major areas and specific questions about benefits that should be available through the human resources or personnel departments where a person works. These include such issues as the particular benefits to which an employee is entitled and how to get services; which practitioners and types of treatment are covered (or not covered) by the plan; contractual limitations under the plan; how to appeal authorization decisions or complain about the care provided; what information is or is not subject to confidentiality and how to protect that right; choice of professional provider; and treatment decisions. The *Wyatt v. Stickney* case, in effect, created a patient's bill of rights. For example, one of the rights ithat mandated is the right to privacy and to refuse potentially hazardous or unusual treatments.

Resources:

American Psychological Association. (March 21, 1997). Text of Mental Health Bill of
　　　Rights. Available: URL http://helpingapa.org/rights.html.

Wyatt v. Stickney, 334 F. Supp. 1341 (1971).

Are "normal" people entitled to receive treatment? (LL 18-6)

The textbook discusses the patient's right to receive as well as to refuse treatment. But what about the basically "normal" person who feels a need to seek therapy for help with improving his or her quality of life? Is the "average" person entitled to receive therapy as well? If so, who should pay and what are that person's rights in a therapeutic situation? According to the American Psychological Association, access to "appropriate, high quality mental health care" is essential for our country's health. Approximately 11 million Americans suffer from depression each year costing our nation more than $40 billion, over half of which is due to absenteeism and reduced productivity at work. Approximately half of Americans between 15 and 54 years old have psychological problems during their lives, and each year about a quarter of the population experiences a psychological disorder and fewer than one-third of these seek professional help. The APA also estimates that over half of the visits made to primary care physicians have psychological bases. In light of this prevalent and expensive phenomenon, it would make sense to offer psychological assistance when the problems first arise, rather than to wait until they intensify. There are also significant economic benefits. Two studies cited by the APA, one beginning in 1989 with BellSouth, the other starting in 1993 at Delta Air Lines, Inc., found that while employees were significantly more likely to use the mental health services that were provided, both companies experienced impressive savings in terms of health care costs. Based on such findings, the APA suggests insurance reforms that offer easily accessible mental health services for anyone needing them, but also cautions that "s managed care proliferates, patients must be protected from abuses through managed care standards and other safeguards" ("Psychological Services," p. 3). Under the auspices of the United States Department of Health and Human Services, a "mental health report card" has been suggested for the benefit of the consumer (MHSIP, 1996). Such a "report card" is designed primarily "to help consumers [including those with serious mental illnesses] choose among various mental health services and systems" (p. 4) to achieve specific outcomes such as reduction of symptoms, increased productivity, greater independence, and development of support systems. In an effort to design the report card, data will be collected from a variety of sources including, among others, therapist surveys and consumer self-reports. The goal is to make the consumer a partner in reforming health care by developing an effective way to select those services that will provide an optimal option for each consumer to meet his or her specific needs.

Resources:

American Psychological Association. (March 27, 1997). <u>Psychological Sciences</u>: Essential to American's health. Available: URL http://www.apa.org/practice/reforrn.html.

U.S. Department of Health and Human Services, Substance Abuse and Mental Health Services Administration, Center for Mental Health Services. (1996). Consumer oriented mental health report card. The final report of the Mental Health Statistics Improvement Program (HSIP) Task Force on a consumer-oriented mental health report card. Available: http://www mentalhealth.org/resource/pubs/mc9660.htm.

463

Using mental health as a political tool (LL 18-7)

There are several places in the world that use or used commitment to manage political dissidents. The former Soviet Union was found to have committed those that disagreed with the state to psychiatric facilities. There is good evidence to suggest that this practice occurs in Cuba and the rate of psychiatric abuse in Cuba may be more significant than in the former Soviet Union. Political activists have been committed to psychiatric hospitals where they are diagnosed and "treated," often times with ECT and psychotropic drugs. One interesting technique was to use against a person his or her own protestation of not having a particular disorder. The person who rejects the state's diagnosis is considered to lack insight. This lack of insight into their psychiatric disorder is seen as consistent with the disorder and therefore reinforces that "fact" that they have the disorder. Therefore, more intense therapy is called for.

Resources:

Brown, C. J., & Lago, A. M. (1991). The politics of psychiatry in revolutionary Cuba. New Brunswick, NJ: Transaction Publishers.

Fulford, K. W. N., Smirnov, A. Y. U., & Snow, E. (1993). Concepts of disease and the abuse of psychiatry in the USSR. British Journal of Psychiatry, 162, 801-810.

Shaw, C. (1992). The World Psychiatric Association and Soviet Psychiatry. In R. VanVored (Ed.). Soviet psychiatric abuse in the Gorbachev era. Amsterdam: International Association on the Political Use of Psychiatry.

Talking Points (TP)

Notable cases involving insanity defense (TP 18-1)
In recent years, there have been several high visibility court trials involving issues presented in this chapter. Kenneth Bianchi was charged with being the Hillside Strangler; he claimed to have had multiple personalities, a defense that failed, and was found guilty of murder. Lorena Babbit cut off her husband's penis and was found not guilty by reason of temporary insanity since she had experienced great physical and sexual abuse. Erik and Lyle Menedez's defense in their murder trial was that they were subject to years of abuse by their father, whom they killed. The text describes the John Hinckley, Jr. case and his attempt to assassinate President Ronald Reagan. For nearly a week, Susan Smith told the public that her two small sons were kidnapped. Ultimately she confessed to drowning them. Her defense team argued that her background of abuse caused her to commit the crime. While she did not use the insanity defense, the case is of interest. John Du Pont, the heir to a huge family fortune, murdered a former Olympic wrestler. He was found guilty, but mentally ill, since he was diagnosed with schizophrenia. Recently, a thirty-five year old teacher, Mary Kay LeTourneau, was sent to jail for second-degree rape. She had sex with one of her sixth grade students, who fathered her child. Upon release she was found with him disobeying a court order. LeTourneau was ordered back to prison. She claimed that her hypomania made her take the risks. Would an insanity defense be effective in her case?

Who is crazy? (TP 18-2)
Insanity defense and insanity are legal terms and need to be understood in that context. Students have a hard time understanding why, for example, cold-blood murderers or child abusers are not insane. Many people do not understand the legal issues that led to the determination that serial killer Jeffrey Dahmer was sane. The crux of the matter rests in how the law defines insanity and how the general public defines insanity. In some sense, anyone who kills or abuses another person is crazy, but whether a person is insane or sane is entirely a legal question.

Perceptions of the insanity defense (TP 18-3)
Students often share the popular misconception that many criminals are acquitted of their crimes because of the insanity defense. Have students discuss their perceptions regarding the abuse of the insanity defense. You may also want the students to write down their guesses at the percentage of cases where the defendant pleads insanity, the number of these cases in which the defendant is acquitted, and what kinds of sentences these acquitted defendants receive.

The O. J. Simpson criminal and civil cases (TP 18-4)
It might be helpful for students to remember the Simpson criminal and civil cases as they try to understand standards of proof. In the civil case, the prosecution had to provide evidence that Simpson committed the murders of Nicole Brown Simpson and Ronald Goldman beyond reasonable doubt. In other words, the jury had to be 90 to 95% sure that Simpson committed the crime. As your students will remember, the jury believed

that there was reasonable doubt and found him not guilty. In the civil case where the Goldman family was asking for damages, the standard of proof is a preponderance of the evidence, or 51% sure. Using this standard, the jury was at least 51% sure that Simpson committed the crime.

Culture and insanity (TP 18-5)
The textbook has discussed how psychological disorders are influenced by the cultures in which they occur. A question to ask your students to consider: Given culture's influence on defining abnormality, should there be cultural differences in what constitutes insanity?

It's society that is insane (TP 18-6)
Thomas Szasz suggests that individuals are not insane--society is. Discuss the ramifications of such a view in terms of treatment and diagnosis. What are the different cultural variables that must be considered when defining abnormality from a societal perspective? Ask for examples from students of different cultures about how they attempt to define abnormal behavior.

Ethical dilemmas (TP 18-7)
An adult female discloses to her therapist that she has been engaging in exhibitionism with children for some time. Discuss what moral, legal, and ethical obligations her therapist has in terms of disclosing to legal authorities, family, and parents of affected individuals. Does the Tarasoff ruling apply? If so, how? A teenage member of a family being seen for therapy confides in their therapist that she is pregnant and is planning to get an abortion. Discuss with the class whether the therapist has any moral, legal, or ethical justification to disclose this to her parents.

Other important legal issues in psychology (TP 18-8)
There are several types of court cases for which psychology can provide insight and research, and, of course, testimony. For example, a number of cases have gone to trial regarding alleged implanting of false memories of abuse. Psychologists are often consulted in criminal cases in selecting a favorable jury. In child custody and child abuse cases, psychologists are often called to testify as expert witnesses. Psychologists and their research are often called upon to help the legal system illuminate these types of cases and to provide support for court decisions.

Cross-Cultural Teaching

Activities and Demonstrations (ACT/DEMO)

Analyzing a case study: Competency to stand trial (ACT/DEMO 18-1)
Objective: To understand the insanity defense
Materials: Case material of *Salvi v. Commonwealth of Massachusetts*
Procedure: In this activity, students will examine the evidence in the form of psychiatric testimony in the double murder trial of John Salvi. At issue is whether Salvi murdered two people for political or religious reasons or because of a severe mental disorder. The Resource URL presents the (1) transcript of the two-and-a half-hour interview of Salvi by defense psychiatrist Dr. Phillip J. Resnick (January 15, 1995), (2) A day-by-day summary of the four-day competency hearing (July 1995). Present the material (or excerpts since it is quite lengthy) to students who are placed in small groups. Consider asking two students to read it out loud, acting the parts of Salvi and Resnick. Each group is to summarize the testimony and then arrive at a decision with regard to competency to stand trial.
Discussion: As the interview is read, point out important elements such as type of confidentiality, leading questions, mini mental state exam. Based on the evidence, what was Salvi's mental state? What diagnosis would be appropriate?

Resource:
http://www2.pbs.org/wgbh/pages/frontline/salvi/texthome.html

Role playing abnormal behavior in the courts (ACT/DEMO 18-2)
Objective: To demonstrate the types of behaviors associated with abnormal psychology in the courts.
Materials: Descriptions of cases, include the most startling local or regional cases. National cases such as the Jeffrey Dahmer case can also be used.
Procedure: Have small groups of students select one of the cases. Have the group role play the jury in the case. Tell the students that they have at least overnight to prepare for their role playing and that they will be expected to role play the jury deliberations in front of the class. If an individual is too shy or anxious to do this assignment, let him or her write a short paper instead. Have individual students or a student volunteer from the groups role play the disorder.
Discussion: Ask the students how they developed their role and who they used as a model. Was there any influence from the media? If so, what specific individuals did they use as models? How has the media changed the way we view sanity in the courts?

Class debate: Confidentiality (ACT/DEMO 18-3)
Objective: To debate ethical issue of confidentially
Materials: None
Procedure: This activity is a series of two cases on an issue important to clinical psychology and law. Case A involves the importance of confidentiality to the therapeutic relationship. Present the scenario that a therapist learns that the client intends to harm another person who has physically abused his elderly father. Students should be assigned one side or another to debate the ethical, legal, and practical aspects of this issue. Case B

involves a young man who is HIV positive receiving therapy. He has not told his girlfriend of his HIV status. Again, debate the relevant aspects of this case.
Discussion: You may wish to have the debate format in small groups, each with several students on both sides of the issue. Summarize the arguments on both sides relating the debate to the Tarasoff case (see Melton, 1988; Hoffman, 1991)

Resources:
Hoffman, M. A. (1991). Counseling the HIV-infected client: A psychosocial model for assessment and intervention. Counseling Psychology, 19, 467-542.

Melton, G. B. (1988). Ethical and legal issues in AIDS-related practice. American Psychologist, 43, 941-947.

Guest speakers (ACT/DEMO 18-4)
Objective: To illustrate the material from a real-world perspective
Materials: None
Procedure: Invite a Ph.D./J.D. level psychologist to discuss current ethical issues in the field. These should include areas such as patients' rights, changes in psychologists' rights to practice, and the use of drugs to control behavior. A judge, public defender, or prosecuting attorney would also be an interesting guest speaker.
Discussion: Beforehand, instruct students to review this chapter and be prepared to ask questions of their guest speakers. Afterwards, ask students to compare and contrast the speakers' presentations.

Films and Videos

Abnormal Behavior. A Mental Hospital. MCG. A documentary about treatment in a mental hospital. Gives students an overview of treatment concerns and diagnostic issues.

An Ounce of Prevention The World of Abnormal Psychology. ANN/CPB.. Discusses prevention in abnormal psychology.

Committed in Error.- The Mental Health System Gone Mad. FHS. This is the story of a man who spent 66 years incarcerated and forgotten in mental health institutions, although there was never anything wrong with him. This story takes place in Britain, but it could as easily have happened in the U.S., where similar errors have occurred.

Crime and Insanity. PSU. NBC white paper examines the problems associated with releasing mental patients after they have been determined to no longer be a danger.

Diverting the Mentally Ill From Jail. FHS. Documents the problems of incarcerating the mentally ill in jails and the benefits of placing them into community-based mental health programs.

Larry. FHS The subject was mistakenly institutionalized and now must struggle to overcome years of cruel treatment.

Madness The Brain. ANN/CPB. Compelling human portraits of schizophrenics and their families are featured, dramatically illustrating the effects of a split between the thinking and feeling parts of the brain. Scientists' efforts to pinpoint the brain's anatomical changes are chronicled.

Mistreating the Mentally Ill. FHS. There are 250 million seriously mentally ill people the world over and no society, rich or poor, has devised a humane system of care. This program focuses on the United States, Japan, India, and Egypt, examining how each culture sees mental illness and treats the less accepted members of society. It concludes that the problem is not merely due to a shortage of funds, but can be attributed to the indifference of society to the mentally ill.

New Race and Psychiatry. FHS. The issue of race within psychiatry is at its most apparent in the psychiatric hospitals and institutions where, as one doctor who appears in this program puts it, "there is an over-representation of black people." There is also a problem of misdiagnosis and mistreatment because some medical staff don't understand why people from different cultures behave contrary to their expectations. This program looks at the issues of racism in mental health care, and at some black self-help groups that offer alternatives to the conventional psychiatric practices that have failed to meet the needs of the black community.

Out of Sight, Out of Mind. PBS. Episode two traces the rise and fall of the asylum, from the establishment of asylums during the Enlightenment, through the high point of Victorian reformist optimism, to the decline of the asylum in the twentieth century. The hour concludes by raising the impact of the pharmacological revolution of the 1950s and 1960s and civil rights reforms of the 1960s as reasons for the current policy of deinstitutionalization.

The Scandal of Psychiatric Hospitals. FHS. While mentally ill patients are being discharged because their insurance benefits have expired, perfectly healthy Americans are being locked up in mental hospitals while the hospital draws their insurance. This program shows how one group of hospitals herded up patients and held healthy Americans unnecessarily hostage; it also shows how bona fide psychiatrists are tempted or duped and how law enforcement agencies are trying to restore psychiatry to its role as a healing profession, not a business.

To Define True Madness. PBS. This first episode examines past misconceptions and modern myths: how mental illness has been confused with neurological disease, moral judgments, deceptive appearances, and cultural stereotypes. The program discusses how mental illness looks to others now and in the past, how it has been misrepresented in art and literature, how it feels to those who experience it, and how it is diagnosed by doctors and psychiatrists.

Using Movies and Mental Illness as a Teaching Tool

Many of your students will have already seen *One Flew Over the Cuckoo's Nest*, and those that haven't seen it should. It is one of the finest films of all time, and a wonderful springboard for class discussions of personality disorders, legal and forensic issues, politics and power in psychiatric hospitals, electroconvulsive therapy, psychosurgery, and the right to refuse treatment.

All students in an abnormal psychology class should watch *Cuckoo's Nest* in its entirety while they are taking the course. If vignettes are used in the classroom, the instructor may want to consider excerpts from *Chattahoochee* (i.e., the shooting episode that leads to arrest and eventual confinement), some of the courtroom scenes from *Nuts*, or the ECT scenes from *An Angel at My Table* or *Francis*. Films like *A Fine Madness* illustrate the abuse of psychiatric power that sometimes occurred with lobotomies.

Another classic film that will be of interest but perhaps unknown to a new generation of students is *A Clockwork Orange*. The novel and film both raise important philosophical questions that we have still not entirely resolved. The film serves as an excellent vehicle to take students to some of the ethical and policy issues they will confront as citizens.

Specific ethical dilemmas associated with psychotherapy and duel relationships are present in films like *Prince of Tides* and *Mr. Jones*. *Rampage* addresses the not guilty by reason of insanity (NGRI) defense and its potential for abuse. In general, students enjoy viewing these films and discussing and debating the ethical and legal issues they raise.

Movie	Link to Chapter	Page Reference to Wedding and Boyd
• Nuts	civil commitment (p. 531)	p. 165
• One Flew Over the Cuckoo's Nest • Chattahoochee • Equus • The Snake Pit	patient rights (p. 537)	p. 163 p. 163 p. 171 p. 172
• Nuts • Chattahoochee	power and mental health (p. 541)	p. 165 p. 163

Classroom Assessment Techniques (CAT)

Memory Matrix (CAT 18-1)
Students should use the handout provided to review the various legal tests for insanity.

Minute Paper (CAT 18-2)
Ask your students to write about an important question they have that remains unanswered.

"I Understand/I Don't Understand" (CAT 18-3)
Ask your students to divide a piece of notebook paper into two. One side is labeled "I understand" and students should write down on this side topics, concepts, and principles they understand. On the other side, labeled "I don't understand," those topics, concepts, topics, and principles that are not understood should be indicated

Suggestions for Essay Questions

- Describe legal tests of insanity presented in the chapter.
- Differentiate between the insanity defense and competency to stand trial.
- If you are mental health professional, what factors should you take into account as standards for civil commitment.
- How did the case *Wyatt v. Stickney* influence patient rights?

Memory Matrix
Classroom Assessment Technique

Legal tests of insanity	Date and historical case	Description	Effect on plea

Chapter 19

Prevention and Social Change

Chapter Map

Section	Instructor Manual Components
What is Prevention?	*The vagrant gaze web site (LL 19-1)* *Primary prevention (TP 19-1)* *"Just Say No!" (TP 19-2)* *Tertiary prevention (TP 19-3)*
The History of the Prevention Movement	
Risk Reduction vs. Facilitation of Resilience	*Resilience in at-risk children (LL 19-2)* *Clinical vs. community psychologist (TP 19-4)*
Risk Reduction Programs • Risk Reduction from a Developmental Perspective • A Model Risk Reduction Program: FAST Track • How Effective Are These Programs?	*Confidentiality and prevention (LL 19-3)* *Principles of successful early intervention (LL 19-4)* *Noise exposure creates environmental stress (LL 19-5)* *Work site wellness promotion program (TP 19-5)* *Guide to community resources (ACT/DEMO 19-1)* *Researching prevention programs (ACT/DEMO 19-2)*
Mental Health Promotion	*Service learning as social change (TP 19-6)*
Social Change	*Background knowledge probe (ACT/DEMO 19-3)*

Chapter Outline

I. Introduction
  A. Since the 1960s some have thought that best way to form a mentally healthy society was to change social institutions for the better
    1. One aspect of social change is **prevention**, a focus on keeping disorders from beginning in the first place by changing the environment, family, or individual
    2. Many advocates of social change are also pioneers of the prevention movement
  B. Prevention has enjoyed a renaissance in 1990s

II. What is Prevention?
  A. **Primary prevention** is preventing mental disorders from developing in the first place
    1. Create environments that are conducive to mental health
    2. Make individuals strong enough to avoid risk factors
    3. Teach skills to people that allow them to cope with risk factors
    4. Designed to impact an entire population
  B. **Secondary prevention** focuses on reducing risk for mental disorder in individuals who are most likely to develop that disorder
    1. High-risk population must be identified
    2. An intervention is applied to that population
    3. **Universal prevention** targets entire population as everyone would benefit from intervention
    4. **Selective preventive interventions** are aimed at subgroup whose risk is higher than average
    5. **Indicated preventive interventions** focuses on individuals who have early signs of disorder or biological marker indicating risk for disorder
    6. Goals of prevention have broadened
    7. **Mental health promotion** can be thought of as enhancement of individual's well-being
    8. Prevention covers full range of interventions and can occur inside variety of setting

III. The History of the Prevention Movement
  A. During 1960s people started to think about prevention and related issues
  B. National Institute of Labor Education (1963) recommended establishment of community mental health centers, giving access to human facilities near neighborhoods
  C. Important books led to some proposed changes
    1. Patient care and diagnoses had little relationship to another; SES determined type of treatment received

475

2.   Mental health professional should be accessible to all people
D.   Barriers emerged to proposed changes
        1.   Joint Commission on Mental Health and Illness (1961)
                recommended continued emphasis on treatment and rejected
                primary prevention
        2.   Implementation was more difficult in practice than in theory
        3.   Community mental health movement disappeared by mid 1970s
E.   Secondary prevention has become dominant
        1.   Early interventions with high-risk populations become most
                promising method
        2.   Focus on social context produced **community psychology,** which
                examines communities rather than individuals
F.   Despite good intentions, the transition from scientist-practitioners to social
        change agents never articulated well
        1.   Clinical psychology unable or unwilling to move from a defect
                model of mental illness to a contextual model
        2.   Goal of contextual model is to eliminate mental illness but also to
                create mental health
        3.   Primary prevention assumes that mental health and illnesses were
                caused largely by environmental stress
        4.   In 1990s a growing emphasis on biological causation seen in
                prevention field

IV.   Risk Reduction vs. Facilitation of Resilience
        A.   Prevention programs tend to be implemented in schools, homes, and
                communities of high-risk individuals focusing on early intervention
        B.   In 1990s primary prevention has come to mean strengthening people
                resilience, which is their ability to cope with stressful environments
        C.   Compared to risk reduction, increasing resilience refers to working with
                population to help people cope more effectively with such environments
        D.   Prevention means both risk reduction and facilitating resilience in general
                population

V.   Risk Reduction Programs
        A.   With regard to schizophrenia, research indicates continued use of
                medications plus relapse reduction programs
        B.   Risk Reductions from a Developmental Perspective
                1.   Many early interventions involve children and adolescents
                2.   Secondary prevention can continue into adulthood
                3.   The skills needed to prevent new or recurring disorders shift at
                        each stage of life
                4.   Risk Reduction in Infants
                        a.   Physical health influences mental health

476

b. High quality care during pregnancy and postbirth and improved parenting decrease risk of violence during adolescence

5. Risk Reduction in Young Children
   a. Acquiring language skills and learning impulse control reduce young children's risk for later mental illness
   b. Head Start is most famous early childhood program

6. Risk Reduction for Elementary-Age Children
   a. Academically deficient or socially incompetent children are by fourth grade at high risk for several psychological disturbances
   b. Family conflict, bad parenting, neglect contribute to risk
   c. Most programs focus on children
   d. One program has successfully taught children important skills
      i. Social competence
      ii. Communicating more effectively with teachers
      iii. Preventing antisocial behavior

7. Risk Reduction in Adults
   a. Many types of intervention with adults show promise in reducing risk of various mental disorders
   b. It is easier to prevent marital problems than to treat them once they have developed
   c. Occupational programs help people cope with stress of losing a job and finding a new one
   d. Support groups for adults who provide care for aging parents are helpful in reducing risks

8. Risk Reduction in Elderly People
   a. Challenges of aging all generate health risks
   b. Programs for facing bereavement received great deal of attention and appears to be effective

9. A Model Risk Reduction Program: FAST Track
   a. FAST track is multifaceted risk reduction program for conduct disorders
   b. Program is designed to prevent young mothers from developing depression, which is related to conduct disorders
   c. Targets groups in schools, families, neighborhoods, and other sources of risk
      i. Attempts to get parents involved in child's school system from first day
      ii. Focuses on reading
      iii. Fosters development of friendships through social skills

                iv.   Directly teaches children how to express emotions in nonaggressive ways

                v.   Makes sure every child has same-sex role model

        d.   Results of project will not be clear until children are teenagers, but does seem to keep families in program

        e.   Cost of program may be prohibitive on a nationwide basis

    10.   How Effective Are These Programs?

        a.   Only well-replicated positive benefits are for programs with children and adolescents

        b.   The clinical significance of these programs is still an open question

VI.   Mental Health Promotion

    A.   Mental health is not just absence of mental illness

        1.   Mentally healthy person functions well physically, socially, and spiritually

        2.   Purpose of mental health promotion is to enhance competence, self-esteem, resilience, and sense of well-being rather than to prevent mental disorders

    B.   Efficacy of these programs is unknown

        1.   Many aspects of health promotion do not fall into category of prevention

        2.   Some programs may be harmful

    C.   Concepts of wellness have been historically associated with primary prevention focused on the individual

VII.   Social Change

    A.   Prevention science has created a continuum of interventions

    B.   Primary prevention now emphasizes programs based on overcoming risk and bolstering resilience within individuals, not on social change

    C.   Universal prevention programs have many goals

        1.   Foster better relations between parent and child

        2.   Train participants in problem solving

        3.   Teach individuals how to modify their own environments

        4.   Make use of the term empowerment, meaning helping traditionally powerless groups take control of their lives

    D.   Some have suggested that progressive social change is unlikely to be initiated by groups with interest in preserving status quo

    E.   Many argue that abnormal psychology is inherently political

    F.   Major criticism is that there are not enough prevention programs because of lack of funds

Chapter Boxes

- The Penn Optimism Project
  - A. Many young people experience depression by age 21
  - B. The time to intervene in majority of cases would be prior to age 15
  - C. Effective prevention programs for adolescent depression are just being developed
  - D. Penn Optimism Project reported some success in preventing the incidence of depressive symptoms in fifth and sixth graders
  - E. Program based on cognitive therapy for depression and problem-solving skills

- Prevention of Smoking by the Mass Media and Schools
  - A. Single risk behavior most responsible for disease and mortality in United States is cigarette smoking
  - B. Best way to avoid effects of smoking is never to begin the habit
  - C. During 1970s and 1980s educational programs to discourage adolescent smoking focused on hazards of smoking and how to resist pressures from peers; preventing smoking tended not to last into later adolescent years
  - D. Media messages maintain effects of school-based prevention programs
  - E. Effect is to change students' perceptions about the acceptability of smoking

- Preventing Childhood Disorders
  - A. It is hard to guard children against psychological disturbances as long as they are exposed to social conditions that breed such problems
  - B. In children, some measure of psychological disturbance is due to heredity
  - C. Large percentage of American children are being exposed daily to environmental conditions that foster psychological disorders
  - D. We need to invest more in genetic counseling, prenatal care, and control of environmental toxins

Learning Objectives (LO)

By the time on have finished studying this chapter, you should be able to do the following:

1.   Define and give examples of primary, secondary universal, selective, and
      indicated prevention, and distinguish between disorder prevention and health
      promotion (546-551).

2.   Trace the history of disorder prevention / health promotion from the 1960s to the
      present, making reference to the community mental health movement and
      community psychology (550-553).

3.   Describe and give examples of risk reduction programs for infants. preschoolers,
      school-age children, adults. and the elderly, and cite data illustrating the need for
      such programs (553-557).

4.   Summarize proposals for mental health promotion measures and discuss how such
      measures might be carried out (557-558).

5.   Describe how prevention is approached in terms of social change, and summarize
      the debate between those who would promote well-being through social change
      and those who would do it by enhancing the ability of the individual to cope with
      the existing environment (558-559).

Lecture Leads (LL)

The vagrant gaze web site (LL 19-1)

Consider developing a "visual" lecture. There is a web site that includes the photography of the homeless of New York City; disposable cameras were given to people who were panhandling on the streets. They were asked to take pictures of things that were important to them. They were also paid $20. The photographs on the web site convey what it means to be homeless, as well as giving the homeless a venue for creativity and self-expression. Consider downloading these photos and presenting them as you discuss the issues raised in Chapter 19.

Resource:
http://www.geocities.com/~mattcook/

Resilience in at-risk children (LL 19-2)

The concept of resilience has captured much attention in recent years. Many children who possess multiple risk factors (e.g., poverty, poor health care) for various psychological and physical disorders, and drop out of school, succeed in school and mature into competent adults. There are certain characteristics of children, families, and schools that increase the likelihood children develop resilience. These characteristics are often summarized in three themes: relationships that are caring and supporting, high expectations, and meaningful participation. For instance, school and teachers in particular have great potential to foster resilience in these at-risk youths. The literature strongly suggests the importance of a "favorite teacher" from whom at-risk students can get guidance and support.. High expectations, often communicated by teachers and school, are critical in developing resilience. In fact, high expectations are related to higher academic success and lower rates of teen pregnancy, drug abuse, and dropping out. Finally, students who experience significant involvement and responsibility in school tend to develop resilience. In the classroom, involvement occurs when students engage in active, hands-on learning, cooperative learning, service learning, and cross-age mentoring.

Resources:

Benard, B. (1991). Fostering resiliency in kids: Protective factors in the family, school, and community. San Francisco: Far West Laboratory for Educational Research and Development.

Edmonds, R. (1986). Characteristics of effective schools. In U. Neisser (ed.)., The school achievement of minority children: New perspectives. Hillsdale, NJ: Lawrence Erlbaum.

Garmezy, N. (1991). Resiliency and vulnerability to adverse developmental outcomes associated with poverty. American Behavioral Scientist, 34, 416-430.

Werner, E., and R. Smith. (1989). Vulnerable but invincible: A longitudinal study of resilient children and youth. New York: Adams, Bannister, and Cox.

Werner, E., and R. Smith. (1992). Overcoming the odds: High-risk children from birth to adulthood. New York: Cornell University Press.

Confidentiality and prevention (LL 19-3)

It is reasonable to assume that before individuals at risk can benefit from prevention programs they must learn to trust mental health care and primary care professionals. At particular risk for psychological disorders are adolescents. If they sense a lack of confidentiality and trust with their physicians and other practitioners, their willingness to seek future health care for sensitive problems will be diminished. Ford et al. compared how two types of guarantees of confidentiality influenced adolescents' willingness and openness to discuss sensitive issues. Subjects were 562 adolescents attending three suburban public high schools in California. Subjects were assigned to one of three groups and then listened to an audio vignette of an office visit. In the office visit, the physician asked the patients about their medical history and then prefaced the questions that followed with a statement regarding the questions' sensitive nature. One group of subjects heard the physician give an unconditional guarantee of confidentiality even from the patient's parents. A second group heard a conditional guarantee of confidentiality; confidentiality would be broken if the physician believed that patient was being abused or poised a suicide risk. The third group heard no assurance of confidentiality. Subjects then anonymously completed a questionnaire assessing their willingness to share personal, sensitive information to the physician depicted on the audiotape. In addition, subjects indicated their willingness to seek future health care from that physician. Results indicated that subjects who were given assurances of confidentiality were more likely to disclose personal information (46.5%) compared to no assurances (39%). Subjects who received assurances of confidentiality were also more likely to seek health care in the future (67%) than those not receiving the assurance. Subjects who received an unconditional confidentiality were the most likely to seek health care (72%). The authors conclude that physicians who assure confidentiality are more likely to receive disclosure and health care visits from adolescents.

Resource:

Ford, C. A., Millstein, S. G., Halpern-Felsher, B. L., & Irwin, C. E., Jr. (1997). Influence of physician confidentiality assurances on adolescents' willingness to disclose information and seek future health care. Journal of the American Medical Association, 278, 1029-1034.

Principles of successful early intervention (LL 19-4)

In a review of early intervention programs, Ramey and Ramey present six principles of effective programs. Principle 1: Principle of developmental timing--Effective programs tend to provide intervention early in a child's development. Principle 2: Principle of program intensity--Programs with significant active contact between staff, parents, and children were more effective. Principle 3: Principle of direct provision of learning experiences--Programs that give children direct learning experience, rather than indirect learning experiences through parental training, are more effective. Principle 4--Principle of program breadth and flexibility--Larger effects are generally seen in programs that provide comprehensive services such as assistance with food, housing, health care, and employment. Principle 5: Principle of individual differences in program benefits--Individual children respond differently to early interventions suggesting some type of person-environment interaction. Principle 6: Principle of ecological dominion and environmental maintenance of development--Any gains that are not continually supported tend to disappear. Effective programs recognize this tendency and provide appropriate support services.

Resource:
Ramey, C. T., & Ramey, S. L. (1998). Early intervention and early experience. American Psychologist, 53, 109-120.

Noise exposure creates environmental stress (LL 19-5)
A two-year study was conducted by Evans et al. to examine the effects of chronic exposure to aircraft noise among 217 third- and fourth-graders living near an international airport in Germany. Prior to the airport's opening baseline measures on blood pressure and stress hormone levels were collected. After 18 months of airport operations the same measures were taken. The results indicate increases in blood pressures and stress hormone levels, specifically epinephrine, cortisol, and norepinephrine. The authors point out that high level of stress hormones may lead to heart disease, high cholesterol, and low immune-cell count. There is some evidence that chronic noise can also have a detrimental impact on reading and listening skills.

Resource
Evans, G. W. et al. (1998). Chronic noise exposure and physiological response: A prospective study of children living under environmental stress. Psychological Science, 9, 75-77.

Talking Points (TP)

Primary prevention (TP 19-1)
An apple a day keeps the doctor away is an example of primary prevention.

"Just Say No!" (TP 19-2)
A primary prevention program was developed during the Reagan administration to address drug abuse. It was the "Just Say No!" campaign. Ask students to consider if a simply slogan was or could be effective?

Tertiary prevention (TP 19-3)
In addition to primary and secondary prevention, there is a third level of prevention, tertiary prevention. This level provides support and assistance to those who are returning to the community after treatment or hospitalization. A good example of this level of prevention would be halfway houses where patients are given some structure as they make the transition from an institution to the community.

Clinical vs. community psychologist (TP 19-4)
Here's a difference that distinguishes the approach and training of clinical psychologists and community psychology. Typically, the clients are typically brought to clinical psychologists. The community psychologist takes a more active role and seeks out clients.

Work site wellness promotion program (TP 19-5)
Your college or university is likely to have a wellness program that emphasizes both physical and psychological wellness. Briefly present this program as an example of an institutional prevention program.

Service learning as social change (TP 19-6)
The recent emphasis on service learning is a nice example of education's attempt to participate in social change. Service learning refers to placing students in community sites where they can apply their academic knowledge to real-life and to help others. Consider asking students to tell about their service learning or volunteer activities.

484

Cross-Cultural Teaching

protests against the **Vietnam war**, and the "**consciousness raising**"...	p. 546
Prevention is enjoying a **renaissance**.	p. 547
following it up with **postnatal mental health care**...	p. 547
smoking appear "**cool**"...	p. 551
There were the **blue prints** to create a society...	p. 552
No **road map** was ever provided for clinical psychologists...	p. 552
there is a **constellation** of risk factors...	p. 556
These programs exist in schools, in **HMOs**...	p. 557
proposed talking "**baby steps**"...	p. 559

Activities and Demonstrations (ACT/DEMO)

Guide to community resources (ACT/DEMO 19-1)
Objective: To identify available community resources
Materials: None
Procedure: After students form small groups, inform them that their task is to develop a presentation that would summarize community resources. Assign certain types or functions of community agencies to the groups. For example, one group may want to focus on children or women or aged, literacy, violence, food and nutrition, health (e.g., immunization), education, or environmental issues (e.g., drinking water, recycling, cleaning up). The report should give others a sense of the history of agency/program, goals of agency/program, structure and organization of agency, and the staff of the agency/program. In addition, the report should examine how the agencies/programs focus on prevention/treatment, emphasis of strengths and competencies of clients, respect for diversity of clients, empowerment, focus on social change, and building sense of community. Sources should include interview of staff and clients, articles, and pamphlets.
Discussion: After all groups have given their presentation ask for volunteers to collate the information into some coherent form and publish it or post it to a web site. You may wish to augment this activity by requiring students to identify additional funding sources for these agencies/programs.

Researching prevention programs (ACT/DEMO 19-2)
Objective: To involve students in a library literature research of a prevention program
Materials: None.
Procedure: This project requires that the instructor divide students into groups of four to five members each. Students in each group are asked to select a prevention program. In conjunction with other group members, they are to do an extensive literature review of that disorder. Students are asked to write a 5 to10 page literature review and to present an oral report to the class on their disorder.
Discussion: This project has several positive aspects. First, it gets students involved with an actual prevention program. Second, it familiarizes students with the use of library facilities when writing research papers. Third, this project acquaints students with the journals and literature of the field of abnormal psychology. Finally, this project provides students with an update of the field of prevention.

Background knowledge probe (ACT/DEMO 19-3)
Objective: To assess the breadth and depth of knowledge that your students have developed
Materials: Background Knowledge Probe Handout
Procedure: To create closure, re-administer the Background Knowledge Probe that you gave students at the beginning of the term.
Discussion: The responses can be very helpful to you for revising the course. It will also help students to get a sense of just how much they have learned.

Films and Videos

Abnormal Behavior. A Mental Hospital. MCG. A documentary about treatment in a mental hospital. Gives students an overview of treatment concerns and diagnostic issues.

An Ounce of Prevention. The World of Abnormal Psychology. ANN/CPB. Discusses prevention in abnormal psychology.

Committed in Error- The Mental Health System Gone Mad. FHS. This is the story of a man who spent 66 years incarcerated and forgotten in a British mental health institutions, although there was never anything wrong with him.

Diverting the Mentally Ill From Jail FHS. the problems of incarcerating the mentally ill in jails and the benefits of placing them into community-based mental health programs.

Larry. FHS. The subject was mistakenly institutionalized and now must struggle to overcome years of cruel treatment.

New Race and Psychiatry. FHS. The issue of race within psychiatry is at its most apparent in the psychiatric hospitals and institutions where, as one doctor who appears in this program puts it, "there is an over-representation of black people." There is also a problem of misdiagnosis and mistreatment because some medical staff don't understand why people from different cultures behave contrary to their expectations.

Out of Sight, Out of Mind. PBS. Episode two traces the rise and fall of the asylum, from the establishment of asylums during the Enlightenment, through the high point of Victorian reformist optimism, to the decline of the asylum in the twentieth century. The hour concludes by raising the impact of the pharmacological revolution of the 1950s and 1960s and civil rights reforms of the 1960s as reasons for the current policy of deinstitutionalization.

The Scandal of Psychiatric Hospitals. FHS. This program shows how one group of hospitals herded up patients and held healthy Americans unnecessarily hostage; it also shows how bona fide psychiatrists are tempted or duped and how law enforcement agencies are trying to restore psychiatry to its role as a healing profession, not a business.

To Define True Madness. PBS. This first episode examines past misconceptions and modern myths: how mental illness has been confused with neurological disease, moral judgments, deceptive appearances, and cultural stereotypes. The program discusses how mental illness looks to others now and in the past, how it has been misrepresented in art and literature, how it feels to those who experience it, and how it is diagnosed by doctors and psychiatrists.

Using Movies and Mental Illness as a Teaching Tool

There are few films appropriate to the specific content of this chapter. We recommend finishing up the semester by letting your class see and discuss, in its entirety, one of the major films discussed during the semester. *A Clockwork Orange* (137 minutes) and *One Flew Over the Cuckoo's Nest* (133 minutes) are excellent ways to end the course, although some students may feel the violence in *A Clockwork Orange* is a bit gratuitous.

Classroom Assessment Techniques (CAT)

One-Sentence Summary (CAT 19-1)
Ask student to summarize a specific piece of information in this chapter by responding to the question, "Who does/did what to whom, when, where, how and why?"

Focused Listing (CAT 19-2)
Select an important point from this chapter (e.g., primary prevention, secondary prevention, universal prevention) and ask students to write five words or phrases that describe the point.

Minute Paper (CAT 19-3)
Ask your students to write about an important question they have that remains unanswered.

Suggestions for Essay Questions

- ❑ What role does prevention play in abnormal psychology?
- ❑ Contrast primary prevention and secondary prevention.
- ❑ Describe the FAST track program presented in the chapter.
- ❑ How might psychology promote social change?

Background Knowledge Probe
Handout

For each term, indicate your degree of understanding using the following scale:

1 - I have heard of this
2 - I have heard of this, but can't really say what it means
3 - I have heard of this and have some general idea of what it means
4 - I have heard of this and could explain it to someone

medical model	1	2	3	4
psychiatrist	1	2	3	4
norms	1	2	3	4
deinstitutionalization	1	2	3	4
DSM-IV	1	2	3	4
test-retest reliability	1	2	3	4
comorbidity	1	2	3	4
mental status exam	1	2	3	4
medical model	1	2	3	4
ABAB design	1	2	3	4
incidence	1	2	3	4
defense mechanism	1	2	3	4
id	1	2	3	4
diathesis	1	2	3	4
genotype	1	2	3	4
monozygotic twins	1	2	3	4
panic disorder	1	2	3	4
generalized anxiety disorder	1	2	3	4
dissociative amnesia	1	2	3	4
migraine headache	1	2	3	4
premorbid adjustment	1	2	3	4
mania	1	2	3	4
antisocial personality disorder	1	2	3	4
detoxification	1	2	3	4
paraphilia	1	2	3	4
positive symptoms	1	2	3	4
flat affect	1	2	3	4
clanging	1	2	3	4
expressed emotions	1	2	3	4
Alzheimer's disease	1	2	3	4
might terrors	1	2	3	4
PKU	1	2	3	4

Appendix A
List of Film and Video Sources

The following is a list of resources where films and videos may be rented or purchased:

AIM - Association of Instructional Materials, 600 Madison Avenue, New York, NY 10022

AEF - American Educational Films, 132 Lashky Drive, Beverly Hills, CA 90212

AVC - Audio-Visual Center, Indiana University, Bloomington, IN 47401

CBS - Columbia Broadcasting System, 51 West 52nd Street, New York, NY 10019

CDI - Cambridge Documentary Films, P.O. Box 385, Cambridge, MA 02139

CM - Concept Media, P.O. Box 19542, Irvine, CA 92714

CPB - Annenberg/CPB Project, P.O. Box 2345, South Burlington, VT 05407-2345

CRM - CRM Films, Del Mar, CA 92014

EMC - Extension Media Center, University of California, Berkeley, CA 94720

FI - Focus International, Inc., 3 East 54th Street, New York, NY 10022

FSH - Film Series for the Humanities, Box 2053, Princeton, NJ 08540

HR - Harper & Row, 10 East 53rd Street, New York, NY 10022

HRM - Human Relations Media (current address not available)

HSC- Health Science Consortium, 103 Laurel Avenue, Corroboro, NC 27510

IU - Audio-Visual Center, Division of University Extension, Indiana University, Bloomington, IN 47401

MEDCOM Inc. - 1633 Broadway, New York, NY 10019

MG - Media Guild - Box 881, 118 South Acacia, Solana Beach, CA 92075

McGraw-Hill - 575 Boylston Street, Boston, MA 02116

MIT - MIT Teleprograms, Inc., 420 Academy Drive., Northbrook, IL 60062

NAMH - National Association for Mental Health, Film Library, 267 West 25th Street, New York, NY

NMAC - National Medical Audiovisual Center, 2111 Plaster Bridge Road, Atlanta, GA 30324

PBS - PBS Video, 1320 Braddock Place, Alexandria, VA 22314-1698

PCR - Psychological Films Distribution Center, 1215 East Chapman, Orange, CA 92669

PSU - Penn State University, Audiovisual Services, 17 Willard Building, University Park, PA 16802

PSCHF - Psychological Films, 189 North Wheeler Street, Orange, CA 92669

PTL - Public Television Library, 475 L'Enfant Plaza, SW, Washington, DC 20024

RP - Research Press, Box 3177, Department J, Champaign, IL 61821

TLF - Time-Life Multimedia, 100 Eisenhower Drive, P.O. Box 648, Paramus, NJ 07652

UA - United Artists Studios, 729 7th Avenue, New York, NY 10019

UCEMC - University of California Extension Media Center, Film Distributor, 2223 Fulton Street, Berkeley, CA 94720

UT - University of Texas, Film Division, Austin, TX 78712

Wiley - John Wiley & Sons, 605 Third Avenue, New York, NY 10016

WNET-TV - 356 West 58th Street, New York, NY 10011

Appendix B
Integrating Multimedia in the Psychology Classroom

Part I: Building Your Own Course Web Page

Why invest the time?

Here are **four** compelling reasons:

➤ **It opens another channel of communication with your students**. Many students do not have the confidence to raise questions in class. Some lack the confidence to ask questions directly during scheduled office hours. A course web site with built in e-mail links can address these challenges. It provides students with a means of asking questions in a non-threatening environment

➤ **It can be a means of incorporating more real life applications into the course via links to news stories on the web**. Most print based publications also have a significant on-line presence. If you find something in a newspaper, magazine, journal or periodical that you think adds relevance and interest to a topic you are covering, check to see if there is an electronic version of the article and link to it.

➤ **It can improve student performance**. A recent article in Chronicle of Higher Education focussed on the work of Professor Gerald Schutte at California State University, Northridge who found that students in the on-line section of his statistics course performed better on average than his regular lecture students. The answer, it seems, lies in the peer collaboration that takes place in an on-line environment. "Because students in the virtual class had no face-to-face contact with their professor, they compensated by working together in study groups. Dr. Schutte concluded that that collaboration had helped the students learn their lessons more effectively."

➤ **It can save paper (trees)**. Think about how many handouts you are currently making and distributing in class. What if students could access your course web site and download these for themselves?

What to put on it

Developing a successful web site has more to do with good design and planning than with lots and lots of content. Content is important though and putting your lecture notes on your web site is one valuable resource that will benefit you students. Other things you may want to include are:

Lecture Outlines
Weekly Readings and References
Assignments
Links to valuable web sites
Quizzes
Contact Information – Voice Mail, E-mail, , Office Hours
Personal Information - Research Interests, Current Projects

Putting this all together in an attractive and intuitive manner can be challenging but it is important. Your web site is a reflection of you and your course – it should have your personality.
This can make a big difference in the success of the site. We won't get into serious design discussions here, we'll leave that for the advanced class. However, the site should be clean and uncluttered, easy to navigate, be visually pleasing, not too dark, avoid distractions (animated gif's like flashing lights) and heavy graphics (graphics files that are large require a long time to download). The design can be the difference between a site that is just a mild success and one that becomes an integral part of the course.

Tips & Tricks

♦ Make the site part of the class, not an extension
♦ Distribute assignments via the web site
♦ Place weekly tests or quizzes on the web site
♦ Use it as a communication tool

Maintenance & Updating

This is one of the greatest challenges with web sites, but it is important. These are "living" documents. They need proper care and maintenance and require regular updates and the occasional face-lift to keep them fresh. If your web site is going to become an integral part of your course you need to keep it up-to–date and dynamic. Students need proof that each time they come to class "virtually" they are not going to see the same "virtual" lecture.

Developing a Site with McGraw-Hill's Page Out

PageOut! is an easy and intelligent HTML authoring tool designed specifically for faculty interested in developing their own course Web pages. With built-in style templates, the **PageOut!** program leads you through the development of the key components of successful course web pages. Simply type the required information into the appropriate text windows or copy and paste information from other word processing programs. When the information is complete, save the course file, and then click on the "Publish" command to create the HTML files. The files can then be File Transferred Protocoled to their appropriate web space or e-mailed to a systems administrator for posting to the web.

PageOut! creates graphically pleasing and professional web pages for faculty and requires no experience or knowledge of HTML programming. It is an ideal program for faculty who want to create an on-line presence for their course without the anguish of learning and writing html code. **PageOut!** is free to adopters of McGraw-Hill textbooks and learning materials.

Program Instructions:

1. To start the program, choose **PageOut!** from the Programs group in the Windows95 Start menu.

2. Choose an item from the Style menu to select a template for the course web site

3. Customize the template by typing information in the program text fields. Information is divided into 6 groups separated by tabs.

4. Click on the **Home Page** tab and type the name of the course (e.g. Developmental Psychology) in the Course Title field. Type the section (e.g. 101) in the Course Section field.

5. Click on the **Syllabus** tab and type the syllabus information in these fields: Required Materials, Course Goals, Policies and Procedures, Course Schedule.

6. Click on the **Lecture Notes** tab. This is where you would type in lecture notes that are organized by date. In the Page Description Text field, type a description of the information contained in this page (e.g. Week 1: Lecture and Discussion Topics). In the Date field, type the date for the class meeting that will cover these lecture notes. In the Notes field, type the topics covered, required reading, and other items that usually go in the daily lesson plan. Click the ADD button to add more lecture notes. Click on the Previous and Next buttons to view and edit existing lecture notes.

7. Click on the **Bookmarks** tab. This is where you would put useful web links and their URL's (web addresses). You can add links to web sites and pages that contain information about their course. These links can also go to sites that help the students learn more about the Internet. In the Description field, type the name or description of the web link (e.g. McGraw-Hill Web Site). In the URL field, type the web address for the web link (e.g. http://www.mhhe.com) Click the ADD button to add more web links. Click on the Previous and Next buttons to view and edit existing web links.

8. Click on the **Instructor** tab to type the instructor's contact information. Type the name in the Instructor's Name field. In the Page Description Text field, type a short description of the information contained in this page (e.g. Please use the following information to contact me regarding assignments and course materials.). Type the instructor's office hours, phone number, fax number and e-mail address in their corresponding text fields. Use the Additional text field to type in any extra information about contacting the instructor (e.g. If you are unable to attend a session, please contact me prior to the session.).

9. Click on the **Assignments** tab to type information on exams and assignments. In the Page Description Text field, type a description of the information contained in this page (e.g. This page contains times, dates, and the materials covered in exams.). In the Exam Name and Date field, type the name of the exam and the date on which it will be taken. In the Materials Covered field, type a description of the materials (e.g. chapter or page numbers) covered by the test or assignment. Click the ADD button to add more tests or assignments. Click on the Previous and Next buttons to view and edit existing ones.

10. Choose Save As from the File menu to save the current course section information. Type the name of the course and click OK. This will allow you to edit the site at a later date. Note: To view or edit an existing site, choose Open from the File menu, select the course name and click OK.

11. Choose Publish from the File menu. Click to select all of the checkboxes in the Publish dialog box. Click on the "..." button to specify a disk or directory to save the HTML (Web) pages and copy their associated graphic files. Click Publish to create the course web pages.

12. After you have published the pages, you must put them out on a Web server so that people can access them. If you have a school Web site, it is recommended that you contact your System Administrator or Webmaster for help in putting your **PageOut!** HTML pages online. If you or your institution does not have a Web server, it is recommended that you sign up for an on-line service or get a dial-up Internet account from a local Internet service provider. Most of these accounts have a small amount of server space for registered users, and a prescribed way of getting your pages/graphics onto the site.

Part II: Presentation Manager – Managing the Media

The McGraw-Hill Presentation Manager CD-ROM allows you to maximize the supplemental media that accompanies our Introductory Psychology texts. The Presentation Manager provides you with an easy to use interface through which you can design and deliver multimedia presentations for use in your class. With hundreds of Digital Images, Animations, PowerPoint slides, Lecture outlines, and Video clips, the Presentation Manager makes it easy for you to get the most out of our various media by allowing you to customize your own presentation and incorporate your own material.

The Presentation Manager CD-ROM organizes the instructor's support material into selected resource areas, for example, Instructors Manual w/ Lecture Outlines and Overviews, Activities and Projects, Image Bank, PowerPoint Slide Presentations, PRISM Interactive Exercises, Computerized Test Items, and Video Clips . An Instructor can work in each individual area, view and select the materials available. Once familiar with the available resources you can then operate in the Presentation Manager. This is the resource that really drives the program. The Presentation Manager allows you to develop a presentation utilizing slides, graphics, and video. The best thing about this resource is that you are not limited to utilizing the content of the CD-ROM to author your presentations. You can even take your own graphics and video and add them right into your presentation.

To begin building the presentation, just open a contact sheet and the presentation dialog boxes within the Presentation Manager window. Adding elements to the presentation is easy; just click and drag the element you wish to add, and drop it on the grid found in the left quarter of the presentation dialog box. If you wish to add your own elements to a presentation, simply select Add Images from the File menu. Once you have all the resource items in the position that you wish, you may view the presentation by selecting Presentation Preview from the Windows menu.

If you have the desire to incorporate multimedia technology into your lectures, the Presentation Manager will provide you with a powerful tool. Also, the Presentation Manager can also be used to link together the course material in an intuitive and helpful way for professors who simply wish to organize supplemental materials for the textbook, all in one small disk.

The Presentation Manager Resources

All of the available resources are listed in the Resources selection box. When you click on a resource, its description will appear in the Resource Description box at the bottom of the form. You can launch the resource by double clicking the item in the Resources list box or by clicking the Launch Resource button with the desired resource selected. Resources will normally include: Instructor's Manual, Computerized Test Bank, PowerPoint slides, and the Presentation Manager program.

Presentation Manager uses three forms to prepare and show lecture support presentations:

Asset Libraries:
These forms contain thumbnails of available images and videos. An asset library for each chapter of the textbook is included on the CD. You can copy and modify these asset libraries or create your own. You will use these as sources to build your presentations.

Presentation Builder Forms:
You assemble and sequence images and videos on the Presentation Builder form. You can use Drag and Drop, cut, copy, paste and move tools to arrange and rearrange your presentations.

Presentation Preview:
The Preview full screen window displays your presentation for your students. All images are displayed at their actual size in the sequence set in the Presentation Builder. Videos begin play as soon as they appear.

Other features include:

Print: To print Asset libraries and Presentations. The File - Print menu item will print the active asset library or presentation as a set of thumbnails with file names. The pages will be numbered and the name of the asset library or presentation will appear at the top of each page. You can use the setup option in the Print dialog box to select portrait or landscape page orientation.

Make HTML: To make an HTML document of your presentation so that it can be viewed with a Web Browser like Netscape Navigator or Microsoft Internet Explorer.

Status Bar: The Status Bar provides a constant stream of information about the resources being displayed and about the tools the mouse pointer is passing over. When the mouse pointer is positioned over screen elements the status bar will display actions that are available to you. It will also advise you of any actions being taken by the program.

Clip Form: The Clip Form displays details about the resource available for pasting. You can edit the name of the resource or add notes to the resource. The clip form contains a thumbnail and other information about resources that have been cut or copied and which now can be inserted in or appended to other asset libraries or presentations. The Clip is always available. Normally it is in minimized form. Click on it, and restore it to its normal size to view its contents.

There are several ways to put resources on the Clip. One of the easiest is to right-click on an image, either on an asset library or in a presentation. Right clicking is the same as Copying using the Edit-menu item, then displaying the Clip form. When you put an item on the Clip by right clicking you can modify the name of the item or the notes that accompany the item. If you do edit the resource information you must press the Update button to save it.

Whenever you put something on the Clip, the current contents are lost. So if you are cutting and inserting or appending, be sure to insert or append before you put something else on the Clip.

Presentation Viewer: You can use a combination of Export and the Presentation Viewer to create your presentation on one computer and play it back on another.

Asset libraries

Asset libraries provide a way to organize images and video clips visually so that you can easily review them and add them to your presentations.

McGraw-Hill has already made up an asset library for each chapter in the textbook. These asset libraries are locked so that you may always have them for reference.

You can make a copy of any of them giving the copy a new name like "Chapter 01 - Fall97". Then you can add or delete other visual resources to the asset library that apply.

Here are some things to do with or to an asset library and the actions to use:

Create a new Asset Library: Use the File - New Asset Library menu item to create a new blank asset library. The asset library is named Untitled until you give it a name as you save it using the Save Asset Library As menu command.

Open an existing Asset Library: Use the File - Open Asset Library menu item to open an existing asset library. When you click on this command a dialog box will be displayed, listing all of the asset libraries on your system. You can select an Asset Library by starting to type its name in the text box at the top of the form. The program will try to match what you type with the name of an asset library and select the closest match. Or you can scroll down the list and click on the asset library you want. Once an asset library is selected, click on the OK button to display it in the workspace. You can also remove unwanted asset libraries by selecting the one you want to delete and then clicking on the Delete button.

Add an Image to an Asset Library from a File: Use the File - Add Images menu item to import an image or video into the active asset library. You can use the following types of images with the Presentation Manager:

- JPEG (*.jpg) the McGraw-Hill images are of this type
- Bitmap (*.bmp) Windows native image format
- ZSoft (*.pcx) Corel Paint and other popular paint programs use this type of file
- TIFF (*.tif)
- Video (*.AVI) Video clip files

There is a drop down list box at the bottom left third of the form that allows you to restrict the types of files displayed in the file list box. By default all still image files will be displayed. If you are looking for Video files select files of type AVI in the drop down list. On the right third of the form is a preview picture box. If you check the Preview check box any time you select an image file in the file list box, a small version of the image will appear in the Preview image box.

If you select a video clip you can play it in the Preview box as well. When a video clip is selected additional controls appear below the Preview box:

- Pause: to stop at the current frame of video
- Play: to play the video clip from the current location
- Scroll Bar: to scan through the video clip.

The end arrows step one frame at a time; the bar next to the arrows step 10 frames at a time and you can drag the button to any place in the clip. When you select a video clip to add to your asset library, you can also select the frame that will be frozen to become the thumbnail. Use the Preview video controls to display the frame you want as the thumbnail. When you press OK, that frame will appear as the thumbnail on the asset library. If you do not preview the video the asset library will display the 20th frame of the video (many video clips fade up from black so the first frame would be blank.)

You can select more than one file to be added to the active asset library. There are two ways to make multiple selections:

❑ **Range:** To select a range of files Click on the first file to select it. Then scroll so that you can see the last file in the range. It can be above or below the file you already selected. Hold down the Shift key and click the last file in the range you want with the mouse. All of the files selected will be highlighted in the list and the file names will appear in the text box above the list.

❑ **Non-sequential:** To select several files that are not in sequence, Click on the first file you want, then hold down the Control key while you click on the rest of the files you want. All of the selected files will be highlighted and appear in the text box above the file list box.

Save an Asset Library: Use File - Save Asset Library As to give an asset library a new name or to save a new, untitled asset library. If you make changes to one of the asset libraries provided by McGraw-Hill you will not be able to save it without changing its name. Names are limited to 64 characters. You can use almost any printable characters and spaces. You can view the list of existing names by clicking on the Show List button. You can replace an existing asset library by selecting its name from the list. Then clicking OK. Since the name already exists and duplicate names are not permitted you will be asked to confirm that you want to replace the existing asset library. If you try to Save a new asset library, the Save Asset Library As form will be displayed automatically so that you can provide a name for your untitled asset library.

Close an Asset Library: Click on the System Menu box at the left end of the title bar of the asset library. When the system menu pops up click on the "Close" item.

The Presentation Builder

The Presentation Builder form is where you arrange your final presentation. McGraw-Hill has already made up a presentation for each chapter in the textbook. These presentations are locked so that you may always have them for reference. You can make a copy of any of them (use File - Save Presentation As), giving the copy a new name like "Chapter 01 - AM Section"

There are two layouts for the presentation form:

• *Image layout:* displays the current image in the large central picture box. You can view information about the current image in the panel below the main image. A thumbnail to the left of the main image displays the next image and the thumbnail on the right displays the previous image.

• *List layout:* Displays a list of all of the image filenames in the central box with the current image file location highlighted. The current image is displayed in the thumbnail on the right and the image available for pasting is the thumbnail on the left. The image information box below the central list box contains information about the current image.

In both layouts you will find a panel with a sequence of numbers in it that represents the presentation. Each number represents the image that occupies that position in the sequence. You can use this model of the presentation for dragging and dropping images into a specific position or as a way to quickly navigate from one part of the presentation to another. When you click on a number, it becomes the current image.

The buttons on the right of the central panel perform editing functions. Use the buttons below the central panel to move through the presentation.

Here are some things to do with or to a presentation using the Presentation Builder Form:

❖ **Create a new presentation**: Use the File - New Presentation menu item to create a new blank presentation. The presentation is named Untitled until you give it a name as you save it using the Save Presentation As menu command.

❖ **Open a presentation**: Use the File - Open Presentation menu item to open an existing presentation. When you click on this command a dialog box will be displayed, listing all of the presentations on your system. You can select a presentation by starting to type its name in the text box at the top of the form. The program will try to match what you type with the name of a presentation and select the closest match. Or you can scroll down the list and click on the one you want. Once a presentation is selected, click on the OK button to display it in a Presentation Builder form. You can also remove unwanted presentations by selecting the one you want to delete and then clicking on the Delete button.

❖ **Switch between Layouts**: The Image List button toggles the central display between the Presentation List and the Current image. The button is located below the central display panel and to the right of the navigation buttons. It will be labeled to indicate what the central display will become if the button is clicked. The thumbnails on either side of the central display are also changed when the buttons is clicked.

❖ **View the image in a certain position**: Use the navigation buttons to step one image at a time to the desired position. The image will appear in the Current image box. Click on the desired image position in the image number panel. Click on the image file name in the Resource Location List panel if visible.

❖ **View an image full size**: Double click on the image thumbnail, its position in the image number panel, or its location in the Resource Location List or use the Actual Size menu item.

❖ **Play a video**: Double click on the video's thumbnail, its position in the image number panel, or its row in the Resource Location List or use the Actual Size menu item.

❖ **Add an image or video to a Presentation**: Drag the image from an asset library and drop it in position on the image number panel or on the Resource Locations List if visible. Use the Insert, the Replace or the Append buttons or menu items.

❖ **Remove an image from a presentation**: Select the image you want to remove by making it the current image. Click the Remove button or press the Delete key.

❖ **Move an image to a nearby earlier position**: Select the image you want to move as the current image. Click the Move Up button until the image is in the desired position.

❖ **Move an image to a nearby later position**: Select the image you want to move as the current image. Click the Move Down button until the image is in the desired position.

❖ **Move an image to a distant position**: Select the image to be moved as the current image. Click the Cut button. Select the image in the position you want the cut image to appear. Click the Insert button. The current image will be shifted down to make room for the image you have moved.

❖ **Edit the caption for an image**: Select the image you want to edit as the current image. Right click on it in the Current image box. This will open the Clip window where you can edit the name (caption) or the notes. Be sure to click the Update button to save your changes.

❖ **Add an image you created from your hard drive**: You must first Add the image to an Asset Library then you can drag it into the presentation.

❖ **Save a presentation**: Use File - Save Presentation As to give a presentation a new name. If you make changes to one of the presentations provided by McGraw-Hill you will not be able to save it without changing its name. Names are limited to 64 characters. You can use almost any printable characters and spaces. You can view the list of existing names by clicking on the Show List button. You can replace an existing presentation by selecting its name from the list. Then clicking OK. Since the name already exists and duplicate names are not permitted you will be asked to confirm that you want to replace the existing presentation.

You can create variations on the same presentation by loading the basic presentation, then make changes and save it with a variation of the original name. For example:

Basic Presentation: Chapter 01 - Standard
Variation 1: Chapter 01 - AM Section
Variation 2: Chapter 02 - PM Section

If you try to Save a new presentation, the Save Presentation As form will be displayed automatically so that you can provide a name for your untitled presentation.

Close a Presentation Builder form: Click on the System Menu box at the left end of the Presentation Builder title bar. When the System menu pops up click on the word "Close."

Presentation Preview

Use the Presentation Preview item in the Windows menu to show your presentation. The images and videos of the active presentation window will be displayed in sequence. You can navigate through your presentation using any of three sets of controls:

The Navigation bar at the bottom of the screen. The Preview Navigation bar contains the controls needed to show your presentation.

The Presentation Selection List allows you to directly access any image in the presentation. The Presentation Selection List displays a list of all of the images in the presentation. You can jump directly to any image by clicking on it in the list.

The Image Control allows you to advance and back up through the presentation without any distracting controls being visible. You can use the Presentation image itself as a control panel. The key is where you click the image. If you click the image on the . . .
Left you will view the previous image
Right you will step forward one image
The vertical position of the mouse pointer does not matter.

You can Exit Preview by clicking on the Exit button on the Preview Control Bar

Part III: Total On-line Course Management with
The McGraw-Hill Learning Architecture
http://www.mhla.net

Designed to manage the delivery and support of education over the Internet and campus Intranets using the World Wide Web the MHLA is a complete solution for delivering educational content over networked environments. The MHLA allows instructors to administer the course or courses, assess the student's progress, facilitate communication, and allow students to apply their knowledge.

The MHLA successfully combines the following features:

Course and class management
- You can assign quizzes, post homework assignments, even track your students' progress with just a few clicks of the mouse. You can easily add your own material if you wish.
- Much like a filing cabinet, Learning Architecture stores such materials as your class roster, grades, and homework assignments. You can post announcements and assign homework to the whole class or to individual students.
- If a student has trouble understanding a topic, he or she can use the McGraw-Hill Learning Architecture's message system to ask the instructor or a fellow student for help. Students can even work together in assigned discussion groups.

Content creation and management
You can use the content supplied by McGraw-Hill without any additional authoring or you can easily customize the material. You can delete content, add your course syllabus, provide Internet links, and integrate original material.

On-line quizzing and testing
Students can take true/false, multiple-choice, and fill-in-the-blank quizzes with the option of automatic grading. Essay tests can be administered as well by using e-mail to send and receive answers. Assignments can be customized to each student based upon testing/quizzing performance.

Secure individualized access requiring only a standard web browser
Students need only a computer with a standard Web browser to navigate through dynamic pages of text, graphics, exercises, PowerPoint slides, and more. If they should have difficulty with a topic, they can use a built-in message system to e-mail the instructor or fellow students with questions.

Gateway to other sites on the WWW

New 1998 Advanced Features Include:

Testing

- **List Matching**   Will be able to associate two unordered lists

- **Image Maps** Will be able to indicate where Chicago is on a map

- **MCQ Images**   Will be able to indicate which picture is correct

- **Multiple Choice**   We will now have the option to have a list of possible answers as check boxes and the student will be required to "check all that apply".   The instructor has the option of assigning points to each answer (allowing some points for getting some of the answer correct) or assigning an overall score, which requires the student to get all answers correct.

- **Date/Time Limits**   This will allow tests to be controlled based on time. Primarily this will affect when you can take the test (e.g. you can take the test between the 1st and the 5th but not before or after), when you can get the results (e.g. not until after the weekend) and how long you have to do the test. (e.g. you have 30 minutes). Instructors can specify the maximum time the student is allowed to complete the test in minutes. When taking a timed test, the student will be warned that after the time limit has expired, any response submitted will not be accepted and the test will be marked as "not completed". A live timer may run while the test is being taken. Other ways date and time boundaries can be set:

  - A starting date and time (i.e. you cannot take this test before 1pm on 1/1/98)
  - A completion date and time (i.e. you must have submitted this test by 5 p.m. on 1/31/98
  - A date and time after which results will be available (e.g. even though this is an auto-corrected test you will not be able to view your score until after 9 p.m. on 2/4/98

- **Other New Testing Features:**
Will provide the option of "question at a time" as well as "all questions together" option. This will allow the student to view only one question at a time and to step backwards and forwards through the questions before submitting the entire test.
The instructor can now define a "passing score" or a set of grades (A, B, C, etc.) Pass/Fail can also be assigned.
The instructor can specify that after X attempts, a student is not allowed to take the test again until XX minutes/days/hours have passed.

Reporting

- **Summary Reports:** Instructors may get summary reports on the current progress of students through their material and monitoring of grades. This will include reports by course, student, tests, and questions.
- **Test Reports:** By selecting a test from the list of all tests assigned, a summary listing will be provided listing each assigned student, whether or not they have attempted the test and if they have, display the score, grade, percentile, date and time of each attempt.

Frames

  - **Optional Frames:** The ability for the toolbar and the contents to be optionally displayed in a frame.

- **Content Frames:** Content developers (MHHE!) will now be able to develop/create courses which utilize frames.

Searching

- **Users:** MHLA users can search for other users on whole or partial names.

- **Content:** A user will now be able to search titles as well as within the body of content.

<u>On-line Registration</u>

Self-Enrollment: Students can now register themselves, or enroll in additional courses. This can work in a few different ways:

- *Immediate* - As soon as all required fields are filled in, a student is granted immediate access.

- *On Approval by* - When the enrollment form is completed, it is sent to the administrator/instructor who can approve or deny.

- *No* - Self-registration is not allowed, but the course remains visible in the list of available classes.

- *Hidden-* Course is not even seen on the list of classes for which one can register.

Email

- **External addresses:** In Personal Preferences, the user will now have the option to select MHLA or SMTP/Internet as their preferred mail in-box. If MHLA is selected, then the internal email system works as it does now. If SMTP/Internet is selected, then the user must specify an Internet address. Any incoming mail will then be sent automatically by MHLA to that email account.

Exploring the McGraw-Hill Learning Architecture

Here are some step-by-step instructions on how to navigate the instructor authoring capabilities of MHLA.

1. Log in with the   Username: instructor
                              Password: instructor
2. Click on *Utilities*
3. Click on *Create/Edit Course*
4. Here, an instructor could type in the name of a course and start from scratch, or...list the courses that he/she is teaching then work within that existing course. Click on *list*.
5. A list of all the available courses pops up. Click on the course (demo) with which you wish to work. (e.g. Lahey, <u>Introduction to Psychology,</u> 6/e.)
6. A table of contents that mirrors the table of contents in the text is displayed. The instructor can choose to remove any chapters not covered in the course by clicking remove (the student will not see removed chapters) or the instructor can go in and edit a chapter. Click *on edit* next to your demo chapter. (Lahey is chapter 5).
7. Now the table of contents within the chapter appears. You have the option to remove any of these sections. Again, this would take them out of the student's view.
8. Now, as for the testing: go to a multiple-choice quiz. (e.g. *Review Questions.*) Click on *edit*.

9. You can change the title, the number of questions to be done, check to be auto-corrected, indicate whether the student can take the quiz multiple times, only once, or as many times as they want and only the last score is submitted, etc.
10. They can type an intro to the test;
11. They can edit, delete, reorder, or add new questions.
12. Scroll down near the bottom to the *New Question* buttons.
13. Click on the *Pick One* button
14. Type a Title for the Question. Example: **My Question**
15. Assign the point value
16. Type in the question. Example: **Today is Monday**
17. Indicate how the answers should appear (across, down, or pop up) by clicking on the box. Most of our possible answers are set-up to go down.
18. Type the possible answers. Example: **True, False**
19. Click the radio button next to the answer that's correct
20. In the boxes next to the possible answers you can provide good feedback to students.
21. Scroll to the bottom of the page and hit *Submit* to save the question.
22. Click on *Preview* to see how the student would view the question.
23. Click on your Netscape *Back* button.
24. Now you should be back on your *Edit Question* page, hit the *Parent* button at the bottom. (*Parent* always takes you to the next level up in the system.)
25. Your question should be added on to the bottom of the test questions.
26. Now, scroll down to the bottom and look at the "Add Coursework" and "Notify Instructor" buttons. A professor can set parameters to be auto notified if a student is doing well or poorly. They can then assign additional coursework based upon a student's performance.

Now....Let's add some of our own notes to MHLA!

1. Click your *Parent* button until you reach the table of contents for the chapter in which you are working. You should see Learning Objectives, Key Terms, PowerPoint Presentation, etc.
2. Scroll down until you see the word *Add* with some icons to the right. There is a little folder (to add a folder of materials)

a page (to just add a single page)

a page with a pencil (to add a test/quiz)

and a folder with a page (to add other material existing within MHLA to your course, or to bring back in a chapter or element within a chapter previously removed).

Click the *add page* icon (the second one).

In the title box, name the page **My Notes**.

3. Go to the big box and type something.
4. Click on the *Preview* button to review what a student would see.
5. Click *Submit*, Then *Parent* to see that your notes have been added in the chapter table of contents.

Now, let's bring in a Word document.

6. Minimize your Netscape (the little minus symbol in the top right hand corner) and go open MS Word.
7. Type something in your Word document. Change the text fonts and just type some stuff.
8. Click on File and choose *Save As HTML*; if that feature does not pop up under File, then click on *Save As...*and choose HTML as the file type.
9. Make sure you save this in a place where you can find it again. I save mine to the desktop.
10. Close out of Word and maximize your browser.
11. Scroll down to the bottom of the screen and click on *HTML Upload*.
12. Click on the "browse" box and locate the word/html file you just created. Select it and hit *Open*. You'll now see that it has appeared in the box to the left of browse.
13. Click *Submit* to bring it in.
14. You may see some error messages pop up. [Ignore them]. TopClass has a strict HTML reader.
15. Scroll down and show it entered your message into the box with the HTML coding.
16. Now scroll further down and click the *Preview* button to see how it will appear to the student.
17. In your navigation bar, there should be an icon that looks like a page with a yellow pencil on it...it means edit. Click on the icon and your HTML page should pop back.

18. Click *Submit*, then the *Parent* Button and you will see the new page that you added.
19. That's it!!

No matter how you integrate multimedia in your course, it is sure to have a significant and positive impact on how your students learn. McGraw-Hill wishes you every success in moving the psychology classroom into the information age, and we welcome your feedback.